Vocal Fold Physiology

Acoustic, Perceptual, and Physiological Aspects of Voice Mechanisms

Edited by

Jan Gauffin, D.M.Sc., and Britta Hammarberg, D.Sc.
Royal Institute of Technology
Stockholm, Sweden

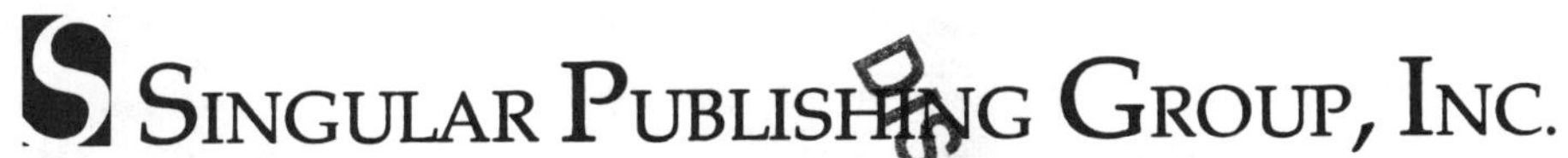
Singular Publishing Group, Inc.

Singular Publishing Group, Inc.
4284 41st Street
San Diego, California 92103

Library of Congress Cataloging in Publication Data
Main entry under title:

Phonatory mechanisms : physiology, acoustics, and assessment / edited by Jan Gauffin and Britta Hammarberg.
p. cm.
Includes bibliographic references and index.
ISBN 1-879105-51-9 : $45.00
1. Speech—Physiological aspects. 3. Larynx—Physiology.
I. Gauffin, Jan. II. Hammarberg, Britta.
QP306.P56 1991
617.7'dc20 91-26091
CIP

Contents

Foreword

The science of voice has advanced dramatically in recent years. Multi-national, interdisciplinary cooperation is responsible for much of the progress. *Vocal Fold Physiology: Acoustic, Perceptual and Physiological Aspects of Voice Mechanisms*" is the sixth volume in a series of publications that document much of the finest work produced in the last decade. Previous volumes include the following: 1) Stevens, K. N. and Hirano, M. (eds.): *Vocal Fold Physiology*, University of Tokyo Press, Tokyo, 1981. 2) Bless, D. M. and Abbs, J. H. (eds.): *Vocal Fold Physiology: Contemporary Research and Clinical Issues*, College-Hill Press, San Diego, California, 1983. 3) Titze, I. R. and Scherer, R. C. (eds.): *Vocal Fold Physiology: Biomechanics, Acoustics, and Phonatory Control*, the Denver Center for the Performing Arts, Denver, Colorado, 1983. 4) Baer, T, Sasaki, K., and Harris, K. (eds.): *Laryngeal Function in Phonation and Respiration*, College-Hill Press, San Diego, CA, 1987. 5) Fujimura, O. (ed.): *Vocal Fold Physiology: Voice Production, Mechanisms and Functions*, Raven Press, New York, 1988.

The new volume makes available the latest and finest research on acoustic, perceptual, and physiological aspects of the voice, presented by leading scientists from around the world. Minoru Hirano's section on phonatory mechanisms provides new perspectives and directions for vocal fold assessment. The sections on voice source acoustics and parametrization edited by Kenneth Stevens and Christine Shadle offer particularly important insights on laryngeal modelling and voice source behavior. The section on physiology edited by Osamu Fujimura includes particularly timely neuro-otolaryngologic information. The section on assessment of laryngeal function edited by Jan Gauffin, Britta Hammarberg, and Christy Ludlow is especially valuable to clinicians, as well as to researchers, highlighting clinical correlation and value of technologically sophisticated assessment.

Like its predecessors in this series, *Vocal Fold Physiology: Acoustic, Perceptual and Physiological Aspects of Voice Mechanisms* is an invaluable addition to the literature. It provides fascinating and useful information for any voice scientist, laryngologist specializing in voice, or speech-language pathologists.

Robert Thayer Sataloff
Professor of Otolaryngology
Thomas Jefferson University

Introduction

The contributions to this volume are based on presentations delivered at the Sixth Vocal Fold Physiology Conference, which was held in Stockholm, July 30 to August 3, 1989. The subtitle, "Acoustic, Perceptual, and Physiological Aspects of Voice Mechanisms," of the present issue enhances the relation between voice production mechanisms and acoustics of the voice and also between the acoustic characteristics of the voice and our auditory image of the voice.

The 36 chapters in this volume have been divided into four parts according to topic and to order of presentation at the conference. These are:

I. Phonatory Mechanisms
II. Voice Source Acoustics and Parameterization
III. Physiology
IV. Assessment of Laryngeal Function

Phonatory Mechanisms

This part mainly concerns observations of vocal fold vibrations. Due to the inaccessibility of the larynx, direct observations of the vocal folds are difficult to make. By using tracheotomized subjects and a fiberscope connected to a video camera, however, Hirano and coworkers were able to video record the vibrating vocal folds from below. Such observations can give useful information needed for a better understanding of the mechanisms behind the vocal fold vibrations, especially the function of the mucous membrane. The wave motion of the mucous membrane was also studied by Fukuda and coworkers, using X-ray tracking of lead pellets in canine larynges.

A new instrumentation for ultrasound laryngography is reported on by Kaneko and coworkers. With this new equipment they were able to demonstrate the phase relations between the upper and lower margins of the vibrating vocal folds.

This part also includes an investigation by Gray of injury to the mucous membrane area in canine vocal folds due to intense prolonged phonation.

Voice Source Acoustics and Parameterization

The main theme of this part is numerical simulations and modelling of the voice source. The high level of activity within this area of research is reflected by the large number of contributions, some presenting new methods applied from other areas.

In the chapter by Stevens, a theoretical framework is suggested drawn on the interaction between laryngeal adjustments and vocal tract constriction for obstruent consonants in speech. The conditions for vocal fold vibrations or noise production is analysed and suggestions are offered for how the speech mechanisms are utilized in production of various classes of voiced and voiceless obstruent consonants. The theories are tested in a computer model of vocal fold vibrations also, described in the chapter by Bickley.

The two-mass model used in computer simulation of the vocal folds is a so-called lumped-element model. A more abstract approach is taken by McGowan in his chapter about phonation from a continuum mechanical point of view. He also discusses the issues of energy balance and stability in the airflow and some aspects of the mucousal wave motion.

Three additional chapters deal with computer simulations of different aspects of voice production. The first of these, by Fant and Lin, is a mathematical description of the glottal voice source which could be used as a natural sounding source in speech synthesis or as an analysis tool. The issue of acoustic interaction between the sub- and supra-glottal cavities is discussed. Also the rationale for choosing the specific model, and how the model can be used to analyse the dynamics of the source in natural speech are treated. Examples of using the model for analysis of voice dynamics in speech is given in the study by Gobl and Karlsson.

The mathematical tools for calculation of the flow through the glottis and the forces acting on the vocal folds are not yet fully developed. A promising attempt to solve this very difficult problem is illustrated by Liljencrants in his chapter on numerical simulation of glottal flow. His method seems to give realistic results but the accuracy of the simulation remains to be explored. Two such model experiments are included in this part. Shadle and coworkers used flow visualization by smoke in both a static and dynamic model using a shutter like glottis. The jet formed at the exit of the glottis could be verified and the influence of the acoustic load by the vocal tract is discussed. The second model experiment is reported on by Sherer and Guo. From their measurement of the pressure drop across the model of the glottis for different flow and vocal fold shapes, a general equation is proposed, describing the pressure-flow relation for a wide range of laryngeal configurations.

A non-invasive, clinically useful method to analyse vocal function is discussed in the contribution by Rothenberg and Nezelek. They propose a system for an airflow-based analysis which provides an easily used and robust method for obtaining from the oral airflow waveform those parameters which are most significant in clinical applications. They discuss how the pitfalls inherent in standard inverse filtering can be by-passed.

A systematic development of a body-cover model for fundamental frequency regulation is outlined in the chapter by Titze. His aim is to clarify and quantify three primary ways of regulating fundamental frequency: by the cricothyroid muscles, by the thyroarytenoid muscle and by changing lung pressure.

The classic problem of explaining the intrinsic fundamental frequency (F0) of vowels is discussed by Vilkman and coworkers and by Honda and Fujimura. It seems clear that biological mechanisms can explain such acoustic characteristics of speech, but also that we learn such characteristics in the course of language acquisition, and we may amplify them and use them as communicative features when they are established as perceptual cues.

Physiology

The work reported on in this part concerns measurements of neural activities either in the brain or in the laryngeal muscles, and addresses the neurophysiological organization of phonatory control.

Larson and coworkers studied brainstem mechanisms involved in vocalization in monkeys. The authors compare results of recordings made in a midbrain area with those made in the medulla. The study by Yoshida and coworkers is an attempt to clarify the postganglionic sympathetic innervation of the larynx in cats.

The remaining papers in this part deal with EMG measurements in speech muscles. A method for quantitative analysis of the EMG interference pattern, called "turns/amplitude analysis," is used in the study by Lindestad and coworkers for evaluating the role of the cricothyroid (CT) and the thyroarytenoid (TA) muscles for fundamental frequency control in females and males, singers and nonsingers. F0 control is also the focus in the chapter by Niimi and coworkers.

Ludlow and coworkers report on the relationship between vocal fold movement and laryngeal activation during speech. The authors focus on onset and offset of phonation and examine the activity in the TA and CT muscles on both sides and the posterior cricothyroid muscle.

Assessment of Laryngeal Function

Most contributions in this part fall into two areas: (1) approaches with multiple simultaneous measures, i.e. visual observation of vocal fold vibration/closure patterns in combination with acoustic and perceptual evaluations; and (2) assessment of perceptual voice features using either synthesis or quantifiable acoustic measurement. Both normal laryngeal function and laryngeal dysfunction are considered. In the first chapter, however, Blaugrund and coworkers take another approach and describe a technique of manually evaluating the larynx prior to laryngeal framework surgery.

Hirose and coworkers report on a new method of digitally imaging vocal fold vibration. The system is capable of simultaneous recording of high-speed digital images of the vibrating vocal folds, the audio signal, and the electroglottographic signal. Applications of the system seem promising for the analysis of pathological vibratory patterns, as in cases with recurrent laryngeal nerve paralysis, vocal fold polyp, and other organic vocal lesions.

Another approach combining visual observation with acoustic and perceptual evaluations is attempted in a study on normal adult speakers by Södersten and coworkers. Glottal closure patterns during fiberscopy were evaluated in relation to degree of perceived breathiness, hypo- and hyperfunction, and to acoustic data, such as the level of the fundamental relative to the first formant level.

In the chapter by Imaizumi and coworkers perceptual experiments were performed to examine the naturalness of voice quality in a glottal source model.

A similar approach of using analysis and synthesis techniques to study voice quality is attempted by Lee and Childers. The authors used the Liljencrants-Fant-model (see chapter 7) for the synthesis of four phonation types: modal, vocal fry, falsetto and breathy voice. For the synthesis of breathy voice, turbulent excitation had to be added to the model. The chapter by Kasuya and Ando also deals with analysis and synthesis of breathy voice, using Klatt's model with a modification for hypofunctional voice quality.

The search for quantifiable acoustic properties of the voice is the theme of the contribution by Koike and Kohda, who apply the cepstrum technique for evaluating voice function after surgery on benign lesions in the larynx. Milenkovic and coworkers try to determine acoustic characteristics of vocal fold nodules by computer analysis of the acoustic speech waveform, together with perceptual evaluation.

As in many chapters in this part, the aim of the contribution by Hertegård and Gauffin is to develop and evaluate methods for quantification of glottal voice source behaviour for clinical purposes. By using inverse filtering, the authors try to analyse the relationship between glottal airflow parameters and breathiness, as a sign of insufficient vocal fold closure.

Each paper presented at the conference was followed by a discussion. The comments during these discussions contributed greatly to the stimulating atmosphere and fruitful exchange of ideas evidenced at the conference. Everyone participating in these discussions are gratefully acknowledged. Unfortunately, due to limited space these discussions could not be included in this volume.

Jan Gauffin and Britta Hammarberg

Acknowledgments

This volume is a collection of papers presented at the Sixth Vocal Fold Physiology Conference held in Stockholm, July 30 to August 3, 1989. The series of conferences was initiated by the Voice Foundation and we wish to thank Dr. Wilbur J. Gould for his foresight in doing so. Besides the grant from the Voice Foundation, the Sixth Conference was sponsored by the National Swedish Board for Technical Development (STU), the Swedish Council for Planning and Coordination of Research (FRN), the Swedish Medical Research Council (MFR), and the Bank of Swedish Tercentenary Foundation (RJ).

The most important credit should go to our colleagues who have contributed to this volume as authors and section editors. Our fellow members of the organizing committee, Gunnar Fant, Björn Fritzell (Chair), and Johan Sundberg should also be acknowledged together with the secretary of the conference, Si Felicetti.

We also wish to thank Thomas Murry and Marie Linvill at Singular Publishing Group, Inc. for their encouragement and kind cooperation in the final preparation of the manuscript.

Jan Gauffin and Britta Hammarberg

Section Editors

Jan Gauffin	Department of Speech Communication and Music Acoustics Royal Institute of Technology Box 70014 S-100 44 Stockholm Sweden
Britta Hammarberg	Department of Logopedics and Phoniatrics Karolinska Institute Huddinge University Hospital S-141 86 Huddinge Sweden
Minoru Hirano	Department of Otolaryngology Head and Neck Surgery School of Medicine, Kurume University 67 Asahi-Machi, Kurume-shi, 830 Japan
Christy L. Ludlow	Speech and Voice, NIDCD Bldg. 10, Rm. 5D38 9000 Rockville Pike Bethesda, MD 20892 U S A
Christine H. Shadle	Department of Electronics and Computer Sciences University of Southampton Southampton SO9 5NH England
Kenneth N. Stevens	Room 36-511 Research Laboratory of Electronics Massachusetts Institute of Technology Cambridge, MA 02139 U S A

Contributors

1

Vibratory Behaviour of Human Vocal Folds Viewed from Below

Minoru Hirano, Tetsuji Yoshida, and Shinzo Tanaka

Dept. of Otolaryngology-Head and Neck Surgery, Kurume University, Kurume, 830 Japan

The vibratory behaviour of the vocal folds has been investigated by many investigators using stroboscopy (Baer, 1975; 1981; Kirikae, 1943; Schönhärl, 1960), ultra-high-speed photography (Fukuda et al., 1983; Hirano, 1975; Hirano et al., 1981; 1983; Hiroto, 1966; Kakita et al., 1983; Moore and von Leden, 1958; Timcke et al., 1958; 1959) and X-ray stroboscopy (Fukuda et al., 1983; Isogai, 1981; Saito, 1977; Saito et al., 1981; 1983; Tsuzuki, 1984). Many aspects of vocal fold behaviour during vibration have been elucidated, at least phenomenologically, through these previous investigations. Most previous observations of vocal fold behaviour, however, have been based on views of the larynx from above.

Matsushita (1969; 1975) appears to have been the first to succeed in taking ultra-high-speed motion pictures viewing vibration of the vocal folds of normal excised human and canine larynges from below. Baer (1975) and Yumoto (1988) investigated vibratory behaviour of the lower aspect of the vocal folds of excised canine larynges.

The purposes of this paper are to present vibratory behaviour of in vivo human vocal folds viewed from below and to supplement our knowledge of vocal fold vibration.

SUBJECTS AND METHODS

Two tracheotomized patients, a 67-year-old female and a 55-year-old male, with normal voice and normal vocal folds, served as subjects. Both subjects had received general anaesthesia for maxillary sinus carcinoma surgery and that for surgery for lower gingival carcinoma, respectively. Tracheostomy had been performed for endotracheal intubation prior to the general anaesthesia.

A fiberscope (Olympus ENF type L) connected to a stroboscope (Pentax LS-IA, modified version) was inserted into the subglottic space through the tracheostoma. The subjects were instructed to sustain vowels at different pitch levels. They were also asked to perform non-phonatory activities including inspiration, expiration, swallow and cough. The fiberscopic images were recorded on video tape by means of a video camera (Hitachi DK-5050) and a video recorder (Sony VO 5800).

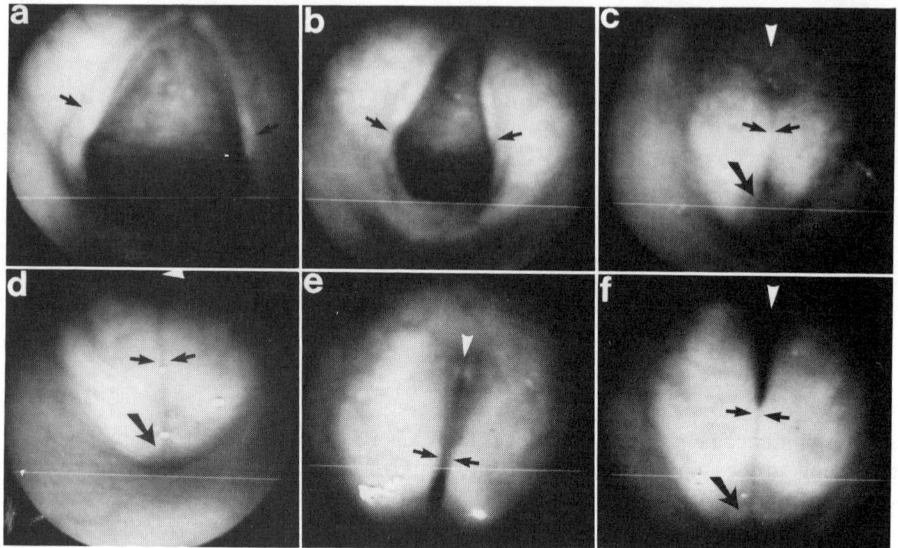

Fig. 1. Glottic configuration for (**a**) inspiration, (**b**) expiration, (**c**) swallow, (**d**) cough, (**e**) phonation near the habitual pitch, 180 Hz and (**f**) high-pitch phonation, 339 Hz. Thick arrows indicate a conic space in the posterior glottis; thin arrows, the location of the tip of the vocal process; and white triangles, the location of the anterior commissure.

The video images were closely examined and selected phonatory samples were subjected to frame-by-frame analysis. The frame-by-frame analysis was performed on printed images obtained from a color video printer (Hitachi VY-100).

GLOTTIC CONFIGURATION FOR VARYING GESTURES

Figure 1 shows glottic configurations for inspiration, expiration, swallow, cough and phonation viewed through the tracheostoma with regular light.

During inspiration, the glottis was wide open (Figure 1a). The tip of the vocal process was located not at the vocal fold edge but slightly lateral and superior to the edge. As a result, a small canopy formed above the vocal process, as had been reported previously (Hirano et al., 1987). During expiration, the glottis became narrower than it was during inspiration (Figure 1b).

During swallow, the glottis was tightly closed and the membranous vocal folds were markedly shortened (Figure 1c). In the posterior or intercartilaginous portion, closure took place not at the level of the glottis but above the glottic level. As a result, a conic space was formed in the posterior glottis. The glottis was also closed very tightly during cough (Figure 1d). The closure was again associated both with shortening of the membranous vocal fold and with a conic space in the posterior glottis.

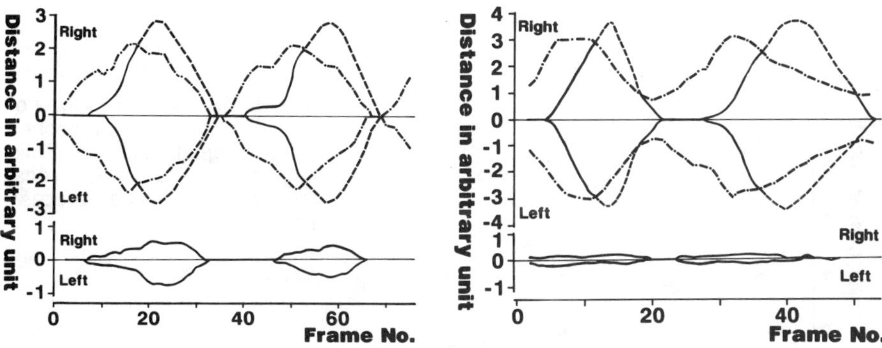

Fig. 2. Trajectory of the upper portion (solid and dashed lines) and lower portion (dotted and dashed line) of the membranous vocal fold (top curves) and of the tip of the vocal process (bottom curves) for the female (left) and male (right) subject.

Phonation at the habitual pitch level was associated with a closed membranous glottis (Figure 1e). The closure was not as tight as that observed for swallow and cough. The posterior glottis was slightly open. This finding has been frequently observed in normal female adults. In high-pitch phonation, the membranous vocal folds were stretched and the posterior portion of the larynx was closed at a level above the glottis (Figure 1f). A conic space was again observed in the posterior glottis. A conic space in the posterior glottis during swallow, cough and phonation is a phenomenon that was first described by Minningerode (1962) and has been extensively studied by Hirano and his co-workers (Hirano et al., 1986; 1987).

VIBRATORY BEHAVIOUR OF THE VOCAL FOLD

Figure 2 shows results of frame-by-frame analysis for a sustained /e/ vowel near the habitual pitch and loudness level of each subject. It was possible to trace movements of the upper and lower portions of the vocal folds. The two portions were thought to be the structures referred to as the upper and lower lips in previous observations seen from above. The movement of the upper portion lagged that of the lower portion. The two portions traced were not of specific points on the mucosa, but were of the apparent crests of the waves travelling in the inferior-superior direction. The glottis was completely closed at the upper portion in both subjects, whereas at the lower portion, complete closure did not take place in the male subject. The closed phase at the lower portion observed in the female subject was shorter than that at the upper portion.

The dashed lines in Figure 2 depict estimated movements of the upper portion of the vocal fold edge. The estimation was based on superior views reported in previous literature (Hiroto, 1966).

The tip of the vocal process was observed more clearly in the view from below than in the usual view from above. The tip of the vocal process was involved in vibration in both subjects. The opening of the glottis at the tip of the vocal process lagged the opening of

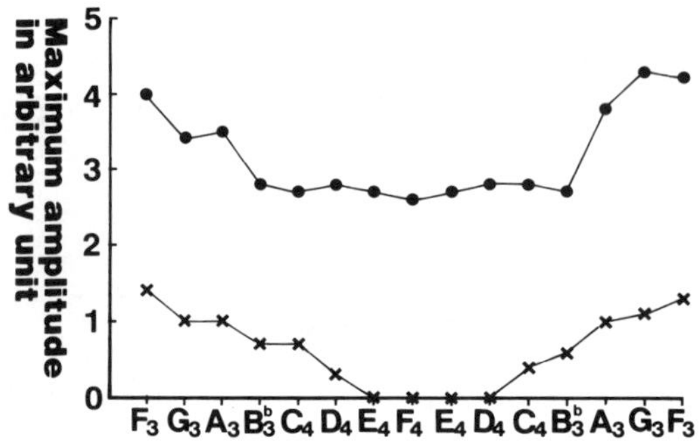

Fig. 3. Maximum amplitude of vibration for different pitches for the female subject. Solid circles: membranous vocal fold, crosses: vocal process tip.

the membranous vocal fold. The delay was more marked for the female subject than for the male.

CHANGE IN VOCAL PITCH

The female subject was able to sing a one-octave scale. The male subject sang a more restricted range of pitches because of lack of familiarity with the task. Figure 3 shows the maximum amplitude of vibration of the membranous vocal fold and of the tip of the vocal process for a one-octave-ascending and -descending scale sung by the female subject.

The amplitude of vibration was negatively correlated with the pitch at both locations. For pitches higher than B_3^b, the change in amplitude at the membranous vocal fold was less marked than for pitches lower than B_3^b.

The tip of the vocal process did not vibrate at high pitches. No posterior glottic chink was observed at high pitches (see Figure 1f).

COMMENTS

It has been demonstrated in many previous investigations that the major phenomena observed in vibratory movements of the vocal fold are waves travelling on the mucosa (mucosal wave) around the vocal fold edge (Hirano, 1975; Hiroto, 1966; Kirikae, 1943; Saito, 1977; Schönhärl, 1960). The waves travel in the inferior-superior direction. The starting point of the mucosal wave was first determined by Matsushita (1975) in his study in which ultra-high-speed photography was used to observe excised larynges from below the vocal folds. According to him, a mucosal upheaval forms below glottis shortly before voice initiation. The mucosal wave begins at the superior border of the upheaval and travels upward. The occurrence of the mucosal wave is located superior to the upheaval. This finding was confirmed by Yumoto (1988) in his ultra-high-speed photographic study of excised canine larynges. The present study has confirmed that a similar phenomenon takes place in living human larynges. The only difference is that, in living humans, the mucosal upheaval is not as marked as that in excised larynges. This may be attributed to the presence of a contracting thyroarytenoid muscle.

It has been noted in previous investigations (Hirano et al., 1973; Saito et al., 1981; Schönhärl, 1960; Yumoto, 1988), that the so-called upper and lower lips on the vocal fold are not unchanging specific points on the mucosa but crests of travelling waves. This was also confirmed in this study.

The vibratory behaviour of the tip of the vocal process has not been investigated extensively. It has been demonstrated that the tip of the vocal process does vibrate (Hirano et al., 1983; Tanabe et al., 1975). During phonation, the tip of the vocal process can be viewed more clearly from below than from above. The glottic opening is delayed at the vocal process relative to the membranous vocal fold. This may indicate that the major force separating the vocal processes is not the subglottic pressure but the lateral excursion of the membranous vocal fold. The vocal process did not vibrate at high pitches in the present study. The same finding was noted in the article by Tanabe et al. (1975). This may be attributed to forceful contraction of the lateral cricoarytenoid and interarytenoid muscles. The forceful contraction of these muscles for high pitches has been electromyographically demonstrated (Hirano, 1988).

In addition, it has been reported that the amplitude of lateral excursion of the vocal fold decreases as the fundamental frequency of phonation increases (Titze and Durham, 1987). The results of the present study agreed with this.

SUMMARY

Vibratory behaviour of the lower aspect of the vocal fold was investigated in two tracheotomized subjects (one female, one male) with the use of videostroboscopy. The results are summarized as follows:

1. The posterior portion of the larynx closes not at the level of the glottis but above the glottis. As a result, a conic space forms in the posterior glottis.

2. The vibratory movements of the lower portion around the vocal fold edge precede those of the upper portion.

3. The tip of the vocal process vibrates at low pitches. Its opening lags the opening of the membranous vocal fold. At high pitches, the tips of the vocal processes remain approximated, demonstrating no vibratory movement.

4 The amplitude of vibration decreases as the pitch increases.

REFERENCES

Baer, T. (1975). *Investigation of phonation using excised larynx*. Ph.D. Thesis, Massachusetts Institute of Technology, Cambridge, MA.

Baer, T. (1981). Observations of vocal fold vibration: Measurement of excised larynges. In: *Vocal Fold Physiology*, edited by K. N. Stevens and M. Hirano, pp. 119-133. University of Tokyo Press, Tokyo.

Fukuda, H., Saito, S., Kitahara, S., Isogai, Y., Makino, K., Tsuzuki, T., Kogawa, N., and Ono, H. (1983). Vocal fold vibration in excised larynges viewed with an X-ray stroboscope and an ultra-high speed camera. In: *Vocal Fold Physiology*, edited by D.M. Bless and J.H. Abbs, pp. 238-252. College-Hill Press, San Diego, CA.

Hirano, M. (1975). Phonosurgery. Basic and clinical investigations. *Otologia Fukuoka*, 21:239-442.

Hirano, M. (1988). Vocal mechanisms in singing: Laryngological and phoniatric aspects. *J. Voice* 2:51-69.

Hirano, M., Koike, Y., Hirose, S., and Morio, M. (1973). Structure of the vocal cord as a vibrator. *J. Otolaryngol. Jpn.* 76:1341-1348.

Hirano, M., Kakita, Y., Kawasaki, H., Gould, W.J., and Lambiase, A. (1981). Data from high-speed motion picture studies. In: *Vocal Fold Physiology*, edited by K.N. Stevens and M. Hirano, pp. 85-91. University of Tokyo Press, Tokyo.

Hirano, M., Matsuo, K., Kakita, Y., Kawasaki, H., and Kurita, S. (1983). Vibratory behavior versus the structure of the vocal fold, In: *Vocal Fold Physiology,* edited by I.R. Titze and R.C. Scherer, pp. 26-39. The Denver Center for the Performing Arts, Denver, CO.

Hirano, M., Kurita, S., Kiyokawa, K,. and Sato, K. (1986). Posterior glottis. Morphological study in excised human larynges. *Ann. Otolaryngol. Rhinol. Laryngol.* 95:576-581.

Hirano, M., Yoshida, T., Kurita, S., Kiyokawa, K., Sato, K., and Tateishi, O. (1987). Anatomy and behavior of the vocal process. In: *Laryngeal Function in Phonation and Respiration*, edited by T. Baer, C. Sasaki, and K. Harris, pp. 3-11. Little, Brown and Company, Boston, MA.

Hiroto, I. (1966). The mechanism of phonation. Pathophysiological aspects of the larynx. *Practica Otologia Kyoto* 39, Suppl. 1:229-291.

Isogai, Y. (1981). An analysis of the vibration of the vocal fold by X-ray stroboscopy. *Otologia Fukuoka* 27:883-930.

Kakita, Y., Hirano, M., Kawasaki, H., and Matsuo, K. (1983). Stereo-laryngoscopy: A new method to extract vertical movement of the vocal fold during vibration, In: *Vocal Fold Physiology,* edited by I.R. Titze and R.C. Scherer, pp. 191-201. The Denver Center for the Performing Arts, Denver, CO.

Kirikae, I. (1943). Über den Bewegungsvorgang an den Stimmlippen und die Öffnungs- und Verschlusszeit der Stimmritze während der Phonation. *J. Otolaryngol. Jpn.* 49:236-262.

Matsushita, H. (1969). Vocal fold vibration of excised larynges. A study with ultra-high speed cinematography. *Otologia Fukuoka*, 15:127-142.

Matsushita, H. (1975). The vibratory mode of the vocal folds in the excised larynx. *Folia Phoniatr.* 27:7-18.

Minningerode, B. (1962). Über die Bedeutung einiger Formvarianten der Kehlkopfhinterwand und ihrer Nachbarschaft für den Verschluss der menschlichen Stimmritze und ihre Beziehungen zur Entstehung pachydermischer Veränderungen in diesem Bereich. *Arch. Ohren- usw. Heilk. u.Z. Hals- usw. Heilk.* 181:9-15.

Moore, P. and von Leden, H. (1958). Dynamic variations of the vibratory pattern in the normal larynx. *Folia Phoniatr.* 10:205-238.

Saito, S. (1977). Phonosurgery. Basic study on the mechanism of phonation and endolaryngeal microsurgery. *Otologia Fukuoka*, 23:171-384.

Saito, S., Fukuda, H., Isogai, Y., and Ono, H. (1981). X-ray stroboscopy. In: *Vocal Fold Physiology,* edited by K.N. Stevens and M. Hirano, pp. 95-103. University of Tokyo Press, Tokyo.

Saito, S., Fukuda, H., Kitahara, S., Isogai, Y., Tsuzuki, T., Muta, H., Takayama, E., Fujioka, T., Kokawa, N., and Makino, K. (1983). Pellet tracking in the vocal fold while phonating. Experimental study using canine larynges with muscle activity. In: *Vocal Fold Physiology*, edited by I.R. Titze and R.C. Scherer, pp. 169-179. The Denver Center for the Performing Arts, Denver, CO.

Schönhärl, E. (1960). *Die Stroboskopie in der praktischen Laryngologie.* Georg Thieme Verlag, Stuttgart.

Tanabe, M., Kitajima, K., Gould, W.J., and Lambiase, A. (1975). Analysis of high-speed motion pictures of the vocal folds. *Folia Phoniatr.* 27:77-87.

Timcke, R., von Leden, H., and Moore, P. (1958). Laryngeal vibrations: Measurements of the glottic wave. Part I. The normal vibratory cycle. *Arch. Otolaryngol.* 68:1-19.

Timcke, R., von Leden, H., and Moore, P. (1959). Laryngeal vibrations: Measurements of the glottic wave. Part II. Physiologic vibrations. *Arch. Otolaryngol.*, 69:438-444.

Titze, I.R. and Durham, P.L. (1987). Passive mechanisms influencing fundamental frequency control. In: *Laryngeal Function in Phonation and Respiration*, edited by T. Baer, C. Sasaki, and K. Harris, pp. 304-319. Little, Brown and Company, Boston.

Tsuzuki, T. (1984). A basic study on the vocal fold vibration from the viewpoint of the layer system of the vocal fold. *Otologia Fukuoka* 30:131-152.

Yumoto, E. (1988). Vocal fold vibration after microsurgery of the larynx. *Jpn. J. Logop. Phoniat.* 29:203-207.

2

Physiological Properties and Wave Motion of the Vocal Fold Membrane Viewed from Different Directions

Hiroyuki Fukuda, Yoshihisa Kawasaki, Masahiro Kawaida, Akihiro Shiotani, Kazuaki Oki, *Tohru Tsuzuki, *Tadashi Fujioka, and **Etsuyo Takayama

*Dept. of Otolaryngology, Keio University School of Medicine, Tokyo, Japan, *Dept. of Otolaryngology, Dokkyo University School of Medicine, Koshigaya Hospital, Tokyo, Japan, **Dept. of Otolaryngology, Tokyo Saiseikai Central Hospital, Tokyo, Japan*

Clarification of the mechanisms of vocal fold vibration is a problem which continues to hold significant fascination for every laryngologist. The traditional means of observing and recording the phonatory behaviour of the vocal folds have been laryngostroboscopy and ultra-high speed cinematography. These methods have indeed clarified the vibratory mechanism to some extent, but they have allowed us to observe vibration on the superior surface of the vocal fold only.

The creation and introduction of X-ray stroboscopy by our laboratory has made observation of vocal fold vibration in the frontal and sagittal planes possible. Our previous studies have led us to the following conclusions:

1. Irrespective of the phonatory condition, the essential principle of phonatory vibration is a travelling wave which moves superiorly and laterally from the lower surface of the vocal fold.

2 The motion of the mucousal cover of the vocal fold plays an important role as a vibratory structure, while the muscular layer is not essential to phonatory oscillation.

In the present study several lead pellets were inserted under the epithelial membrane of the so-called free edge of the vocal folds to serve as a contrast medium. Their vibratory movement was observed from the frontal, lateral, and superior directions in order to derive a more precise description of vocal fold vibratory motion.

METHOD

The larynges of 25 healthy dogs were excised and prepared for the experiment. At least three very small lead pellets (diameter 0.5 mm, length 0.5 mm, mass 0.5 mg) were inserted under the epithelial membrane, equidistant from the anterior and posterior ends

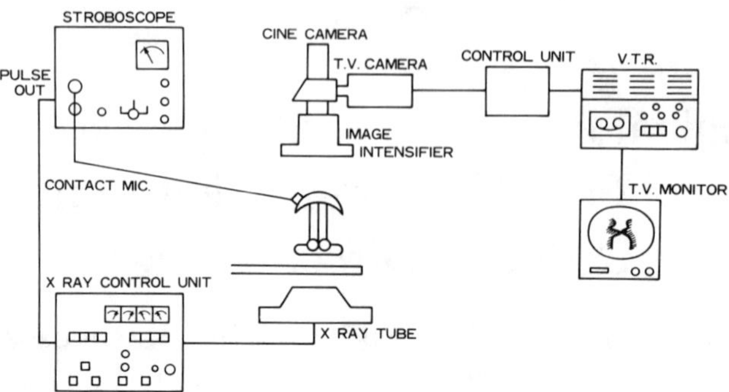

Fig. 1. Block diagram of the experimental instrumentation.

Their vibratory movements during experimentally-induced phonation were recorded by X-ray stroboscopy and fluorocinematography. Because the pellets had been stained black they could be observed visually through the overlying membranous tissue, which allowed us to record their movements with an ultra-high speed camera as well.

Observation of vibration from the lateral direction required the use of a hemilarynx. After the specimen was sectioned in the sagittal plane a plastic window was attached to

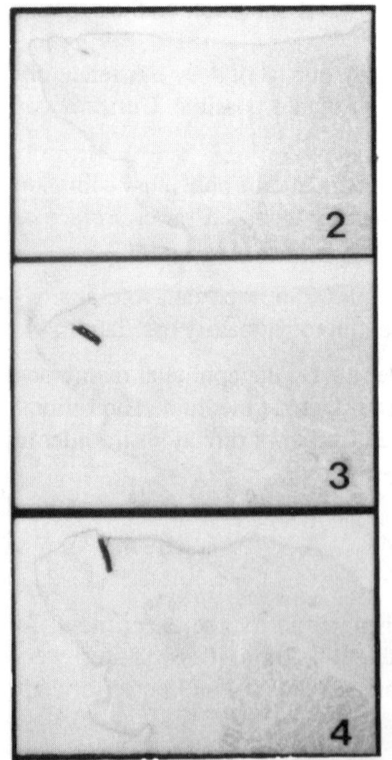

Fig. 2. Histological verification of pellet location.

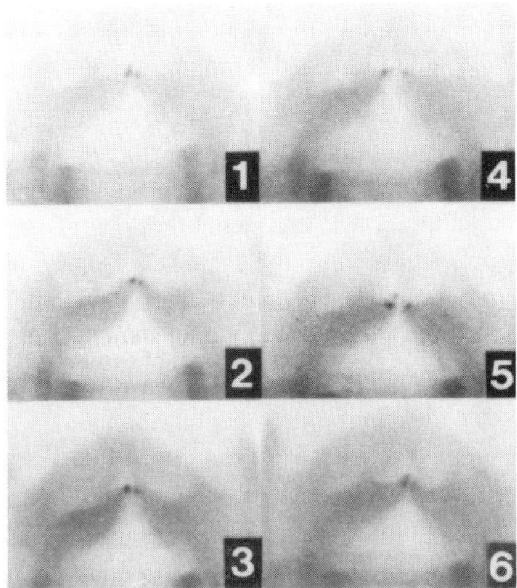

Fig. 3. One cycle of pellet motion, viwed in the frontal plane.

the cut margin to form an airtight space. Voice-synchronized X-ray images were observed by using a pulse signal from a laryngostroboscope to trigger a pulsed X-ray unit.

A block diagram of the experimental instrumentation is presented in Figure 1. Frame-by-frame analysis of pellet motion was achieved with a NAC film motion analyzer, model 42-057. Precise location of the lead pellets was verified histologically at the conclusion of the experimental series (Figure 2).

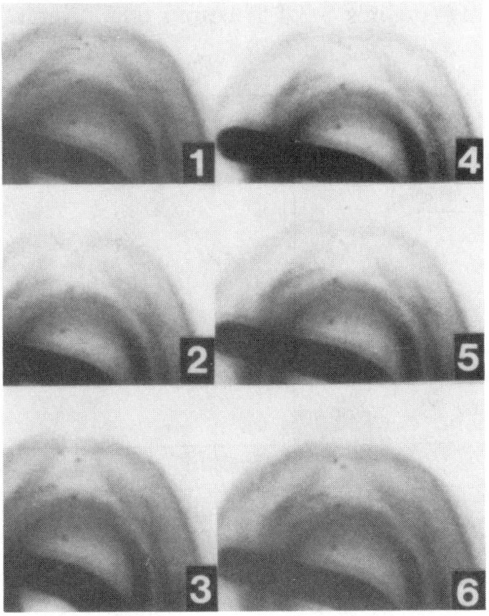

Fig. 4. One cycle of pellet motion, viewed in the plane of the upper surface of the vocal fold.

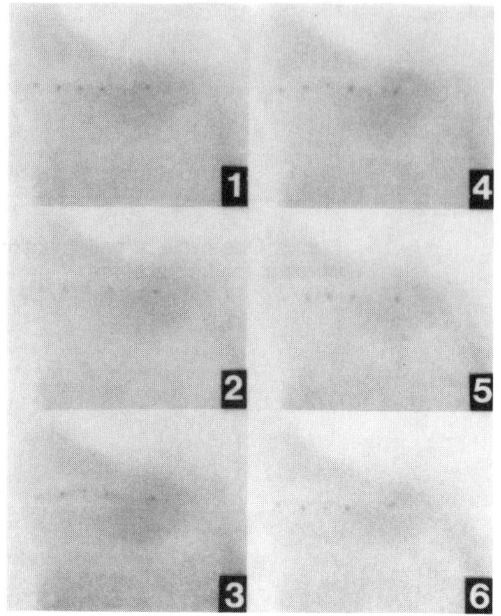

Fig. 5. Lateral view of a single cycle of pellet motion. Anterior is to the left; top of the image is cranial.

RESULTS

X-Ray Studies

X-ray tracking of the lead pellets was successful and revealed the following:

1. In the frontal plane (Figure 3), pellets were found to move upwards (Figures 3-1, 2), proceed laterally and then downwards (Figures 3-3,4,5) before finally returning to

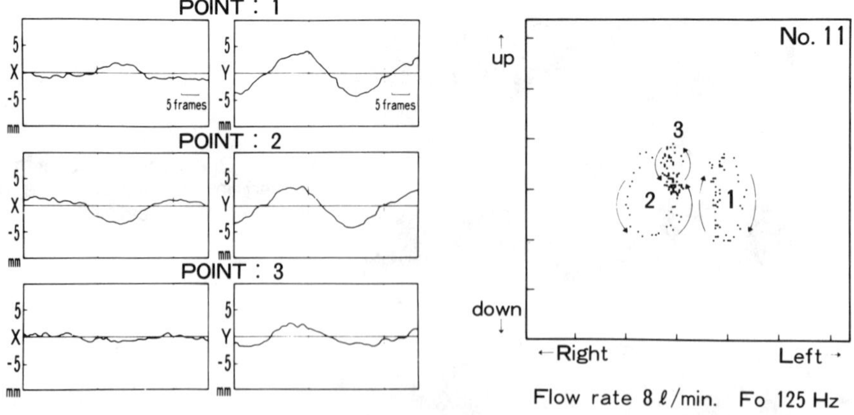

Fig. 6. Trajectories of three points in the frontal plane (left) and the resultant Lissajous figures (right).

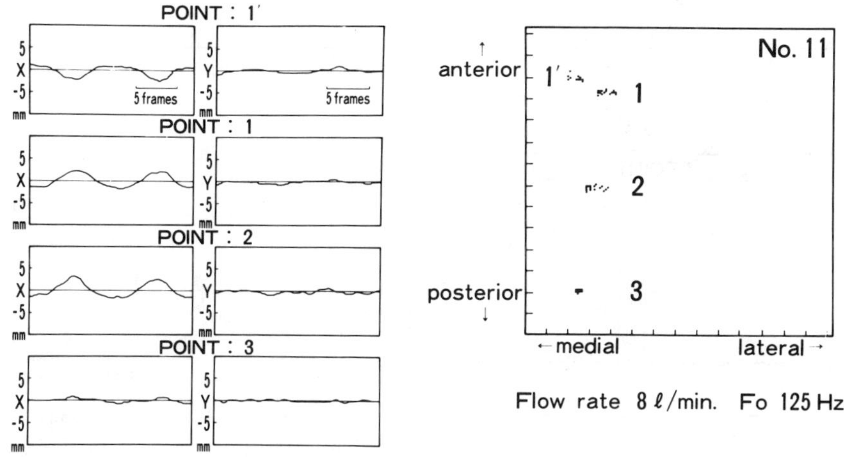

Fig. 7. Trajectories of three points in the plane of the upper surface of the vocal fold (left), and the resultant Lissajous figures (right).

their original location (Figures 3-6). Note that in Figure 3a membranous wave is also observed to move from the lower part, along the free margin, to the upper part of the vocal fold.

2. In the transverse plane, viewed superiorly (Figure 4), the pellets showed lateral motion (Figures 4-1,2) to a maximal lateral displacement (Figures 4-3) before medial motion (Figures 4-4, 5) returned them to their initial position (Figures 4-6). Maximal displacement amplitude was shown by the pellet located in the middle part of the vocal fold, with motion becoming less as pellet position approached the vocal fold ends.
3. When viewed from the lateral aspect (Figure 5) the pellet trajectories were first superior (Figures 5-1,2) and then inferior (Figures 5-4,5) to return to the original location (Figures 5-6). Maximal displacement amplitude was again at the middle part of the vocal fold; pellets at a distance of a quarter from the ends underwent less dis-

Table 1. *Maximal amplitude of displacement of all three points in plane of the upper surface of the vocal fold.*

Exp. No.	Flow rate (l/min)	F0 (Hz)	Amplitude (mm)		
			1	2	3
2	15	130	1.8	4.3	2.1
3	15	76	1.4	2.0	1.9
7	10	240	2.0	6.1	5.0
9	5	120	2.3	2.9	2.3
11	8	125	3.9	5.0	1.8

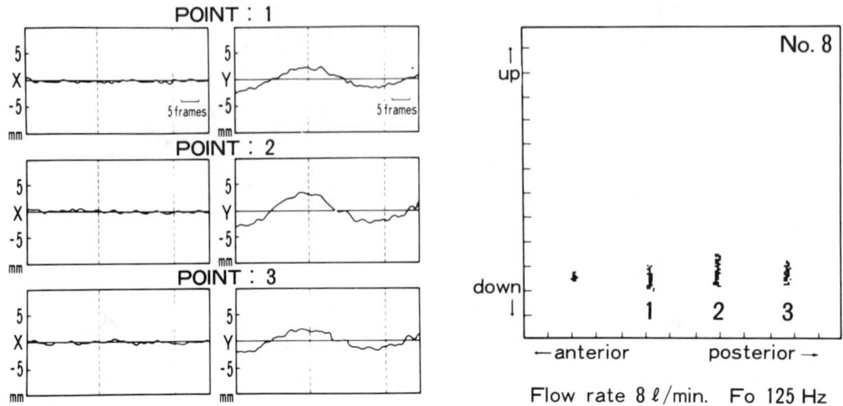

Fig. 8. Trajectories of pellets viewed from the lateral aspect (left) and related Lissajous figures (right).

placement, while the pellets at both anterior and posterior ends failed to show any movement.

Analysis of pellet trajectories

Frontal plane

A trajectory analysis of the motions of points in the frontal plane as accomplished by inserting pellets under the vocal fold epithelium in a different configuration. A pellet at the middle of the length of the vocal fold was designated POINT 2, while POINT 3 was located halfway between POINT 2 and the vocal process. Similarly POINT 1 was established by a pellet halfway between POINT 2 and the anterior commissure, except that it was located contralaterally (on the left vocal fold) in order to avoid overlapped images. Trajectory patterns are shown in Figure 6. The Y-axis scales vertical motion, while the X-axis is horizontal. At each of the three points, vertical motion is much larger than horizontal displacement. The phase of the horizontal component of POINT 1 is, of course, reversed with respect to POINT 2 and POINT 3. The lower portion of Figure 6 depicts the Lissajous figures described by the three points. The trajectory of each is approximately an ellipse whose major axis is oriented vertically.

Transverse plane

Demonstration of motions in the plane of the upper surface of the vocal fold was accomplished in the same manner as described above, except that a new point, designated POINT 1 was added exactly opposite POINT 1, that is, midway between the middle of the vocal fold and the anterior commissure ipsilateral to POINT 2 and POINT 3. The resultant data are illustrated in Figure 7, in which the X-axis represents horizontal displacement and the Y-axis shows anteroposterior motion. There is regular motion in the horizontal (X-axis) plane, but no organized movement in the anteroposterior (Y-axis)

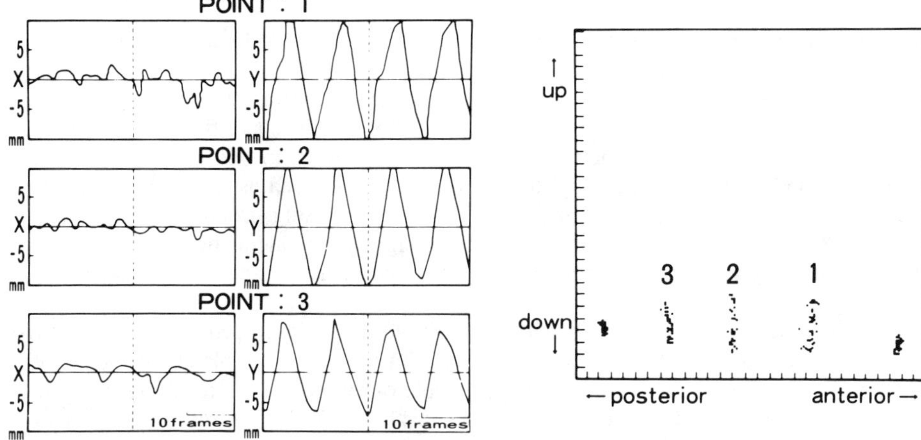

Fig. 9. Motions of the pellets as viewed from the medial aspect resolved by frame-by-frame analysis of ultra-high speed films (left) and the resultant Lissajous figures (right).

direction. Maximal amplitude of horizontal motion (summarized in Table 1) was observed at POINT 2 in each experiment.

Lateral projection

POINTS 1, 2 and 3 were tracked for this analysis. Figure 8 demonstrates that there was regular movement along the vertical, or Y-, axis, but none along the anteroposterior, or X-, axis. Vertical motion was maximal at POINT 2 in each experiment. It thus seems most likely that the pellets do not move in the anteroposterior plane, while there is regular and phasic motion in the vertical plane.

ULTRA-HIGH SPEED FILM STUDY

To permit viewing of vocal fold vibration from the medial direction one thyroid ala was resected and replaced by a transparent plastic sheet. Pellet locations were the same as described earlier. Figure 9 illustrates their trajectories from the medial viewpoint. There is clear and regular motion along the vertical (Y-) axis, but no organized movement in the anteroposterior (X-axis) direction. The associated Lissajous figures collapse to simple linear vertical paths.

CONCLUSIONS AND DISCUSSION

It is generally conceded that observation and analysis of vocal fold vibratory motion is an important key to the clarification of the mechanisms of phonation. Beyond that, such analysis plays a very important role in the estimation of the physical properties of the vocal fold membrane. Wave motion patterns inform us of the stiffness of the membrane: if there is a locus at which such wave motion is absent we may reasonably infer great stiffness at that location. Such a pathological condition might, for example, have its etiology in malignant invasion. Hence, it is important that vocal fold vibration be observed as part of everyday clinic evaluation.

The laryngostroboscope is one of the tools available for such clinical purposes, and ultra-high-speed filming is also of clinical value, although it is not sufficiently convenient for routine use. While these methods unfortunately allow us to observe vibration only from the upper surface of the vocal fold, several authors (such as Baer, 1981; van den Berg 1958; Kirikae, 1943; Schönhärl, 1960; Timcke, 1956 using stroboscopy, and Hirano et al., 1981 and Timcke et al., 1958 and by ultra-high speed cinematography) have used them to investigate vocal fold vibration and have constructed stereostatic images with them.

On the other hand, Saito and his colleagues (1981) has developed an X-ray stroboscopic method that permits observation of vibration in the frontal plane. Using it, they have advanced the idea that the essential principle of vibration is a travelling wave that proceeds upward from the lower surface of the vocal fold. In the present research, we observed vocal fold vibration from superior, frontal, and medial viewpoints using tiny lead pellets under the vocal fold membrane. Ordinary stroboscopic observation as well as auditory perception confirmed that they did not significantly impair normal vibration. Our analyses indicate that the pellets are displaced only in the frontal plane, and never in the anteroposterior direction. The amplitude of membrane motion is greatest at the middle of the vocal fold, and diminishes as one approaches its ends. There is no detectable pellet displacement at the anterior and posterior commissures. In short, the membrane of the vocal fold moves like a child's jump rope, relatively free in the middle and tethered at both ends.

REFERENCES

Baer, T. (1981). Observation of the vocal fold vibration. Measurement of excised larynges. In: *Vocal Fold Physiology*, edited by K.N. Stevens and M. Hirano, pp. 119-133. University of Tokyo Press, Tokyo.

van den Berg, J.W. (1958). Myoelastic-aerodynamic theory of voice production. *J. Speech Hear. Res.*, 1:227-244.

Fukuda, H., Saito, S., Kitahara, S., Isogai, Y., Makino, K., Tsuzuki, T., Kogawa, N., and Ono, H. (1983). Vocal fold vibration in excised larynges. In: *Vocal Fold Physiology*, edited by D.M. Bless and J.H. Abbs, pp. 238-252. College Hill Press, San Diego, CA.

Hirano, M., Kakita, Y., Kawasaki, H., Gould, W.J., and Lambiase, A. (1981). Data from high-speed motion picture studies. In: *Vocal Fold Physiology*, edited by K.N. Stevens and M. Hirano, pp. 85-93. University of Tokyo Press, Tokyo.

Kirikae, I. (1943). Über den Bewegungsvorgang an den Stimmlippen und die Öffnungs- und Verschlusszeit der Stimmritze während der Phonation. *J. Otolaryngol. Jpn.*, 49:236-262.

Saito, S., Fukuda, H., Isogai, Y., and Ono, H. (1981). X-ray stroboscopy. In: *Vocal Fold Physiology*, edited by K.N. Stevens and M. Hirano, pp. 95-106. University of Tokyo Press, Tokyo.

Schönhärl, E. (1960). *Die Stroboskopie in der praktischen Laryngologie*. Georg Thieme Verlag, Stuttgart.

Timcke, R. (1956). Die Synchron-Stroboskopie von menschlichen Stimmlippen bzw ähnlichen Schallquellen und Messung der Öffnungszeit. *Z. Laryng. Rhin. Otolaryngol.*, 35:331-335.

Timcke, R., von Leden, H., and Moore, P. (1958). Laryngeal vibrations. Measurements of the glottic wave. 1. The normal vibratory cycle. *Arch. Otolaryngol.*, 68:1-19.

3

Ultrasound Laryngography: Multiple Simultaneous Recording of Vocal Fold Vibration

Toshio Kaneko, Takeshi Hino, Haruhiko Suzuki, Tsutomu Numata, and Hideaki Tsuchiya

Dept. of Otorhinolaryngology, School of Medicine, Chiba University, Chiba, 280 Japan

Ultrasonoglottography, UGG, was originally developed in our laboratory in 1964. Recent and rapid progress in the area of ultrasound electronics has allowed us to develop new instrumentation for ultrasound laryngography, ULG. At the Fifth Vocal Fold Physiology Conference we reported preliminary results of observations of vocal fold vibration using this method (Kaneko et al., 1988).

UGG uses a single 10 mm probe and a frequency of 2.25 or 5 MHz. The resulting ultrasound beam attains a width of about 10 mm at the free margin of the vocal fold. ULG, on the other hand, uses a linear scanner at a frequency of 7.5 MHz. The beam is electronically focused to an area of 2x2 mm at the surface of the vocal fold. Thus, ULG achieves better spatial resolution than the older UGG. Further, UGG uses A-mode to detect the vocal fold, making it difficult, in practice, to estimate the exact proportions of vocal fold displacement. However, ULG allows monitoring of a vertical section of the larynx using B-mode. This makes it easy to detect the vocal fold, and we can determine exactly which portion of the vocal fold has been recorded by using M-mode.

In the present paper we demonstrate the different vibratory modes of the upper and lower portions of the vocal fold as revealed by ULG. We also contrast the waveforms obtained by ULG to those generated by photoglottography (PGG).

SUBJECT AND METHOD

Analyses were done of a 31 year old male with no known vocal pathology who phonated the vowel /e/ at comfortable pitch and loudness.

The experimental instrumentation is diagramed in Figure 1. Two probes were used for the ULG recordings. One, a small linear-scan transducer with a carrier frequency of 7.5 MHz, was used for the B-mode and high-speed M-mode analyses. The other was a single probe having a diameter of 13 mm that was used for pulsed-transmission examinations. The probes were mounted on a holder and applied to the skin with their central axes

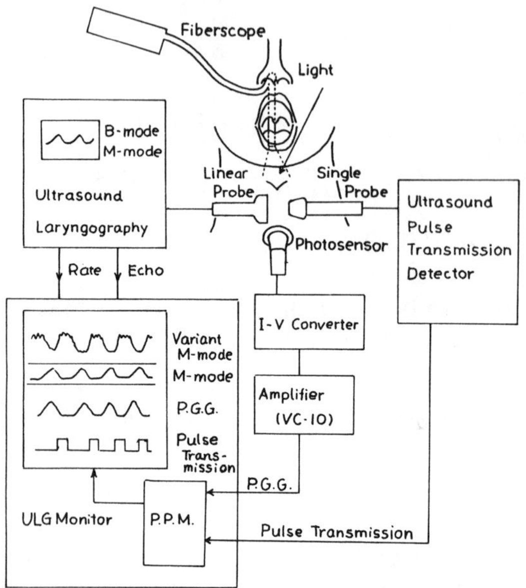

Fig. 1. Block diagram.

aligned. Inter probe distance was adjusted to suit the subject's larynx before the probes were placed on either side of the neck. The linear-scan probe was oriented vertically on the skin of the lateral region of the neck in order to obtain a B-mode coronal section of the larynx. The following recordings were obtained:

1. *High-speed M-mode method.* While observing the ULG B-mode display the cursor position was adjusted to the desired vocal fold level and the display changed to M-mode. The ultrasound pulse repetition rate was set for 10 KHz. The echo and the pulse repetition rate signals were fed to the ULG monitor, allowing it to display M-mode information.

2. *Pulse-transmission method* . The single probe was used to receive the ultrasound pulses transmitted from the opposite side of the larynx during the periods of vocal fold contact. This probe's output was processed by the ultrasound pulse-transmission detector, which produced a 2 V DC output whenever the signal exceeded a threshold value.

3. *Variant M-mode method.* The time window for the variant M-mode was adjusted for either the free margin or the inner layer of the vocal fold by observing the ULG display.

4. *Photoglottography.* The PGG signal was obtained from a flexible fiberoptic light source (inserted *per nasum*) and a photosensor on the neck surface just below the level of the glottis.

All waveforms were displayed simultaneously on the ULG monitor. Single sweeps of the display were photographed with a Polaroid camera.

RESULTS

Modes of Vocal Fold Vibration Recorded by ULG

The M-mode waveform was found to vary as the cursor was moved from the lower to the upper portion of the vocal fold during phonation. Ultrasound is, in theory, totally reflected at the mucous membrane/air interface. In the M-mode, the intensity of the reflected beam modulates the brightness of the display. Total reflection of the beam results in maximal modulation, thus making the air/membrane boundary the brightest feature in the display.

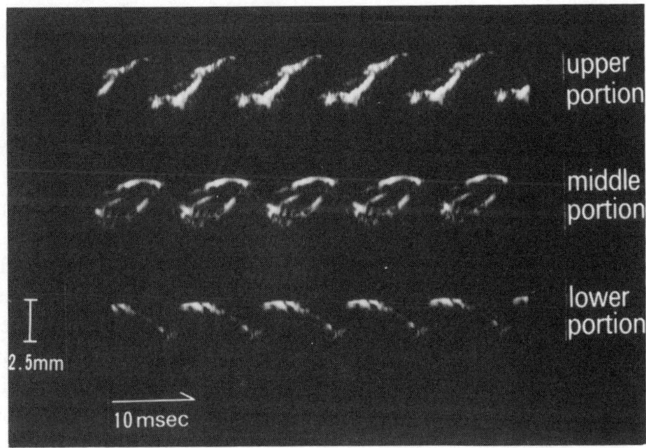

Fig. 2. Recordings of the vocal fold vibration by M-mode method (phonation at 100 Hz).

Figure 2 shows recordings at three vocal fold levels during steady phonation. The top trace is of the M-mode waveforms from the upper portion of the vocal fold. The M-mode image of the free margin of the vocal fold was brightened during the closed and opening phases. During the latter, the trace appeared as a series of ascending lines. The portion of the trace representing the closed phase, however, was dark.

The bottom trace of Figure 2 illustrates the M-mode record of the lower portion of the vocal fold. It is bright during the closed and closing phases of the vibratory cycle. During the latter, the display shows convex curves. The opening phase produced no visible trace in the display.

Finally, the center trace of Figure 2 depicts the M-mode waveform from the middle portion of the vocal fold. The record from this region seems to be a combination of the upper and lower traces in that the ascending lines of the opening phase correspond to those of the upper portion of the vocal fold, while the descending traces of the closing phase correspond to those of the lower portion. It is, therefore, our opinion that the ascending and descending lines obtained from the middle portion of the vocal fold indicate the glottal width of the open phase.

Figure 3 schematizes the M-mode image of Figure 2. Four vertical markers have been added. The first, labelled A, demarcates the point at which vocal fold opening begins. B indicates peak glottal opening and C shows the point at which the glottis is closed. The next opening phase begins at the marker labelled D. If E and F denote the points of maximal opening of the lower and upper portions of the vocal folds, respectively, then the phase difference between the two regions is about 85°.

Simultaneous M-mode and pulse transmission-mode recordings of the upper and lower portions of the vocal fold are illustrated in Figure 4. Closed phases are indicated by upward deviations from the baseline in the pulse transmission records. In these recordings, the closed time of the middle portion of the vocal folds was longer than that of either the upper or lower portion.

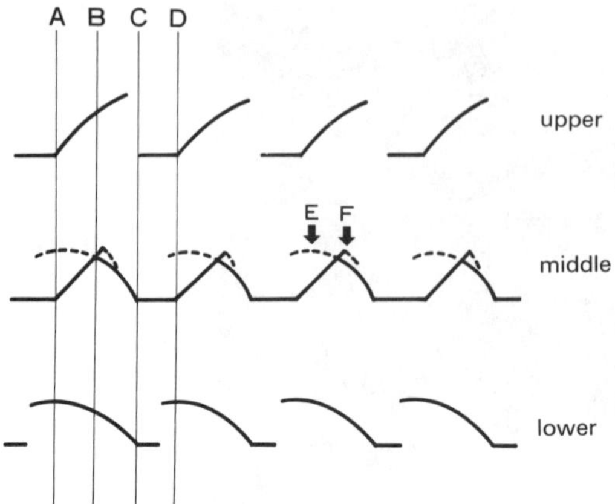

Fig. 3. Schema of the M-mode images.

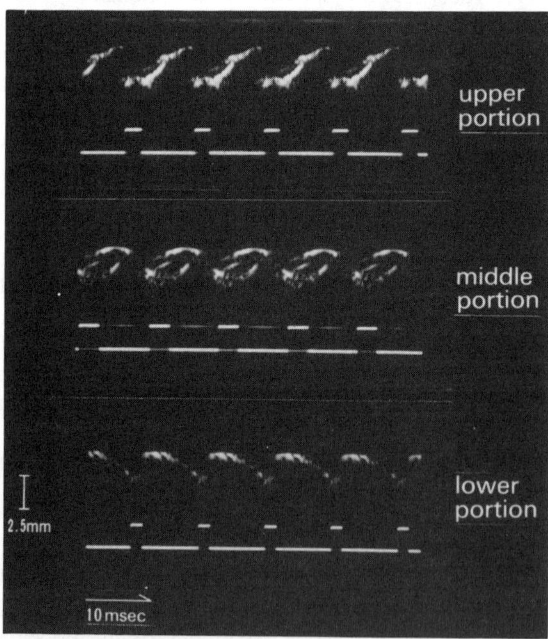

Fig. 4. Simultaneous recordings of the vocal fold vibration by M-mode and pulse transmission method (phonation at 100 Hz).

Figure 5 plots the mean open quotient (OQ) calculated from 40 cycles of the pulse transmission records of each of the three vocal fold regions. The middle region has the lowest OQ.

Simultaneous recordings of M-, variant M-, and pulse transmission-mode data for the middle portion of the vocal folds are shown in Figure 6. Two time windows were used for the variant M-mode recording. One, adjusted to the level at which the vocal folds made contact, was used to observe minute movements of the free margin of the vocal folds during the closed phase. The other was adjusted to the inner layer of the vocal fold. The variant M-mode waveform is plotted with increasing echo energy upward; it shows energy as a function of time. The variant M-mode signal of the free margin of the vocal fold increases abruptly when vocal fold contact begins, and the closed phase is associated with some ripples in the signal. We assume that these ripples are the product of two factors: minute vibrations caused by vocal fold collisions and a reduction of echo energy caused by ultrasound transmission through the contacting vocal folds.

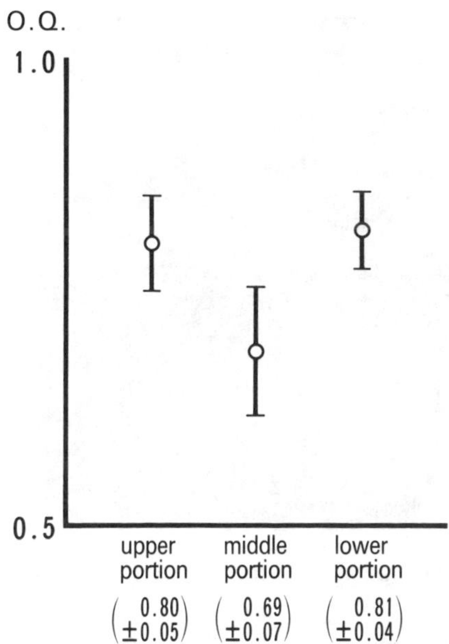

Fig. 5. Open quotient measured by pulse transmission method.

Relationship of PGG and ULG Waveform

ULG waveforms from the middle portion of the vocal folds were compared to the PGG waveforms. Figure 7 shows recordings of about 5 cycles of steady phonation at 103 Hz. From top to bottom, the traces are M-mode, PGG, and pulse transmission modes. Glottal width measured from the M-mode data is practically identical to the width represented in the PGG record. Peak glottal opening in the PGG record, however, was found to occur slightly earlier than in the M-mode trace. The moments of glottal closure in the pulse transmission and the PGG records were the same. In the PGG signal, opening is so gradual that it was difficult to designate a single point to demarcate its start. Furthermore, the PGG signal rises

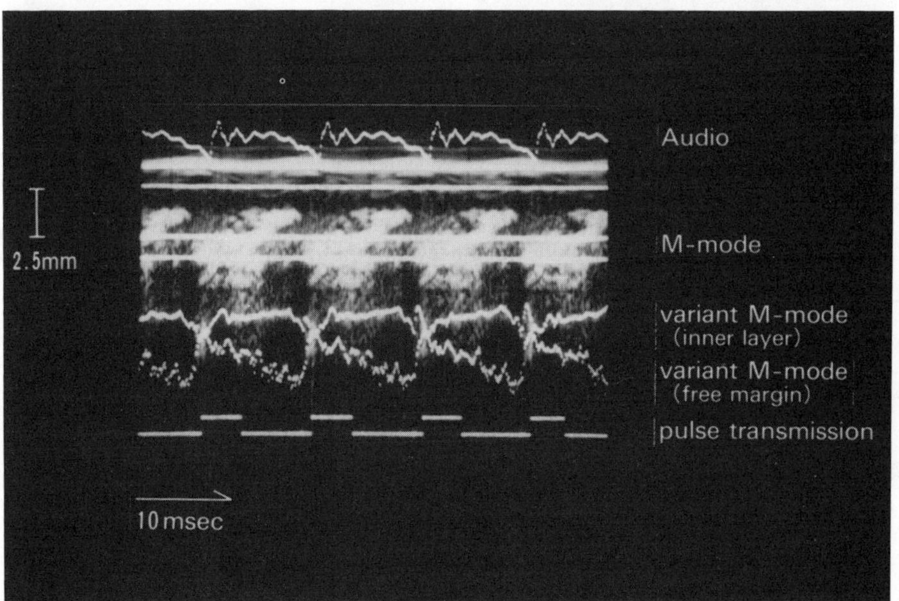

Fig. 6. Simultaneous recording of the vocal fold vibration by M-mode, variant M-mode, pulse transmission and audio signal (phonation at 87 Hz).

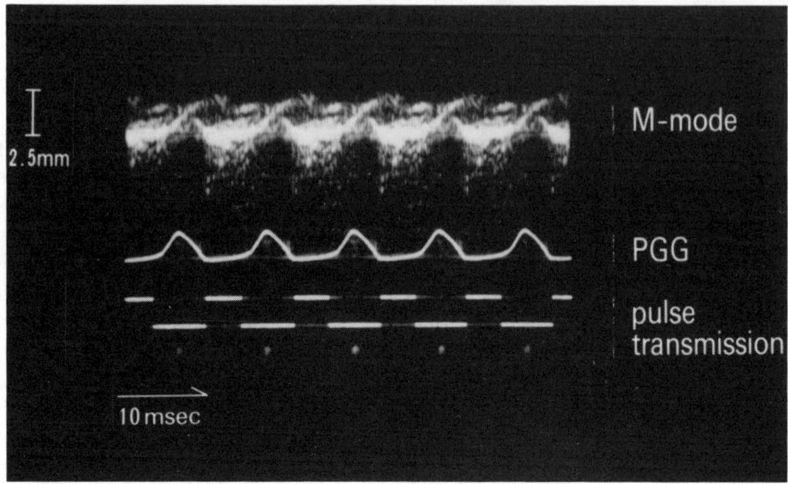

Fig. 7. Simultaneous recording of the vocal fold vibration by M-mode, pulse transmission and PGG.

from baseline at the end of what the pulse transmission trace represents as the closed phase.

CONCLUSION

From our ULG and PGG recordings of the phonation of an adult male, we draw the following conclusions:

1. Three different types of M-mode traces are obtained, depending on whether the upper, middle, or lower portion of the vocal fold is being observed;
2. The open quotient is smallest at the middle level of the vocal folds;
3. Ripples appear in the closed-phase portion of the variant M-mode record;
4. There is good correspondence of the ULG and PGG findings.

REFERENCES

Kaneko, T., Numata, T., Suzuki, H., Hino, T., Komatsu, K., and Masuda, T. (1988). Newly developed ultrasound laryngographic equipment and its clinical application. In: *Vocal Fold Physiology: Voice Production, Mechanisms and Functions*, edited by Osamu Fujimura. pp. 271-278. Raven Press, New York.

4

Basement Membrane Zone Injury in Vocal Nodules

Steven D. Gray

Dept. of Otolaryngology-Head and Neck Surgery, University of Iowa Hospitals and Clinics, Iowa City, IA, USA

The basic structural organization of the vocal fold (the epidermis, the lamina propria, and the thyroarytenoid muscle) (Figure 1) has been studied using light microscopy and histological staining techniques. Hirano and Kurita (1986) found that the superficial layer of the lamina propria (SLLP) differed from the deep layer in the amount of fibre present. The SLLP has fewer fibrous components and is relatively acellular, which makes it very pliable tissue.

Hirano's studies also show that the collagen fibres of the deep layer of the lamina propria intertwine with the thyroarytenoid muscle; from this contact, collagen and elastin fibres construct a network that spans the lamina propria and connects to the epidermis. Our study was designed to show how this fibrous network attaches to the epidermis. We explored the structural characteristics of the attachments and their relationship to pathological conditions of the vocal fold resulting from vocal abuse. The basement membrane zone (BMZ), or area of junction between the epidermis and the lamina propria (Figure 2), includes the sites at which the cell layers are attached while being subjected to stretching, shearing and friction producing forces. The mechanism of attachment is a complex and only partially understood arrangement of proteins and structures. If the epidermal-lamina propria junction is similar to other epidermal junctions, then it is highly probable that type 1 collagen fibres and the elastin fibres do not directly insert into the basement membrane of the epidermis (Katz, 1984).

Dermatological investigators have divided the BMZ into four areas: the plasma membrane of the basal cell of the epidermis; the lamina lucida; the lamina densa; and the sublamina densa or sub-basement membrane zone (Abrahamson, 1986; Katz, 1984; Martinez-Hernandez and Amenta, 1983). Each area has a unique function and consists of attaching structures and proteins found only in the BMZ. Figure 2 shows structures that can be identified and quantified by electron microscopy. The basal cell of the epidermis attaches to the lamina lucida and densa by means of hemidesmosomes, which consist of an attachment plaque (AP) (part of the basal cell membrane secured to the cytoskeleton by tonofilaments); a sub-basal dense plate (DP) in the lamina lucida; and anchoring filaments (AFL), which extend from the attachment plaque through the sub-basal dense plate and into the lamina densa, holding them all together (Figure 2).

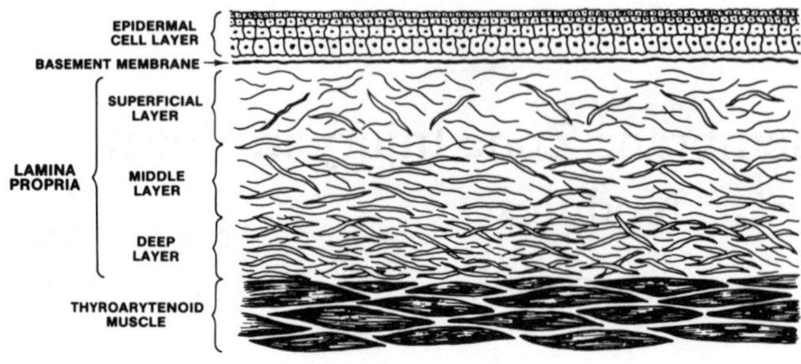

Fig. 1. Structure of the fold. Drawing is not to scale; the lamina propria is thicker compared to the epidermal cell layer than shown.

The sublamina densa sub-basement membrane area contains electron dense structures known as anchoring fibrils (AF) and dermal myofibril bundles (Goldsmith and Briggaman, 1983; Sakai et al., 1986). These structures probably attach to the lamina densa and extend into the lamina propria. Type 1 collagen and elastin fibres do not connect directly into the lamina densa or to the basal cell: however these fibres form a supporting network that extends from the muscle up to the epidermis.

ELECTRON MICROSCOPY

Normal Human Vocal Folds in Basement Membrane Zone

Electron microscopy reveals many structures observed in the normal canine BMZ (Figure 3). Hemidesmosomes are abundant with well developed attachment plaques securing the basal cell to the lamina densa (basement membrane) and the lamina lucida. The thickness of the lamina densa and lamina lucida appear similar to other epidermal-dermal junctions. The lamina densa forms a single-layer, narrow sheet upon which the basal cells sit. Occasional anchoring fibres extend from the lamina densa,

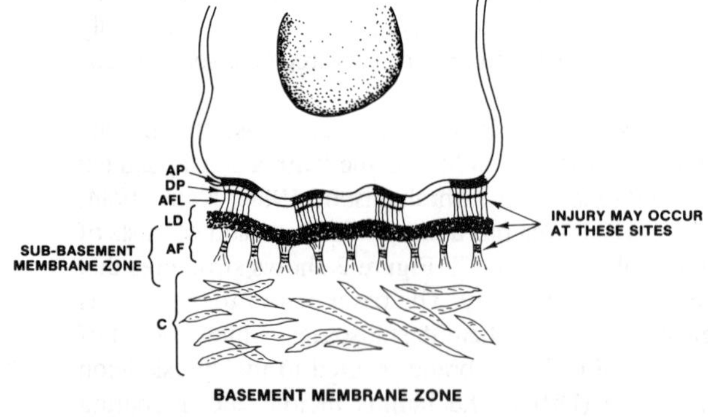

Fig. 2. Basement membrane zone. Basal cells are connected to lamina densa by attachment plaques (AP) in the plasma membrane of the epidermis. Anchoring filaments (AFL) extend from the attachment plaque through the sub-basal densa plate (DP) and attach to the lamina densa, a dark single-layer, electron-dense band just beneath the basal cell layer. The sub-basement membrane zone consists of anchoring fibres (AF) that attach to the lamina densa and extend into the superficial layer of the lamina propria. These fibres are near and may attach to the network of the lamina propria. (Note: the fibrous network of the lamina propria does not directly attach to the epidermis).

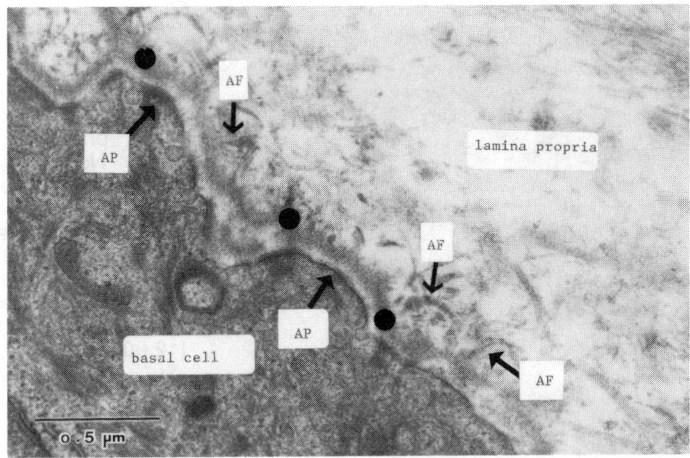

Fig. 3. Normal vocal fold including basal cell basement membrane zone (arrow) and fibres from the lamina propria (10,000 x). A) Canine vocal fold (10,000 x) B) Human vocal fold. Electron micrograph details basement membrane zone (BMZ). LD-lamina densa; AF-anchoring fibers; HD-hemidesmosomes; CF-collagen fibre type 1. Note that in normals the BMZ is contained within 0.5 um of the basal cell membrane. Transition to superficial layer of lamina propria is complete (60,000 x).

making small loops into the SLLP or just ending in the SLLP. Type 1 collagen fibres come up into the sublamina densa area (sub-basement membrane zone). In the normal vocal fold the fibrous network of the lamina propria is very close to the basal cells of the epidermis, being separated only by a single thin layer of specialized proteins and structures. This narrow, thin area contains structures for holding the epidermis to the lamina propria during periods of intense vibration. Since the lamina propria and the epidermis are composed of very different types of tissue, stress at the attachment sites may be unevenly absorbed. Stress during vibration may result in injury to the attachment structures of the BMZ. We tested this hypothesis by subjecting canine vocal folds to intense prolonged phonation.

Canine Vocal Folds Subjected to Vibration

In a previous study the vocal folds of dogs were subjected to intense phonation (60-90 dB at 6 ft.) for approximately 4 hours (Gray and Titze, 1988), after which they were harvested and examined with light and electron microscopy. The following injury patterns were found: 1) detachment of the lamina densa from the basal cells, presumably due to disruption of the anchoring filaments of the hemidesmosomes since the remaining structures (attachment plaques, basal cell membrane and tonofilaments) consistently appeared intact; 2) destruction and disintegration of the lamina densa, or 3) disruption of the sublamina densa layer, specifically the anchoring fibrils (Figure 4). In one case the epidermis became detached from the lamina propria and floated freely. In another, the injury created a space in which interstitial fluid and debris collected. The physiological result was the same with each of these injury patterns: the attaching structures that secured the fibrous network of the lamina propria to the epidermis were destroyed, and

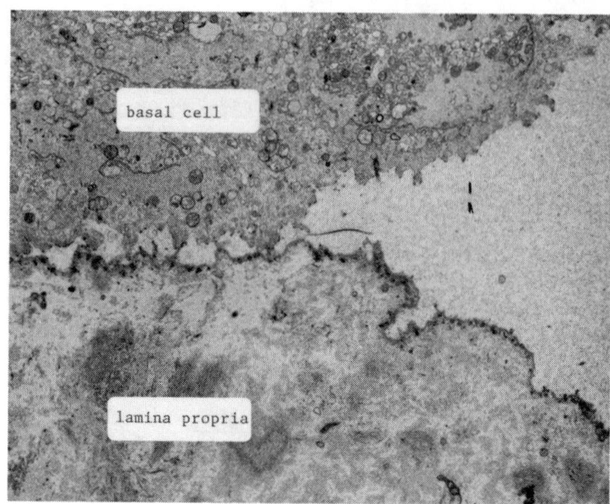

Fig. 4. Canine vocal fold after being subjected to intense phonation for four hours. Note separation of the basal cell layer from the lamina propria. Anchoring filaments, lamina densa, and anchoring fibres have been injured and the lamina propria is detached from the epithelium in this area (12,000 x).

epidermis and lamina propria are less coupled. If the fibrous network is released from the BMZ, it may contract and pull away (Figure 4). An additional consequence of these acute injuries is edema.

Nodules on Human Vocal Folds

In this study we used electron microscopy to examine nodules from four patients who shared the following characteristics:

- the nodules were chronic, having been present for more than six months;
- they failed to improve with voice rest followed by at least 3 months of intensive speech and/or voice therapy and rehabilitation and
- the nodules were located in the middle of the membranous fold.

As we examined the vocal nodules we found pathological conditions in the BMZ. Overall thickness was markedly increased (Figure 5). We were unable to identify single layers of lamina lucida and lamina densa. Although we have not quantified thickness, in some of the nodules typical SLLP histology with type 1 collagen fibres was not found, which suggests that we resected the nodule from abnormal tissue. In another specimen we saw a gradual transition from what appeared to be proliferation of BMZ components to normal SLLP histology.

Examination of the BMZ at higher magnification revealed specific abnormalities (Figure 5). The basal cell membrane and attachment plaques were present but many plaques appeared not to be cemented to the lamina densa since no anchoring filaments were present below the attachment plaques. Normal BMZ architecture was absent and beneath certain parts of the basal cells no lamina densa was present to which they could attach.

Instead of creating a single sheet-like structure beneath the basal cells, the lamina densa appeared convoluted, reduplicated, poorly oriented, fragmented, and did not follow the contour of the basal cell membrane. Abundant anchoring fibres were identified attaching into the lamina densa, more than we had found in normal human vocal folds.

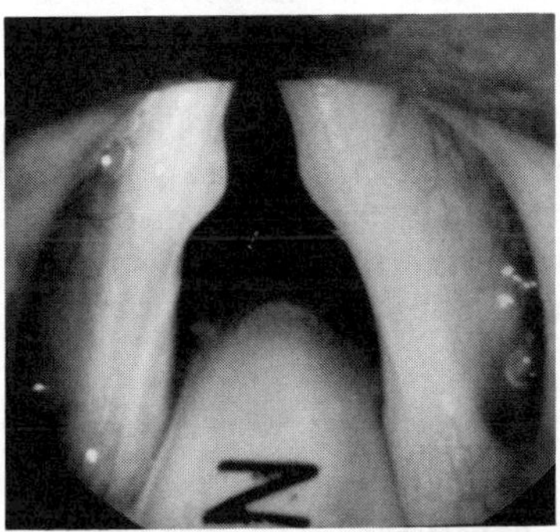

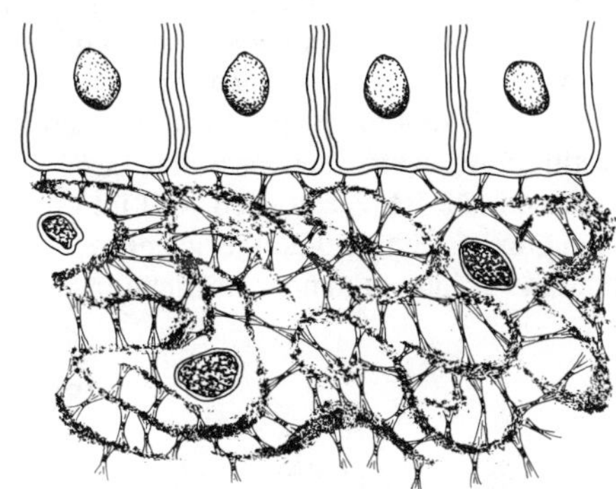

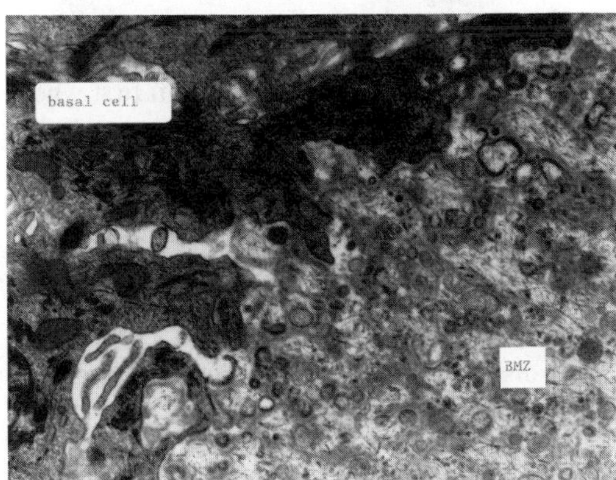

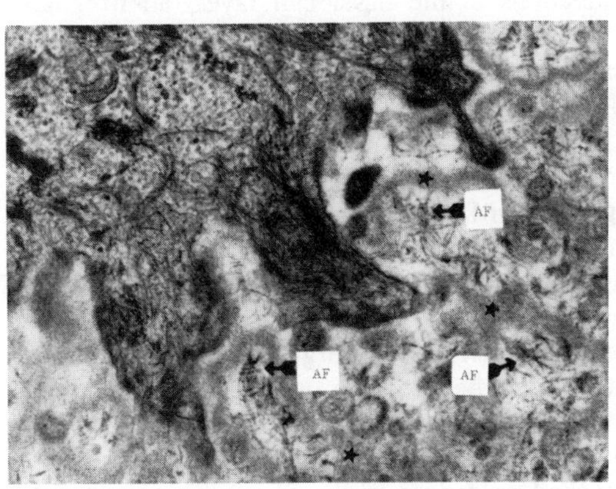

Fig. 5. Human vocal fold nodule. (**a**) Prior to excision. (**b**) Electron micrograph of A. Note thick basement membrane zone below basal cell. Higher magnification shows duplication and convolutions of the lamina densa (basement membrane). Many extracellular organelles are visible (15,000 x). (**c**) Higher magnification of B shows robust anchoring fibres (AF). Note random orientation of anchoring fibers (AF) and lamina densa (LD) (basement membrane) (50.000 x). (**d**) Schematic outline of basement membrane zone in vocal nodule: shaded area represents lamina densa (basement membrane) with anchoring fibres robust and randomly arranged.

However, because of the convolutions in the lamina densa, the anchoring fibres were oriented in all directions and could not attach the lamina densa to the lamina propria. Furthermore many of the anchoring fibres seemed partially formed and rudimentary. The whole BMZ was markedly thickened and in total disarray. No type 1 collagen fibres or elastin fibres were seen near the basal cell membrane. In the human vocal nodules examined, the BMZ extended well into the area where only lamina propria components should exist. Extracellular organelles were abundant and thought to represent BMZ components, although no identification has been made at this time.

DISCUSSION

It is probable that some of the tissue injury due to excessive vocal fold vibration is a result of at least two actions, the shearing forces of vibration and the dampening of the vibratory pattern from the epidermis to the thyroarytenoid muscle. The vocal fold is constructed to withstand these forces, with a woven network of collagen and elastic fibres extending from the muscle to the squamous epidermal covering. The canine experiments were designed to determine which part of this architecture would break down first when subjected to prolonged intense phonation. Although epidermal damage was noticed, the first area of injury to the vocal fold occurred at the junction of the fibrous network and the epidermis, namely the BMZ. Tissue deformation during vibration is greatest at the epidermal cover and lessened quickly as it progressed laterally into the vocal fold (Saito et al., 1983). It would seem that the SLLP and the BMZ are likely areas of injury from phonation.

Electron microscopic findings in vocal nodules indicate that the BMZ had been subjected to repeated injury that resulted in disorganization of the normal structures. Because of these changes it is likely that the BMZ is functionally less able to provide secure attachment of the SLLP to the epidermis, although no research has demonstrated this as yet.

In support of the position that the BMZ is an important area for injury to the vocal fold and development of nodules (Mossallam et al., 1986) reported two cases that showed distorted and attenuated desmosomal junctions at the basal cell layer; an irregular, disconnected, and thickened basement membrane; and sub-basement membrane zone containing abundant precollagenous substances. These findings are consistent with reports of BMZ injury. Kleinsasser (1986) reported that histology of early cases of Reinke's edema showed the epithelium was lifted off the lamina propria under which a collection of fluid developed. He further stated the only pronounced histologic finding in long-standing cases is marked thickening of the BMZ.

In summary, this research would suggest that BMZ injury occurs as a result of vibratory and shearing forces and may play a role in the development of nodules. Ultrastructural histology using electron microscopy of human vocal nodules reveals a thickened BMZ with reduplication of the lamina densa and disorganized anchoring fibres indicating recurrent injury. Chronic nodules may be due to in part a repeatedly injured BMZ which, being unable to heal normally because of repeated disruption, injury, and reseparation of the SLLP and the epidermis, heals in a disorganized fashion while attempting to secure the repeatedly detached epidermis to the SLLP. This aberrantly repaired BMZ may predispose the area to vocal injury at a lower vibration threshold, making resolution of a nodule in the chronic state more difficult to treat. We acknowledge that these findings based on a small number of nodules and normal human specimens, are preliminary. Research will continue in this area as additional specimens become available.

REFERENCES

Abrahamson, D.R. (1986). Recent studies on the structure and pathology of basement membranes. *J. Pathol.*, 149:257-278.

Goldsmith, L.A. and Briggaman, R.A. (1983). Monoclonal antibodies to anchoring fibrils for the diagnosis of epidermolysis bullosa. *J. Investig. Dermatol.*, 81:464-466.

Gray, S.D. and Titze, I.R. (1988). Histological investigation of the hyperphonated canine vocal cords. *Ann. Otol. Rhinol. Laryngol.*, 97:381-388.

Hirano, M. and Kurita, S. (1986). Histological structure of the vocal fold and its normal and pathological variations. In: *Vocal Fold Histopathology: A Symposium*, edited by J.A. Kirchner, pp. 17-24. College-Hill Press, San Diego, CA.

Katz, S.I.(1984). The epidermal basement membrane zone - Structure, ontogeny, and role in disease. *J. Am. Acad. Dermatol.*, 11:1025-1037.

Kleinsasser, O. (1986). Microlaryngoscopic and histologic appearances of polyps, nodules, cysts, Reinke's edema, and granulomas of the vocal cords. In: *Vocal Fold Histopathology: A Symposium*, edited by J.A. Kirchner, pp. 51-55. College-Hill Press, San Diego, CA.

Martinez-Hernandez, A. and Amenta, P.S. (1983). The basement membrane in pathology. *Lab. Investig.*, 48:656-677.

Mossallam, I., Kotby, M.N., Ghaly, A.F., Nasser A.M., and Barakah, M.A. (1986). Histopathological aspects of benign vocal fold lesions associated with dysphonia. In: *Vocal Fold Histopathology: A Symposium*, edited by J.A. Kirchner, pp. 65-80. College-Hill Press, San Diego, CA.

Saito, S., Fukuda, H., Kitahara, S., Isogai, Y., Tsuzuki, T., Muta, H., Takayama, E., Fujioka, T., Kokawa, N., and Makino, K. (1983). Pellet tracking in the vocal fold while phonating-experimental study using canine larynges with muscle activity. In: *Vocal Fold Physiology: Biomechanics, acoustics and phonatory control*, edited by I. Titze and R.C. Scherer, pp. 169-182. The Denver Center for the Performing Arts, Denver, CO.

Sakai, L.Y., Keene, D.R., Morris, N.P., and Burgeson, R.E. (1986). Type VII collagen is a major structural component of anchoring fibrils. *J. Cell Biology*, 103:1577-1586.

5

Vocal-Fold Vibration for Obstruent Consonants

Kenneth N. Stevens

Dept. of Electrical Engineering and Computer Science and Research Laboratory of Electronics, Massachusetts Institute of Technology, Cambridge, MA 02139, USA

An obstruent consonant is produced by forming a narrow constriction in the vocal tract, and by increasing or decreasing the pressure within the vocal tract, relative to atmospheric pressure. Thus the salient characteristic of an obstruent is the appearance of a pressure drop across the vocal-tract constriction.

In the vicinity of the time when there is a constriction, the configuration of the glottis, the configuration of the vocal tract, and the state of the vocal folds can be adjusted so that various amounts of pressure drop appear across the glottal and supraglottal constrictions, and different patterns of acoustic sources are produced at the two constrictions. For some of these adjustments, the vocal folds can vibrate, and for these and other adjustments turbulence noise is generated at one or both constrictions.

In this paper we shall develop a theoretical model for analyzing the interaction between these glottal and supraglottal parameters when various classes of voiceless and voiced obstruents are produced. Predictions from the model are consistent with acoustic and pressure-flow data that have been obtained for these consonants. The proposed analysis builds on the earlier theoretical work of Rothenberg (1968) and of Westbury (1979, 1983), and draws on experimental data of Dixit (1975), and others.

LARYNGEAL STATES FOR OBSTRUENT CONSONANTS

Effect of intraoral pressure on glottal opening

When a supraglottal constriction is formed, together with a relatively constricted laryngeal configuration, a speaker has the option of increasing or decreasing the intraoral pressure by manipulating the size of the volume between the two constrictions, as well as by manipulating the sizes of the glottal and supraglottal constrictions. One consequence of an increase or a decrease in the intraoral pressure is that this pressure creates abducting or adducting forces on the upper surfaces of the vocal folds. The result of these forces is a passive outward or inward displacement of the upper portion of the vocal folds when this part of the glottis is open. Thus, for example, if the vocal folds are in a particular resting configuration with the upper edges slightly separated, and the supraglottal pressure increases from zero pressure (i.e., atmosphere pressure) to 8 cm H_2O, the upper surfaces of the folds will spread apart as a consequence of the passive force. For a normal vocal-fold stiffness per unit length of about $2x10^4$ dynes/cm^2 (Kakita et al., 1981), and assuming a thickness of this upper surface of about 1 mm, the magnitude of the abducting displace-

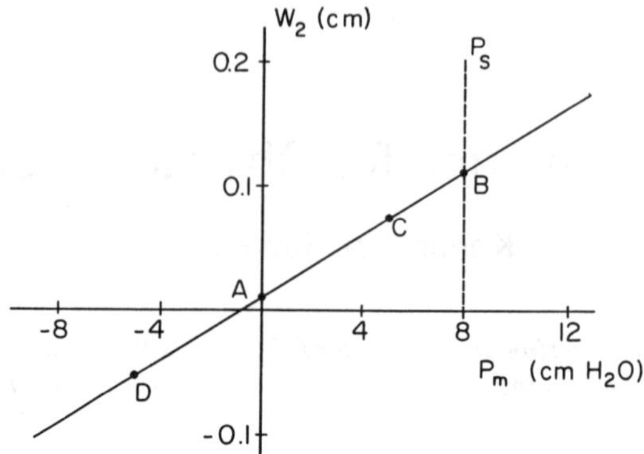

Fig. 1. Illustrating the passive change in the effective width w_2 of the superior edge of the glottis as the intraoral pressure P_m changes. A typical subglottal pressure P_s is shown as a vertical dashed line. Points along the sloping line are discussed in the text. Negative values of w_2 indicate what the vocal-fold position would be if its displacement were not inhibited by the opposing vocal fold. Numerical values are selected to be in the range considered reasonable for a two-mass model of adult vocal folds.

ment of each fold is estimated to be about 0.05 cm. On the other hand, a decrease in the supraglottal pressure below atmospheric pressure will cause an inward displacement of the upper vocal-fold surfaces. The decreased supraglottal pressure can result in complete adduction of the folds, so that there is an inward force that bonds the folds together.

The situation is summarized graphically in Figure 1, which shows a plot of the width w_2 of the upper edge of the glottis as a function of the intraoral pressure P_m. The ordinate represents the resting width for different values of P_m, although under some conditions the vocal folds will vibrate when a subglottal pressure is applied. In this case, w_2 might be considered as an average width around which vocal-fold vibration occurs.

The point *A* on the w_2-axis indicates a hypothetical resting width for the upper vocal-fold surface when $P_m = 0$. We have selected this resting width to be 0.1 mm, although other resting widths are, of course, possible. An increase in P_m causes an increase in the width w_2 as shown by the upward sloping line to the right, and a decrease in P_m causes a decrease in w_2. We show w_2 becoming negative for a sufficiently negative intraoral pressure. This negative width simply indicates a hypothetical position that would be assumed by a vocal-fold surface if there were no opposing surface. The slope of the line is determined by the stiffness of the vocal folds. A nominal stiffness is assumed for the slope in the figure, corresponding to a stiffness per unit length of about 2×10^4 dynes/cm^2.

A dashed vertical line is drawn in Figure 1 at a value of $P_m = 8$ cm H_2O. We shall assume a fixed subglottal pressure of 8 cm H_2O, so that on this vertical line the subglottal and supraglottal pressures are equal. As we traverse from point *A* to point *B* in the figure, the transglottal pressure decreases from 8 cm H_2O to zero. When the transglottal pressure is more than about 3 cm H_2O (i.e., to the left of point *C*, located at $P_m = 5$ cm H_2O), the vocal folds are expected to vibrate, whereas for conditions corresponding to the segment *CB* vocal-fold vibration cannot be maintained. Similarly there is a point *D* to the left of

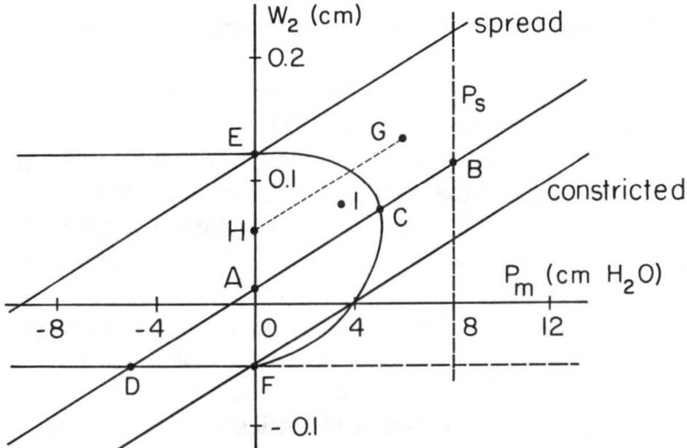

Fig. 2. The chart of Figure 1 is expanded to illustrate a range of laryngeal configurations. Active adjustment of the model yields the spread and constricted configurations as indicated, in addition to a modal configuration considered in Figure 1. Vocal-fold vibration can occur within the contour *ECFD*, but cannot occur outside this contour. The dashed line at the bottom is the boundary line below which the glottis remains closed when a subglottal pressure of 8 cm H_2O is applied. The various labelled points on the chart are discussed in the text.

the starting point *A* where the adducting force due to the negative supraglottal pressure is sufficient to prevent the glottis from opening as a consequence of the forces from the subglottal pressure. This situation is estimated to occur for a value of w_2 of about -0.05 cm.

Effect of active glottal abduction and adduction

The position of the sloping line in Figure 1 can be manipulated up or down by active adjustment of the abducting or adducting laryngeal muscles. Figure 2 shows lines corresponding to two extreme glottal configurations: a spread configuration with a resting width of about 0.12 cm (for zero intraoral pressure), and a constricted configuration with the upper surfaces pressed together to yield a width of -0.05 cm. The middle line is intended to correspond to a modal glottal configuration, and is the same as the line discussed in Figure 1.

Within the w_2 - P_m plane in Figure 2 we can delineate regions within which glottal vibration will occur. We have already noted the point *C* delineating the boundary between the condition of glottal vibration (to the left of point *C*) and the condition of no glottal vibration (to the right of *C*). When the glottis is in a more spread configuration, a greater transglottal pressure (i.e., a smaller P_m) is needed in order to maintain vibration. Finally, when the glottal width exceeds a particular critical value, taken as 0.12 cm in Figure 2, vocal-fold vibration cannot be maintained even with the full subglottal pressure across the glottis (i.e., for $P_m = 0$). This point is labelled *E* in the figure. Likewise, when the glottis is sufficiently constricted, the subglottal pressure cannot force the glottis open, and vocal-fold vibration will not occur. Point *F* in Figure 2 indicates the threshold between vibration and no vibration when the supraglottal pressure is zero. The contour joining points *E*, *C*, and *F* delineates the boundary between the vibrating and nonvibrating conditions for intermediate glottal configurations, in the region where the intraoral pressure is greater than zero.

In the region to the left of $P_m = 0$ in Figure 2, the intraoral pressure is negative. As has been noted above, this condition can be achieved by appropriate expansion of the vocal-tract volume. The region in which vocal-fold vibration can occur has been marked in the figure. The lower edge of this region is a horizontal line that connects with point *F*. For the (negative) value of w_2 given by this line, the subglottal pressure of 8 cm H_2O is not sufficient to push the vocal folds apart independent of the supraglottal pressure. The upper edge of the region is taken to be a horizontal line that connects to the point *E*. To the left of point E, it is assumed that the increased transglottal pressure (i.e., the increased value of $P_s - P_m$ as P_m becomes more negative) can sustain vocal-fold vibration for glottal widths greater than those defined by the line labelled spread.

In summary, then, the chart of Figure 2 identifies a number of different regions that can be traversed for various manipulations of the glottis, the supraglottal constriction, and the intraoral pressure. The region of operation for vowels and other sonorants is the w_2-axis, for which the full subglottal pressure appears across the glottis. Above point *E*, the glottis is sufficiently spread that vocal-fold vibration does not occur, and aspiration noise is generated in the vicinity of the glottis. In a region immediately below point *E*, breathy vocal-fold vibration occurs, with a spread glottal configuration. The region surrounding point A on the vertical axis corresponds to modal vocal-fold vibration. Below point *F* on the w_2-axis, again there is no glottal vibration, whereas the region immediately above *F* identifies a condition of vocal-fold vibration with a constricted glottis, sometimes called pressed voicing. Regions to the right or left of the w_2-axis in Figure 2 can only be achieved when there is some kind of supraglottal constriction.

To the right of the w_2-axis, the intraoral pressure is positive. This half-plane is divided into two regions, corresponding to the presence or absence of glottal vibration. The dividing line between these regions is the contour *ECF*. Also identified at the lower part of the chart is a region where the glottis is closed ($w_2 < 0$), the intraoral pressure is positive, and vocal-fold vibration does not occur. Ejective consonants are produced within this region, usually for values of P_m greater than P_s, i.e., in the lower right-hand portion of Figure 2.

In the left-half plane of Figure 2, where intraoral pressures are negative, there are again two regions - one in which vocal-fold vibration occurs, and the other in which vocal-fold vibration cannot occur, either because the glottis is too spread or is too constricted.

Vertical movement within the chart between and beyond the *constricted glottis* and the *spread glottis* conditions is achieved by active control of the intrinsic abducting and adducting laryngeal muscles. Movements along one of the sloping lines on the chart (either up to the right or down to the left) occur passively as a consequence of changes in the intraoral pressure.

Trajectories in the w_2 - P_m plane

During the production of an obstruent consonant such as a fricative or a stop, the state of the glottis and the intraoral pressure at a given time can be specified by a point in the w_2 - P_m plane of Figure 2. An example of such a point is *G*, which might correspond to a voiceless fricative consonant. When the consonant is released into a following vowel, there is a rather abrupt decrease in intraoral pressure. The duration of this change is usually short enough that there is little change in the glottal configuration due to active manipulation of the adducting or abducting muscles during this time in which the drop in intraoral pressure occurs. The immediate consequence of the consonant release, then, is a rapid displacement of the point *G* along a line parallel to the sloping lines (the dotted line in Figure 2), until it reaches the w_2-axis at point *H*. Vocal-fold vibration commences immediately, and the mode of vibration is determined by where along the w_2-axis the trajectory from *G* comes to rest. Any further adjustment of the glottal configuration following the consonant release is manifested as a vertical movement of the trajectory along the w_2-axis.

For some fricative or stop consonants, the state of the system during the constricted interval lies within the region of Figure 2 where vocal-fold vibration occurs. The sound that is radiated from the talker's head and neck during such a voiced interval is quite different from the sound during a vowel. Consider, for example, a stop consonant corresponding to point *I* in Figure 2. The intraoral pressure is 3.5 cm H_2O and the glottis is slightly abducted since there are passive forces on the glottis due to the increased pressure. If the conditions of glottal flow and glottal configuration corresponding to point *I* are to be maintained over a time interval, it will be necessary to expand the volume of the vocal tract between the glottis and the point of closure (Bell-Berti, 1973; Perkell, 1969). Since the transglottal pressure is about one-half of its value for a vowel, some reduction in the amplitude of the glottal pulses is expected. Both experimental and theoretical considerations suggest that the amplitude of these pulses is roughly proportional to the three-halves power of the transglottal pressure. For point *I* in Figure 2, then, the amplitude of the volume-velocity pulses from the glottis would be about 10 dB below that in an adjacent vowel. Other factors also influence the shape of the glottal pulses. The spectral characteristics of the sound that is radiated from the mouth and neck surfaces of the speaker during the voiced consonantal interval will be quite different from the spectrum for a vowel. In the case of a stop consonant, all of the sound is radiated from the surfaces of the face and neck, whereas for a voiced fricative consonant, some of the radiated sound comes from the mouth opening.

The quantitative details of the chart in Figure 2 have to be worked out, although its general form seems to be based on valid theoretical premises. For example, the exact conditions under which vocal-fold vibration can occur might vary from one individual to another. Also, the slopes of the lines corresponding to different glottal configurations depend on the vocal-fold compliance, which may be nonlinear, and may also vary from one individual to another.

Experimental data showing trajectories in a plane similar to the w_2 - P_m plane have been shown for some vowel-consonant-vowel utterances of Japanese by Yoshioka (1984). His measure of glottal opening was obtained from glottal transillumination records. These data provide some indication of the shapes of the trajectories and the conditions necessary for onset and offset of voicing. Our approach here will be to estimate the expected form of the trajectories for various classes of consonants based on both experimental data and theoretical analyses.

MODELLING CLASSES OF VOICED AND VOICELESS OBSTRUENTS

The various panels of Figure 3 show estimated trajectories for several classes of voiced and voiceless stop and fricative consonants when they occur in intervocalic position. In all cases, we assume that there is a simple closing and opening movement of the vocal tract at a designated point in the oral cavity. The different panels of the figure correspond to different active adjustments of the glottal configuration and of the volume of the supraglottal cavity. For stop consonants (Figures 3a to 3d), the supraglottal closure is complete, whereas for fricatives (Figure 3e) a partial opening remains in the airway.

The form of each of the trajectories in Figure 3 is based in part on theoretical analysis, in part on observations of airflows, pressures, and glottal configurations for consonants, and in part on inferences made from acoustic analysis of consonants, particularly near the boundaries between consonants and vowels. We have drawn on physiological data from Dixit (1975, 1987) for voiced aspirated stop consonants; from Fujimura (1961) for rates of movement at stop consonant releases; from a series of studies from the Research Institute of Logopedics and Phoniatrics in Tokyo, mostly concerned with fiberoptic examination of the glottis for various types of consonants (Sawashima and Hirose, 1983; Fukui and Hirose, 1983; Iwata and Hirose, 1976; Kagaya and Hirose, 1975) and from our own data and those of Klatt et al. (1968) for airflow patterns for different consonants. Our estimates of the trajectories are also based on our own acoustic data for a variety of consonants.

For plain voiced and voiceless stops (Figure 3a), we assume that there is no active adjustment of the glottal configuration. Depending on whether voicing is to occur in the closure interval, the trajectory that is followed is *ABA* for a voiceless stop and *AGA* for a voiced stop. When a stop consonant is voiceless and aspirated, there is a movement toward a spread glottal configuration (point *K* in Figure 3b) in the closure interval. Following release of the consonant, this point returns to the modal vowel state along trajectory *KEA*. Two possible trajectories can be followed in reaching point *K* from the modal configuration at A: an abducting movement (path *AJK*) that terminates voicing in a breathy mode, and an adducting movement followed by glottal abduction (path *ALK*) in which voicing is terminated in a glottalized or pressed mode. In the case of a voiced aspirated stop (Figure 3c), the path must remain within the region in which vocal-fold vibration continues (e.g., point *M* or point *N* in Figure 3c). Possible trajectories for a voiced aspirated stop are thus *AHMPHA* or *AHNQREHA*. The latter path contains an interval (*QRE*), following the consonant release and during the period of aspiration, in which voicing ceases and then begins again. Similarly, trajectories can be drawn (Figure 3d) for laryngealized stop consonants. The consonant can be generated either with continuing vocal-fold vibration (*AWA* or *AVA*), or as a voiceless ejective (*ASTUFA*).

Finally, trajectories for voiced and voiceless fricatives are shown in Figure 3e. For voiceless fricatives, a typical trajectory is *AXYZHA*, with the state remaining in the vicinity of point *Y* for much of the fricative, i.e., outside of the region where vocal-fold vibration occurs. It can be shown that this trajectory gives the expected double-peaked airflow pattern for an intervocalic voiceless fricative consonant (Klatt et al., 1968). In the case of a voiced fricative, the trajectory is *AIA*, although it may happen that vocal-fold vibration ceases during the fricative (Stevens et al., 1987), in which case the trajectory might extend beyond the voicing boundary to point *J*.

DISCUSSION

We have attempted to develop a theoretical framework within which the voicing characteristics of obstruent consonants can be interpreted. For the most part, these consonants are produced with two constrictions in the airway - one in the supraglottal region and one

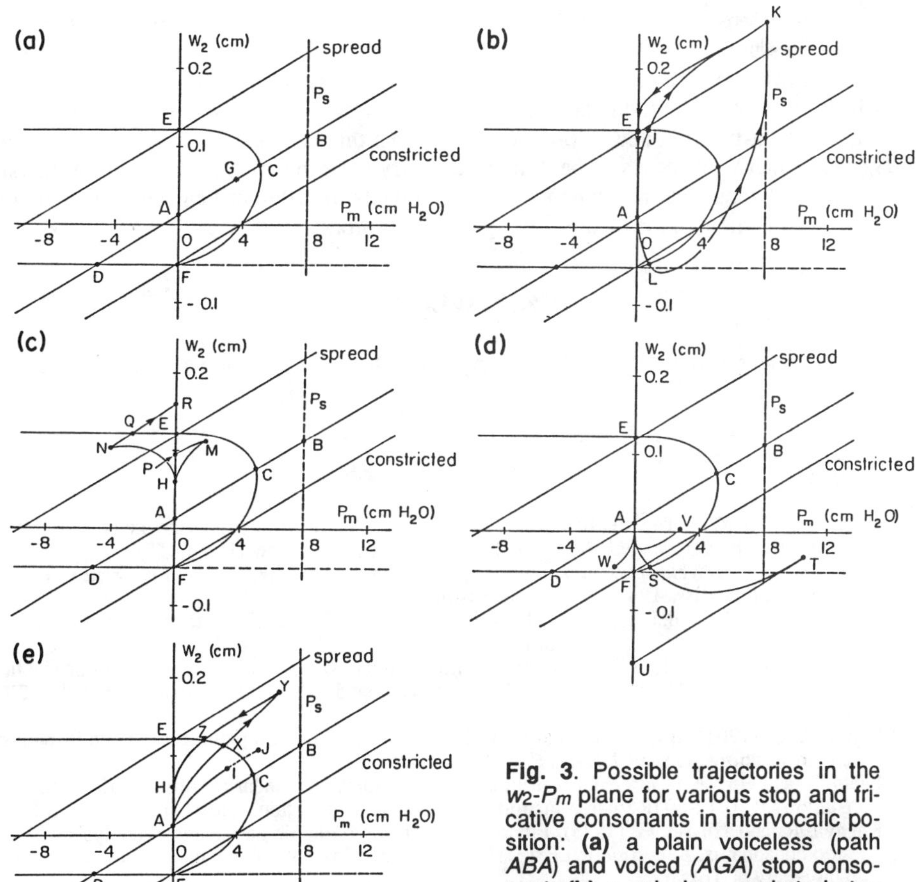

Fig. 3. Possible trajectories in the w_2-P_m plane for various stop and fricative consonants in intervocalic position: **(a)** a plain voiceless (path *ABA*) and voiced *(AGA)* stop consonant; **(b)** a voiceless aspirated stop consonant with a breathy offset for the preceding vowel (*AJKEA*) or a glotta- lized vowel offset (*ALKEA*); **(c)** a voiced aspirated stop consonant with an egressive release (*AHMPHA*) and with an ingressive release (*AHNQREHA*); **(d)** a laryngealized stop consonant that is voiced (*AVA* or *AWA*) or is a voiceless ejective (*ASTUFA*); and **(e)** a voiceless fricative consonant (*AXYZHA*) or a voiced fricative (*AIA*, possibly extending to point *J* if the fricative contains an interval where glottal vibration ceases).

at the larynx. When the supraglottal constriction is sufficiently narrow, the intraoral pressure can be different from atmospheric pressure, whereas the subglottal pressure usually remains relatively constant throughout most of an utterance. The intraoral pressure, and hence the transglottal pressure, can be manipulated by a speaker through appropriate adjustment of the structures surrounding the airways (particularly the vertical position of the larynx, and the pharynx walls), and through control of the glottal configuration and the supraglottal constriction. The changes in intraoral pressure influence the laryngeal sound source in two ways: (1) through passive forces on the glottal walls leading to modifications in the glottal shape; and (2) through increases or decreases in the transglottal pressure.

We have attempted to sketch out the region of the pressure and glottal parameters in which vocal-fold vibration can occur, and we have suggested how different parts of this region might be exploited to produce consonants that can function distinctively in language. Much work needs to be done to quantify these regions, through further physiological and acoustical measurements of consonants in different languages, and through further refinement of the theoretical aspects of the model.

ACKNOWLEDGMENT

This research was supported in part by grant DC00075 from the National Institutes of Health.

REFERENCES

Bell-Berti, F. (1973). The velopharyngeal mechanism: An electromyographic study. *Supplement to Status Report on Speech Research*, Haskins Laboratories, New Haven, CT.

Dixit, R.P. (1975). *Neuromuscular aspects of laryngeal control: With speech reference to Hindi.* Unpubl. Ph.D. diss., Univ. of Texas at Austin.

Dixit, R.P. (1987). In defense of the phonetic adequacy of the traditional term "voiced aspirated." *Proc. Eleventh Int. Congr. of Phonetic Sciences, Tallinn, Vol. 2*, pp. 145-148.

Fukui, N. and Hirose, H. (1983). Laryngeal adjustments in Danish voiceless obstruent production. *Ann. Bull. RILP*, 17:61-71. (Research Inst. of Logopedics and Phoniatrics, University of Tokyo).

Fujimura, O. (1961). Bilabial stops and nasal consonants: A motion picture study and its acoustical implications. *J. Speech Hear. Res.*, 4:233-247.

Iwata, R. and Hirose, H. (1976). Fiberoptic acoustic studies of Mandarin stops and affricates. *Ann. Bull. RILP* 10:47-60 (Research Institute of Logopedics and Phoniatrics, University of Tokyo).

Kagaya, R. and Hirose, H. (1975). Fiberoptic electromyographic and acoustic analysis of Hindi stop consonants. *Ann. Bull. RILP* 13:61-81 (Research Institute of Logopedics and Phoniatrics, University of Tokyo)

Kakita, Y., Hirano, M., and Ohmaru, K. (1981). Physical properties of the vocal fold tissue: Measurements on excised larynges. In: *Vocal Fold Physiology*, edited by K.N. Stevens and M. Hirano, pp. 377-396. University of Tokyo Press, Tokyo.

Klatt, D.H., Stevens, K.N., and Mead, J. (1968). Studies of articulatory activity and airflow during speech, *Ann. of New York Academy of Sciences* 155:42-55.

Perkell, J.S. (1969): *Physiology of speech production: Results and implications of a quantitative cineradiographic study.* MIT Press, Cambridge, MA.

Rothenberg, M. (1968). The breath-stream dynamics of simple-released plosive production. *Bibliotheca Phonetica*, No. 6. S. Karger, Basel/New York.

Sawashima, M. and Hirose, H. (1983). Laryngeal gestures in speech production. In: *The Production of Speech*, edited by P.E. MacNeilage, pp. 11-38. Springer-Verlag, New York.

Stevens, K.N., Blumstein, S.E., and Glicksman, L.B. (1987). Voicing distinction for fricatives: Acoustic theory and measurements. *J. Acoust. Soc. Am.*, Suppl. 1, 82:S16.

Westbury, J.R. (1979). Aspects of the temporal control of voicing in consonant clusters in English. *Texas Ling. Forum*, 14:1-304.

Westbury, J.R. (1983). Enlargement of the supraglottal cavity and its relation to stop consonant devoicing. *J. Acoust. Soc. Am.*, 73:1322-1336.

Yoshioka, H. (1984). Glottal area variation and supraglottal pressure change in voicing control. *Ann. Bull. RILP* 18:45-49. (Research Institute of Logopedics and Phoniatrics, University of Tokyo).

6

Vocal-Fold Vibration in a Computer Model of a Larynx

Corine Bickley

Research Laboratory of Electronics, Massachusetts Institute of Technology, Cambridge, MA 02139, USA

In an earlier paper we described a computer-based model of the interaction between the glottal source and the vocal tract; glottal pulse shapes were computed for various supraglottal constrictions (Bickley and Stevens, 1986). Representation of the behaviour of the mechanical system during intervals when the glottis is closed was not included in the model, and therefore vibration frequency could not be determined. In this report, we present extensions to the basic model which allow sustained vocal-fold vibration in conjunction with an open vocal tract, and which can be used to examine the time course of cessation of vibration in the presence of a constricted vocal tract.

Implementation of computer model of vocal-fold vibration

The implementation of the mechanical component of the model follows traditional lines. A schematic representation of the two-mass mechanical model is shown in Figure 1, along with a low-frequency equivalent circuit representing the acoustic behaviour of the system. Each vocal fold is represented as two coupled masses (Flanagan et al., 1975; Ishizaka and Matsudaira, 1968; 1972). Vocal-fold tissue mass, stiffness, and resistance are included in the model, as are conditions which prevent the masses from overlapping when glottal closure occurs. During glottal closure, a nonlinear stiffness and resistance are incorporated within the model, to represent the behaviour of the vocal folds when they are in contact. The dimensions and values of tissue properties which are used in the model are taken or derived from the literature (Fant et al., 1976; Goldstein, 1980; Hirano et al., 1980; Ishizaka et al., 1975; Kahane and Kahn, 1984; Kakita et al., 1980; Kaneko et al. 1987; Perlman and Titze, 1983), and are listed in Table 1. The pressures within the upper and lower sections of the glottis act as driving forces for the equations of motion. Solution of these equations, written in the form of difference equations, gives the velocity and therefore the displacement of each vocal-fold section at every iteration. Glottal cross-sectional area in turn is calculated from vocal-fold displacement.

The mechanical component of the model is linked to the aerodynamic component through the glottal cross-sectional area. Glottal airflow calculations include kinetic and viscous effects. The effect of displacement of the vocal-tract walls in the case of a closed vocal tract is also included in the model.

Pressure values throughout the glottal and supraglottal system are calculated based on glottal airflow. A kinetic pressure drop is included at the juncture between the trachea and the lower vocal folds. For instances in which the upper folds are more closely

Table 1. *Dimensions and values of tissue properties used in the model*.

Parameter		Value	
Vocal-fold	length (membranous)	1.5	cm
	thickness (upper)	0.1	cm
	thickness (lower)	0.2	cm
	vibrating mass (upper)	0.02	g/cm
	vibrating mass (lower)	0.04	g/cm
	compliance (upper)	10	$\times 10^{-5}$ cm^2/dyne
	compliance (upper surface)	**	cm^2/dyne
	compliance (lower)	4	$\times 10^{-5}$ cm^2/dyne
	compliance (lower surface)	**	cm^2/dyne
	compliance (coupling)	2	10^{-4} cm^2/dyne
	resistance (upper)	6.3	g/cm sec
	resistance (upper surface)	125.6	g/cm sec
	resistance (lower)	3.1	g/cm sec
	resistance (lower surface)	31.4	g/cm sec
Vocal-tract	volume	50.0	cm^3
	wall mass	0.015	g/cm^4
	wall compliance	0.001	cm^5/dyne
	wall resistance	18	g/cm^4 sec

**The compliance of each surface is proportional to the displacement of the corresponding section from the glottal midline, e.g., compliance (upper surface) = $x_u0 \times C_u/th_u$, where x_u0 is the displacement of the upper section from the glottal midline, C_u is the compliance of the upper section, and th_u is the thickness of the upper section.

approximated than the lower folds, a kinetic pressure drop between the lower and upper vocal-fold sections is also calculated. Viscous pressure drops are computed along each glottal section. It is assumed that there is no pressure recovery at the glottal exit. The calculation of the supraglottal pressure depends on the vocal-tract configuration. For an open vocal tract, supraglottal pressure is atmospheric, but there may be an increased intraoral pressure when the vocal tract contains a supraglottal constriction. For a closed vocal tract, the pressure in the oral cavity builds up as air flows into the oral cavity during each pulse. The effect of the mass, compliance, and resistance of the vocal-tract walls and the compliance of the air in the oral cavity are included for the closed-vocal-tract case.

Simulation of vocal-fold vibration for the open-vocal-tract case

The computer model was tested with an open-vocal-tract configuration for various conditions of subglottal pressure and vocal-fold resting position. Figure 2 shows the calculated glottal area, airflow waveform, and derivative of the airflow waveform for a subglottal pressure of approximately 8 cm H_2O and a resting state in which the upper folds are slightly more adducted than the lower folds (the lower folds are separated by 0.022 cm and the upper folds are separated by 0.01 cm). The calculated glottal flow is periodic with a peak amplitude of approximately 730 cm^3/sec. The frequency of vibration is 113 Hz, and the open quotient is approximately 0.6. The expected skewed shape of the glottal

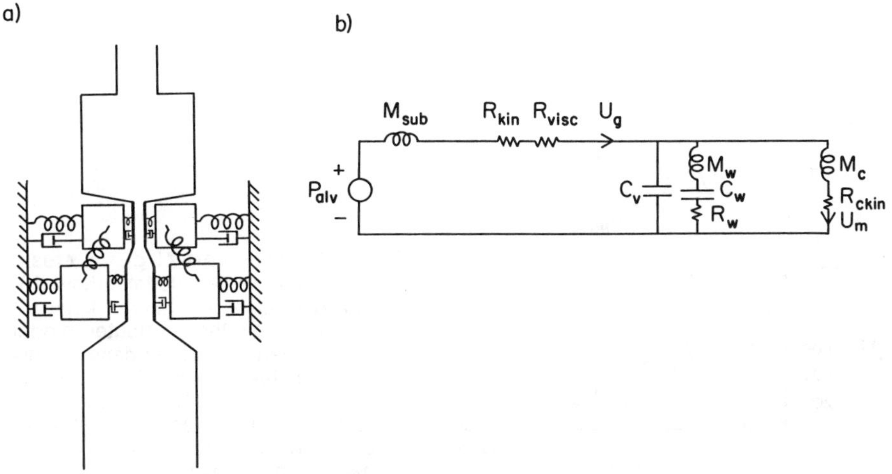

Fig. 1. (**a**) Two-mass model of the vocal folds coupled to a supraglottal system in which the vocal tract can be either open or closed. (**b**) Low-frequency equivalent circuit used for estimating pressure and flows in the vocal tract. See text for discussion of components.

pulse is evident in the figure: the flow is increasing for about 3.4 ms and is decreasing for about 1.7 ms. The bottom panel of the figure shows the time derivative of the glottal flow (dU/dt); the derivative exhibits a negative pulse with an abrupt return to zero in approximately 0.24 ms, in agreement with observed shapes of this derivative waveform.

Vocal-fold vibration is maintained by the model for a range of subglottal pressures. For higher values of subglottal pressure the glottal flow pulses are greater in amplitude, and lower amplitude pulses occur for lower subglottal pressures. Figure 3 shows the amplitude of glottal vibration (on a logarithmic scale) for the model, plotted as a function of the subglottal pressure. Doubling the pressure drop ΔP across the glottis produces an increase in peak glottal flow by a factor of approximately 2.9. When the pressure drop across the glottis falls below a critical value, approximately 3 cm H_2O, vocal-fold vibration ceases, as shown by the abrupt drop in the curve in Figure 3. The dashed line shows values which are predicted from a simple relationship of maximum amplitude proportional to change in pressure raised to the power 1.5.

The glottal resting state also affects vocal-fold vibration. For a configuration in which the resting position of each lower fold is 0.061 cm from the glottal midline and each upper fold rests at 0.055 cm from the midline, the vocal folds vibrate as shown in Figure 4 after steady state is reached. In this case, the vibration frequency is 124 Hz, and the open quotient is 0.77. There are several differences between vocal-fold vibration with this offset resting position (as might be the case with breathy voicing) and the vibration pattern shown in Figure 2 (which is intended to correspond to modal voicing). One difference is that the peak flow is greater for the "breathy" case. Another is that the open quotient is larger. A third difference is that a more gradual termination of the glottal pulse occurs with the "breathy" configuration than with the modal configuration. The time derivative of the glottal flow is shown in the panel at the bottom of Figure 4; in contrast with

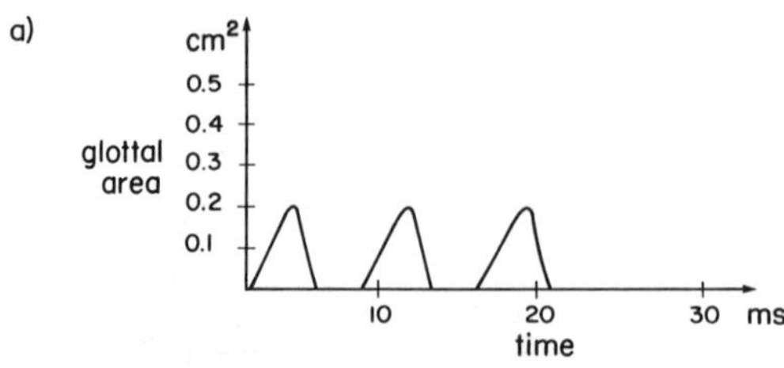

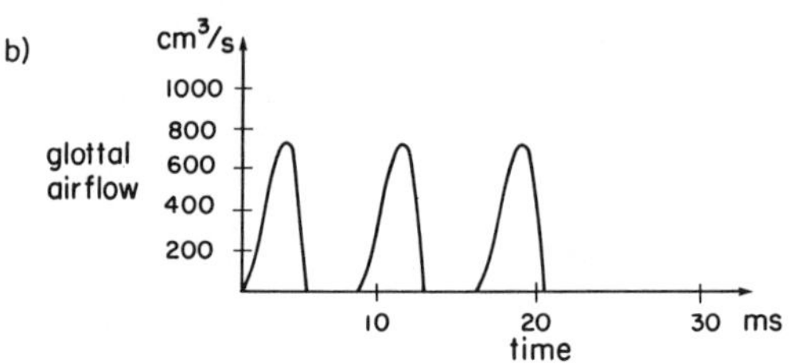

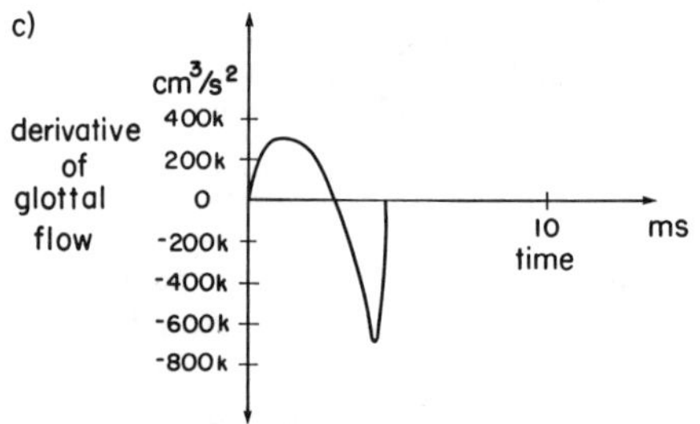

Fig. 2. Waveforms of glottal cross-sectional area (**a**), glottal airflow (**b**), and derivative of glottal flow (**c**) generated by the computer model for the open-vocal-tract case. In this example, the subglottal pressure is approximately 8 cm H_2O, the vocal tract is unconstricted, and the upper folds are slightly more adducted than the lower folds.

the bottom panel of Figure 2, a less abrupt termination (by a factor of about six times) is apparent.

The relative displacement of the upper and lower vocal-fold sections also affects vibration. For a configuration in which the glottal width of the upper section is approximately 0.006 cm or more greater than the width of the lower section, the vocal folds do not vibrate. That is, vocal-fold vibration does not occur if the resting position of the vocal folds has this diverging shape.

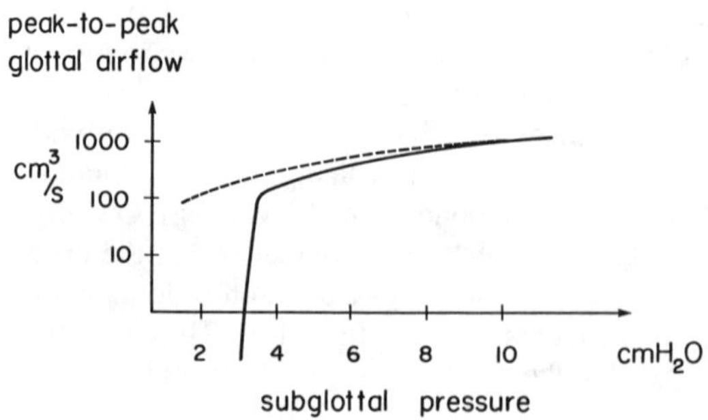

Fig. 3. Relationship between transglottal pressure and peak-to-peak airflow through the glottis during modal voicing with an open vocal tract. The solid line represents the behavior of the model. The dashed line is based on a simple theoretical relationship between maximum amplitude and change in pressure. (See text for discussion.)

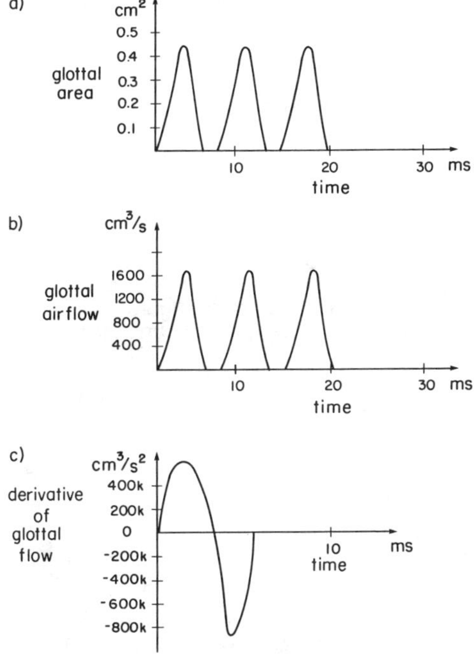

Fig. 4. Waveforms of glottal cross-sectional area (**a**), glottal airflow (**b**), and derivative of glottal flow (**c**) generated by the computer model for the open-vocal-tract case and a subglottal pressure of approximately 8 cm H_2O. The lower folds are separated by 0.122 cm, and the upper folds are separated by 0.110 cm. In this example, the resting positions of the vocal folds are slightly abducted in comparison with the example shown in Figure 2.

SIMULATION OF VOCAL-FOLD VIBRATION FOR THE CLOSED-VOCAL-TRACT CASE

For a closed-vocal-tract configuration, vocal-fold vibration decays after the vocal tract is closed, and the vocal folds come to rest in a position offset from the midline of the glottis. Figure 5 shows glottal area and airflow patterns which result from applying a subglottal pressure of 8 cm H_2O with a closed vocal tract and an initial intraoral pressure of zero. In this example, the lower folds are initially barely separated and the upper folds are touching lightly. One full glottal pulse occurs after closure, followed by some movement of the vocal folds for another 8 ms or so. At this time, the vocal folds are near their final positions, and airflow through the glottis continues at a decreasing rate until the pressure in the oral cavity reaches the level of the subglottal pressure. When flow ceases, the glottal area is approximately 0.2 cm^2. The upper vocal fold comes to rest in a position which is slightly more abducted than that of the lower fold (0.006 cm difference in separation); that is, the supraglottal pressure passively changes the configuration of the vocal folds.

DISCUSSION

Several aspects of the simulation results are in agreement with measurements of speech and with theoretical predictions. The frequency of vibration of the model is within the range of measured fundamental frequencies for adult male voices. (The dimensions

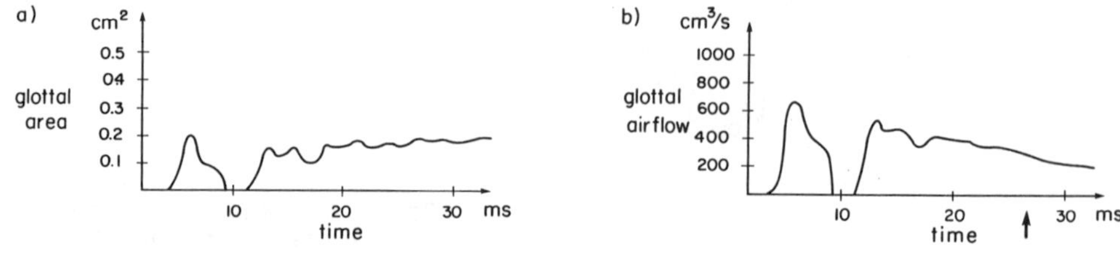

Fig. 5. Glottal cross-sectional area (**a**) and glottal airflow (**b**) generated by the computer model for the case of the vocal tract closing abruptly (at time t=0). In this example, the subglottal pressure is approximately 8 cm H_2O. The vocal folds are configured for modal voicing before the time that the vocal tract is closed. The arrow indicates when the trans-glottal pressure has fallen to approximately 3 cm H_2O.

and tissue property parameters used in the model are typical values for an adult male.) As mentioned previously, the shape of the computed glottal pulses resembles those reported in the literature (see, for example, Fant, 1979; 1983), and the open quotient of the computed pulses is similar to measured values, Holmberg et al., 1988; Price, 1987). The maximum amplitude of airflow also agrees with simple theory which predicts an increase proportional to $\Delta P^{1.5}$, or approximately 2.8 times for a doubling of subglottal pressure.

The open-vocal-tract case with offset vocal folds represents a possible laryngeal configuration for breathy phonation. The increase in open quotient (see Figure 4) in comparison to the simulation of modal voicing (see Figure 2) is in line with measurements of speech. The less abrupt termination of the glottal pulse at closure, which results in a source spectrum with relatively fewer high-frequency components, is also characteristic of breathy voicing, Klatt and Klatt (1990).

For the closed-vocal-tract case, the results of the model are consistent with measurements of speech. When the oral-cavity volume is held constant (except for the passive change in volume due to the compliance of the walls), the model produces vocal-fold vibration for one or two pulses and then ceases vibrating. In the production of voiceless stop consonants, for example, evidence of a short interval of voicing is often apparent after stop closure, assuming that there is no active glottal adjustment; these pulses are reduced in amplitude in comparison with voicing during a preceding vowel. This reduction in amplitude is apparent in the first pulse shown in Figure 5 in comparison with those shown in Figure 2. Observations of speech show that speakers can maintain weak voicing for a longer interval of time than the 20 to 30 ms illustrated in Figure 5. Speech production data offer some explanation of the mechanisms which speakers might use to maintain voicing during a closure interval. Westbury (1983) determined that increases in supraglottal volume are found during production of the voiced stops /b d g/. Ohala and Riordan (1980) suggested that active lowering of the larynx might be used to prolong the voicing interval. Active enlargement of the vocal-tract volume has not, though, been included in the present version of the model.

The results with the model also indicate that vibration of the simulated vocal folds is dependent on the relative positions of the vocal-fold sections. For configurations in which the upper sections are more closely approximated than the lower sections and for cases in

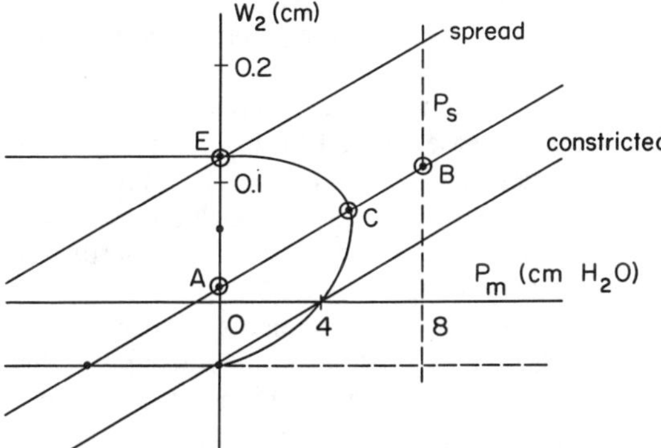

Fig. 6. Several points in the plane of glottal width W_2 versus intraoral pressure P_m discussed by Stevens (this volume). Simulations of the behaviour of the model corresponding to points A, B, C, and E are discussed in the text.

which the resting offsets of the lower and upper sections are nearly equal, vocal-fold vibration can be maintained. If, however, the upper sections are offset from the glottal midline more than the lower sections by some critical amount, vibration ceases. Perhaps speakers use some means of orienting their vocal folds (such as rotating the arytenoid cartilages so as to separate the upper edges of the vocal folds more than the lower edges) to inhibit vibration.

The results of simulations with the model can be identified with the various states in the mouth-pressure-vs-glottal-width space presented by Stevens (20), and reproduced in Figure 6. Point A represents modal voicing with a pressure of 8 cm H_2O across the glottis, atmospheric pressure in the oral cavity, and a resting glottal width of 0.01 cm. The model produces vocal-fold vibration for these conditions at a frequency of 113 Hz and an open quotient of 0.58.

For the case of a spread glottis and open vocal tract, Stevens indicates that vibration should occur for rest position widths of up to approximately 0.12 cm (point E in Figure 6). The model produces vocal-fold vibration for all resting positions in this range. For a resting position corresponding to that of point E, the calculated vibration frequency is 126 Hz and the open quotient is 0.79. However, the model also produces vibration for vocal-fold offsets beyond the range suggested by Stevens. A glottal width of 0.24 cm is needed to prevent vibration. The computed value of 0.24 cm resulted from a glottal configuration in which the vocal-fold sections were maintained in their relative positions with respect to each other, and were simply offset as a pair from the midline of the glottis. It is possible that this sort of displacement is not the movement which would result with natural vocal folds. If rotating the arytenoid cartilages outwards abducts the upper section more than the lower section, then this movement could result in a configuration for which vocal-fold vibration could not be maintained. The frequency of vocal-fold vibration for the model shows an increase for a resting position of the vocal folds that is abducted. This increase is in agreement with measurements of F0 in a vowel that follows the consonant /h/, which show an average increase in F0 at the beginning of the vowel relative to the frequency about 50 ms later (Manuel and Stevens, 1989). However, there is often a *decrease* in F0 at the end of a vowel preceding /h/ (albeit smaller than the increase in the following vowel), and the model does not explain this decrease, unless one postulates a relaxation of vocal-fold tension or a decreased transglottal pressure at this point in the utterance.

For the closed-vocal-tract case, the pressure in the oral cavity increases to the subglottal pressure. Point B in Figure 6 represents this case, and falls outside the region of vocal-fold vibration. The vocal folds of the model cease vibration after 10-20 ms when the oral cavity is closed and the intraoral pressure builds up to the subglottal pressure. Computed vocal-fold oscillation terminates when the pressure drop across the glottis has fallen from approximately 8 cm H_2O to 3 cm H_2O (point C in Figure 6).

A difference between the behaviour of the model and measurements of speech concerns the effect of rest position of the vocal folds on peak airflow during voicing. For the model, increasing the offset of each vocal-fold section from the midline of the glottis, while keeping the relative positions of the sections fixed, increases the peak amplitude of the airflow pulse (cf. Figures 2 and 4). This increase is greater than that observed during the production of voiced aspirated /h/, where the amplitude of the fundamental does not change appreciably in comparison to the fundamental of a preceding or following vowel, (Manuel and Stevens, 1989).

Another possible difference concerns the shape of a glottal pulse in the closed-vocal-tract case. An example of such a glottal pulse is shown in Figure 5. In this case, the glottal area does not decrease monotonically during glottal closure, but rather shows an initial decrease (as expected), followed by an interval during which the glottal area is decreasing less rapidly before finally closing. It is not known whether this pattern of glottal closing occurs in the brief time interval following supraglottal closure in a postvocalic stop consonant.

SUMMARY

A computer model of the interaction between vocal-fold vibration and vocal-tract configuration has been implemented. The model includes two-mass representations of the vocal folds and the behavior of the model has been observed when it is coupled to an open and a closed vocal tract. In many ways, the behavior of the model is consistent with measurements of vocal-fold vibration and inferences of vibratory characteristics which are based on acoustic observations. The model generates periodic glottal pulses when the vocal tract is unconstricted, a sufficient pressure drop across theglottis exists, and the vocal folds are appropriately positioned.

For the cases of modal and "breathy" voicing, there is good agreement between many characteristics of the behavior of the model and measurements of speech. The behavior of the model also seems reasonable in cases in which voicing is inhibited, such as a reduction in the transglottal pressure and changes in the glottal configuration. When the vocal-tract load is changed, the model also produces the expected characteristics. Following closure of the vocal tract to simulate a stop consonant, the model shows a decay in vocal-fold vibration, and the vocal folds come to rest with upper folds more abducted than lower.

We have found that a two-mass model of the vocal folds continues to be a simple but useful research tool. Although some patterns of vocal-fold vibration cannot be adequately simulated with this model, many characteristics of vocal-fold behavior can be successfully modeled. We plan to continue trying to understand the causes for model behavior which differs from measurements of speech. We also hope to use a version of the model to analyze other interactions between the vocal tract and the glottal source.

ACKNOWLEDGMENTS

This research was supported in part by Grant DC00075 from the National Institutes of Health.

REFERENCES

Bickley, C. B. and Stevens, K. N. (1986). Effects of a vocal-tract constriction on the glottal source: experimental and modelling studies. *J. Phonetics*, 14:373-382.

Fant, G. (1979). Glottal source and excitation analysis. *STL-QPSR*, 1:85-107 (Dept. of Speech Communication and Music Acoustics, Royal Institute of Technology, Stockholm)

Fant, G. (1983). Preliminaries to analysis of the human voice source. *STL-QPSR*, 4:1-27 (Dept. of Speech Communication and Music Acoustics, Royal Institute of Technology, Stockholm).

Fant, G., Nord, L., and Branderud, P. (1976). A note on the vocal tract wall impedance. *STL-QPSR*, 4:13-20 (Dept. of Speech Communication and Music Acoustics, Royal Institute of Technology, Stockholm).

Flanagan, J. L., Ishizaka, K., and Shipley, K. L. (1975). Synthesis of speech from a dynamic model of the vocal cords and vocal tract. *Bell Syst. Tech. J.*, 54(3):485-506.

Goldstein, U.G. (1980). *Articulatory model for the vocal tracts of growing children.* Unpublished Ph.D. dissertation, Massachusetts Institute of Technology, Cambridge, MA.

Hirano, M., Kurita, S., and Nakashima, T. (1980). The structure of the vocal folds. In *Vocal Fold Physiology*, edited by K. N. Stevens and M. Hirano, pp. 33-41. University of Tokyo Press, Tokyo.

Holmberg, E. B., Hillman, R. E., and Perkell, J. S. (1988). Glottal airflow and transglottal air pressure measurements for male and female speakers in soft, normal, and loud voice. *J. Acoust. Soc. Am.*, 84:511-529.

Ishizaka, K. and Matsudaira, M. (1968). What makes the vocal cords vibrate. In: *Reports of the 6th Internat. Congr. on Acoustics*, edited by Y. Kohasi, pp. B9-B12. Maruzen Co. Ltd., Tokyo, and Elsevier, Amsterdam.

Ishizaka, K. and Matsudaira, M. (1972). Theory of vocal cord vibrations. *Rep. Univ. Electro-Comm.*, 23-2:107-136 (Tokyo).

Ishizaka, K., French, J. C., and Flanagan, J. L. (1975). Direct determination of vocal tract wall impedance. *I.E.E.E. Trans. Acoust. Sp. Signal Proc.*, 23:370-373.

Kahane, J. C. and Kahn, A. R. (1984). Weight measurements of infant and adult intrinsic laryngeal muscles. *Folia Phoniat.*, 36:129-133.

Kakita, Y., Hirano, M., and Ohmaru, K. (1980). Physical properties of the vocal fold tissue: measurements on excised larynges. In *Vocal Fold Physiology*, edited by K.N. Stevens and M. Hirano, pp. 377-396. University of Tokyo Press, Tokyo.

Kaneko, T., Masuda, T., Shimade, A., Suzuki, H., Hayasaki, K., and Komatsu, K. (1987). Resonance characteristics of the human vocal fold in vivo and in vitro by an impulse excitation. In *Laryngeal Function in Phonation and Respiration*, edited by T. Baer, C. Sasaki, and K. Harris, College-Hill Press, Boston, MA.

Klatt, D. H. and Klatt, L. C. (1990). Analysis, synthesis and perception of voice quality variations among female and male talkers. *J. Acoust. Soc. Am.*, 87(2).

Manuel, S. and Stevens, K. N. (1989). Acoustic properties of /h/. *J. Acoust. Soc. Am.*, Suppl. 1, 86:S49.

Ohala, J. J. and Riordan, C. J. (1980). Passive vocal tract enlargement during voiced stops. *Rep. Phonology Lab.*, 5:78-88 (Univ. of California, Berkeley).

Perlman, A. L. and Titze, I. R. (1983). Measurements of viscoelastic properties in live tissue. In *Vocal Fold Physiology: Biomechanics, Acoustics and Phonatory Control*, edited by I.R. Titze and R.C. Scherer. pp. 273-281. Denver Center for Performing Arts, Denver, CO.

Price, P. J. (1987): Voice quality and the glottal waveform. *Speech Communication Group Working Papers, M.I.T.* V:68-86. (Massachusetts Institute of Technology, Cambridge, MA).
Stevens, K. N. (this volume). Vocal-fold vibration for obstruent consonants.
Westbury, J. R. (1983): Enlargement of the supraglottal cavity and its relation to stop consonant voicing. *J. Acoust. Soc. Am.*, 73(4):1322-1336.

7

Comments on Glottal Flow Modelling and Analysis

Gunnar Fant and Qiguang Lin

Dept. of Speech Communication and Music Acoustics, Royal Inst. of Technology (KTH), Stockholm 100 44, Sweden

At the Royal Institute of Technology, Stockholm, we have a long history of acoustic voice source analysis. Examples of inverse filtered vowels were first published by Fant (1961a) shortly after the pioneering work of Miller (1959). Our first issue of the Speech Transmission Laboratory, Quarterly Progress and Status Report (STL-QPSR 1/1960), contained a brief resume of work by Cederlund et al., who used a four-formant inverse filter system. It was followed in issue 2/1960, by a report by Cederlund and Mártony, and in issue 4/1961, by Mártony on spectral analysis of inverse filtered vowels. An RC-anti-resonance module was described by Fant (1961b). Briess and Fant (1962) performed inverse filtering of a hoarse voice which showed double excitation. Photoelectric glottography in combination with inverse filtering was demonstrated by Fant and Sonesson (1966). An extension to include electrical glottography was reported by Fant et al. (1966).

A complete inverse filter based on RC modules was constructed by Lindqvist-Gauffin (1963) and used in experiments, (e.g., Lindqvist-Gauffin, 1964; 1965) and in a later more extensive study (Lindqvist-Gauffin, 1970), where pulse shape parameters and their variation within an SPL versus F0 frame were discussed. Important work along this line was reported by Gauffin and Sundberg (1980) and by Sundberg and Gauffin (1979).

Mártony (1964) demonstrated a good fit between spectrum analysis of inverse filtered vowels and source spectra derived from spectrum matching. The extensive report on voice source spectra of Mártony (1965) derived from spectrum matching has a renewed interest in view of recent frequency domain analysis (Fant, 1988; Fant and Lin, 1988).

A three-parameter generative model of vocal flow was introduced by Fant (1979a) in support of inverse filtering studies with analog instrumentation (Fant, 1979b; 1980; 1982a; 1982b). These studies included several examples of connected speech with discussions on onset and offset characteristics, stress correlates, and glottal abduction in voiced aspiration. An important step forward in the modelling of glottal flow was obtained by the LF-model introduced by Fant et al. (1985a), see Figure 1. The fourth parameter added was the duration T_a of a finite return phase after the instant T_e of maximum discontinuity. T_a is defined by drawing a tangent to the differentiated flow immediately after T_e and noting its intersection with the zero line. The longer the T_a the more profound is the drop off of the source spectrum, as shown in Figure 2. This effect is equivalent to a low pass filter of the first order defined by a cut-off frequency $F_a = 1/(2\pi T_a)$. A

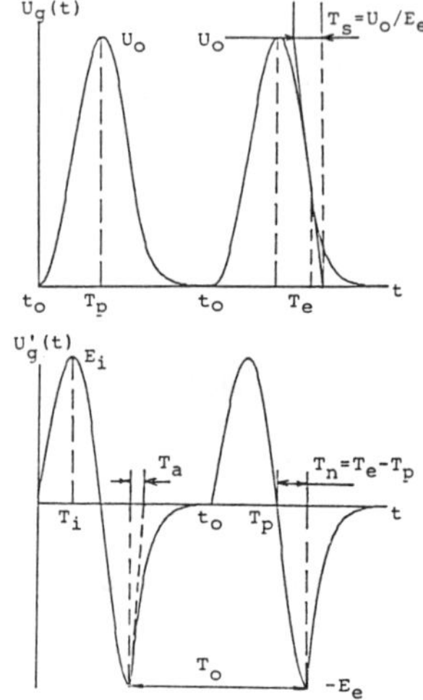

Flow derivatives:

$$U_g'(t) = E_0 \cdot e^{\alpha \cdot t} \cdot \sin(\omega_g \cdot t),$$
$$0 \le t \le T_e;$$

$$U_g'(t) = -\frac{E_e}{\varepsilon \cdot T_a} \cdot \left[e^{-\varepsilon \cdot (t - T_e)} - e^{-\varepsilon \cdot (T_c - T_e)} \right],$$
$$T_e < t \le T_c.$$

$\omega_g = 2 \cdot \pi \cdot F_g;$ $\quad F_g = 1/(2 \cdot T_p);$

$R_g = F_g/F_0;$ $\quad R_k = T_e/T_p - 1;$

$O_q = (T_e + T_a)/T_0;$ $\quad O_q' = T_e/T_0;$

$F_a = 1/(2 \cdot \pi \cdot T_a);$ $\quad R_a = T_a/T_0;$

$T_c = T_0 = 1/F_0.$

Fig. 1. The LF-model: Glottal flow $U_g(t)$ and flow derivative $U_g'(t)$. Note that $T_s = U_0/E_e$ is defined as a closing time.

similar model was described by Ananthapadmanabha (1984) who adopted a parabolic return phase as an alternative to our exponential return phase.

Increased duration of the return phase with its associated low pass spectral effect and a concomitant increase of first formant bandwidth are the main acoustic correlates of glottal abduction. Glottal flow models that do not incorporate these features will fail in description of source dynamics. A substantial part of our present work is directed to the study of connected speech (Carlson et al., 1989; Gobl, 1988; Gobl and Ní Chasaide, 1988; Gobl and Karlsson, 1991; Karlsson 1988). We have gained an understanding of the main structures of voice source dynamics but there still remains much analysis work to support the development of our text-to-speech synthesis rules.

PRODUCTION MODELS - INTERACTION EFFECTS

The LF-model is intended as a tool for linear system function analysis, i.e., source-filter interaction is disregarded. A true speech production model, on the other hand, should incorporate all sorts of interaction phenomena (Fant, 1987). One class of interaction is aerodynamic-mechanical. A supraglottal constriction of a voiced continuant will impede the air flow, reduce the transglottal pressure drop, and perturb the vibratory pattern of the vocal folds (see, e.g., Bickley and Stevens, 1986). Corresponding changes in glottal flow parameters have been observed by Gobl and Ní Chasaide (1988), and by Gobl and Karlsson (1991). The other major class of interaction is referred to as acoustic. It treats the temporal profile of the effective glottal area, $A_g(t)$, as given but takes into account the variation of instantaneous transglottal pressure drop as an interactive component determined by the supraglottal pressure and thus by formant oscillations, which will modify the true glottal flow. In view of the second power relation between transglottal flow and pressure this is a nonlinear process. The first comprehensive study of these effects was that of Ananthapadmanabha and Fant (1982) and Fant and Ananthapadmanabha (1982).

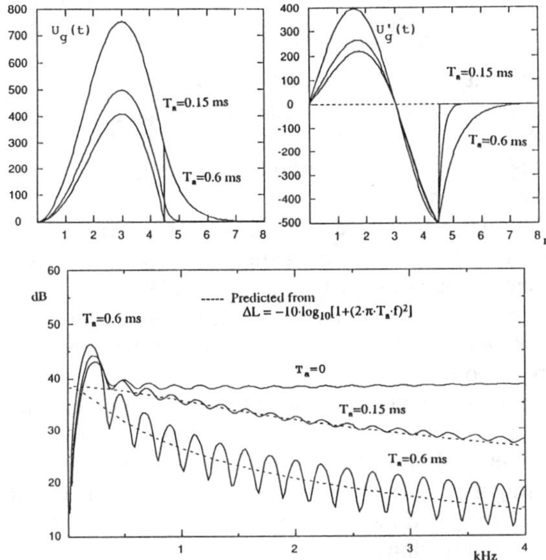

Fig. 2. Wave shapes and spectral changes associated with an increase of the return time parameter T_a.

These have been followed up by studies of Fant et al. (1985b), Fant (1986; 1987), Fant and Lin (1987), Lin (1987; 1990).

Acoustic interaction can be quite important at a high F0 and low F1 of the same order as F0. Fant et al. (1985b) verified theoretically an observation of Rothenberg (1985) that when a soprano sings with an F0 matching F1, the glottal flow pulse is reduced in amplitude by an F1 component of the transglottal pressure producing a minimum in the middle of the flow pulse. This effect may be regarded as an economy of production in addition to the F1 reinforcement efficiency. However, it is interesting to note the systematic trends in relative amplitude of the voice source fundamental comparing female phonations of vowels with low F1. As shown by Fant and Lin (1988, see their Figure 8), a step between two vowels differing in F1, in one such that F1 = F0 and in the other F1 = 1.5F0, was accompanied by a 5 dB increase in the amplitude of the voice source fundamental. This difference could be explained by the same phenomenon of acoustic interaction just mentioned, or it could be an interaction affecting already the vibratory patterns of the vocal folds and a loss of transglottal pressure. A clear separation between aerodynamic-mechanical and acoustic interaction is not possible to attain in the analysis of human speech. Fant and Mártony (1963) found that during the course of the phonation of a vowel with gliding F0, the F2 and F3 amplitudes did not only vary with their Fn/F0 ratios but were synchronized with the F1/F0 ratio. A modelling reconstruction from acoustic interaction performed by Lin (1987) was in part successful.

One of the main aspects of acoustic interaction is pulse skewing, i.e., the tilting of the glottal flow pulse to the right compared to the glottal area function. This inertia effect has been extensively treated by Rothenberg (e.g., Rothenberg, 1981; see also Fant, 1982). Even though the glottal area function may be tilted to the left, the glottal flow attains an asymmetry so that the falling branch has a steepness of 1-4 times of that of the rising branch. The negative to positive peak ratio E_e/E_i of the differentiated flow is thus of the order of 1-4 and typically 2.5. The pulse skewing increases somewhat with overall vocal tract inductance and also with decrease of glottal resistance accompanying low subglottal pressure. However, these tendencies remain to be verified. Since excitation is proportional to the amplitude of the negative peak of the differentiated flow it follows that increased pulse skewing causes an increase of formant amplitudes whilst, apart from some shift of energy from the fundamental to the second and third harmonics, the level of the low-frequency area stays intact. Perceptually the redistribution of low-frequency energy is less apparent than the increase of formant amplitudes.

Interaction effects other than pulse skewing produce extra peaks in the differentiated glottal flow and extra zeros and humps in the corresponding spectrum. These have been verified by inverse filtering (see further Fant et al., 1985b; Fant and Lin, 1987; Lin, 1987; 1990). These are related to the nonlinearity of the glottal impedance shunting the vocal tract network. Multiple excitations within one voice period and the nonlinear superposition from previous periods can also be important.

Another class of interaction is the coupling between the subglottal and the supraglottal system under the conditions of a finite glottis impedance. Such conditions are at hand in a breathy voice and in the glottal open interval. Formant bandwidths, especially B1, tend to increase and a positive shift of F1 during the maximally open phase may be seen. The effective frequency detuning is usually negligible if the main part of the formant oscillation derives from the maximally closed glottal condition.

The first comprehensive study of subglottal formants was that of Fant et al. (1972). The close tie between breathy phonation and subglottal coupling has been pointed out by Klatt and Klatt (1990). Their observations that in breathy phonation subglottal coupling may markedly affect a vowel spectrum by appearance of extra formants and the weakening of other formants have been confirmed by Fant and Lin (1988) who observed an extra formant at 1400 Hz below F2 in the spectrogram of a female vowel /ε/. A vocal tract modelling verified that this was a true subglottal effect. Implication of such interaction on the derivation of glottal flow parameters was discussed by Fant and Lin (1988). One consequence is the ambiguity in the determination of the duration T_a of the glottal flow derivative return phase.

We lack comprehensive perceptual tests of the significance of interaction effects. Even though interaction effects add to the naturalness of synthetic speech, the effects appear to be rather small, especially if a best linear model match is pursued such that pulse skewing and bandwidth shifts are taken into account (see Nord et al., 1984; Lin, 1990).

FREQUENCY AND TIME DOMAIN RELATIONS

A detailed account of frequency domain interpretation and derivation of glottal flow parameters was given by Fant and Lin (1988), see also Fant (1987). We shall here bring out some of the main points and add a few expressions related to alternative sets of descriptive parameters.

Our present work on voice source analysis and synthesis, (see Carlson et al., 1989; Gobl, 1988; Gobl and Ní Chasaide, 1988; Gobl and Karlsson, 1991; Karlsson, 1988), is based on the four parameters of the LF-model, R_k, R_g, R_a, and E_e, which are related to three basic time events: (1) the locations of the flow peak T_p; (2) the discontinuity point T_e at glottal closure (see Figure 1). Both T_p and T_e are defined with reference to a flow

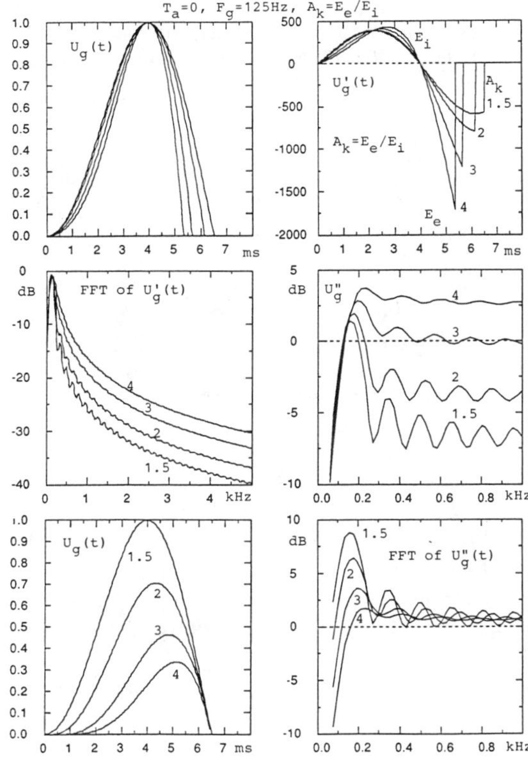

Fig. 3. In the top two rows: LF-flow $Ug(t)$, flow derivative $Ug'(t)$, spectrum of $Ug'(t)$, and spectrum of $Ug''(t)$ at varying Ee/Ei, constant U_0, and $Ta = 0$. In the bottom row: LF-flow and spectrum $Ug''(t)$ when maintaining constant Ee ($Ta = 0$)

onset point; (3) the duration of the return phase T_a, defined by the projection on the time-axis of the tangent to an exponential approximation to the return phase.

The flow derivative E_e at T_e is a scale factor. The voice fundamental frequency $F_0 = 1/T_0$ enters as a fifth parameter. The time locations are now converted into wave shape parameters by the expressions:

$$R_k = \frac{T_n}{T_p}, \text{ with } T_n = T_e - T_p$$
$$R_g = \frac{T_0}{2T_p} = \frac{F_g}{F_0}, \text{ with } F_g = \frac{1}{2T_p} \qquad (1)$$
$$R_a = \frac{T_a}{T_0}$$

These define an open quotient $O_q = \dfrac{1+R_k}{2R_g} + R_a$, or omitting the return phase, $O_q' = \dfrac{1+R_k}{2R_g}$.

One possible change in the set of parameters is to leave out R_k and instead include the closely related parameter E_i/E_e where E_i is the maximum of the flow derivative in the ascending branch, see Figure 3. An alternative is to introduce the peak value of glottal flow U_0 which for R_k greater than 0.25 comes close to

Table 1. *Values of $A_0/A_{k'}$ (column a) and $A_2/A_{k'}$ (column b) in dB as function of R_k and R_g. Remarks: The other model parameters are taken constant values. F_0 = 125 Hz, R_a = 0. The combinations of R_g = 0.7 and R_k = 0.5 or 0.6 have no solutions.*

Rk	0.2		0.3		0.4		0.5		0.6	
Rg	a	b	a	b	a	b	a	b	a	b
0.7	-6.0	-1.3	-1.0	0.0	2.3	0.8				
0.8	-7.6	-1.8	-2.2	0.2	1.5	0.6	4.6	0.7	7.4	1.5
1.0	-10.0	-3.0	-4.8	0.4	-0.6	2.0	2.9	2.5	6.2	2.0
1.25	-14.0	-4.8	-7.8	-0.3	-3.4	2.6	-0.4	4.8	3.9	6.6
1.5	-17.0	-6.8	-11.0	-1.6	-6.0	2.0	-2.0	4.9	1.5	7.5
2.0	-21.0	-11.0	-15.0	-4.8	-10.0	-0.6	-6.4	3.0	-2.6	6.0

$$U_0 = \frac{2T_p}{\pi} E_i \tag{2}$$

The error in this expression is 2% for E_e/E_i = 2 and 11% for E_e/E_i = 4. This follows from the quasi-sinusoidal character of the flow derivative up to $t = T_p$. From T_p to T_e, assuming R_k< 0.4, the area enclosed by the flow derivative may be approximated by that of a triangle, $E_eT_n/2$. For R_a smaller than 0.1 the area enclosed by the return phase is with good approximation E_eT_a. From the requirement of area balance we derive the approximate expression:

$$\frac{E_i}{E_e} = \pi\left(\frac{R_k}{4} + R_a R_g\right) \tag{3}$$

which is valid for R_k smaller than 0.4. By combining eq. (3) and eq. (2) we arrive at:

$$\frac{U_0}{E_e} = \frac{R_k}{4F_g} + \frac{R_a}{F_0} = \frac{T_e - T_p}{2} + T_a \tag{4a}$$

Eq. (4a) holds true within 10% for 0.35 <R_k<0.55 and $R_a \leq 0.05$. It is noted that with a small R_a the range of R_k in which eq. (4a) is valid gets relatively wider. Eq. (4a) can be supplemented to improve the prediction accuracy. For instance, for T_a= 0, eq. (4b) holds within 5% for a range of 0.2 <R_k < 0.55.

$$\frac{U_0}{E_e} = \frac{(T_e - T_p)}{2} + (0.5 - 1.2R_k) \tag{4b}$$

From speech production theory (Fant and Lin, 1988; eq. 5), we find that the amplitude of the voice fundamental in a Fourier series of the source spectrum of the radiated wave at a distance of a cm from the speaker is:

$$A_0 = U_0\, k\, \pi\, F_0 \frac{\rho}{4\pi a} \tag{5}$$

where the constant k = 1 for an opening quotient O_q = 0.5, k = 0.9 for O_q = 0.4 and k = 1.05 for O_q between 0.6 and 0.8.

A further development of the frequency domain analysis presumes that the recorded sound has been submitted to an inverse filtering which can be performed either before the

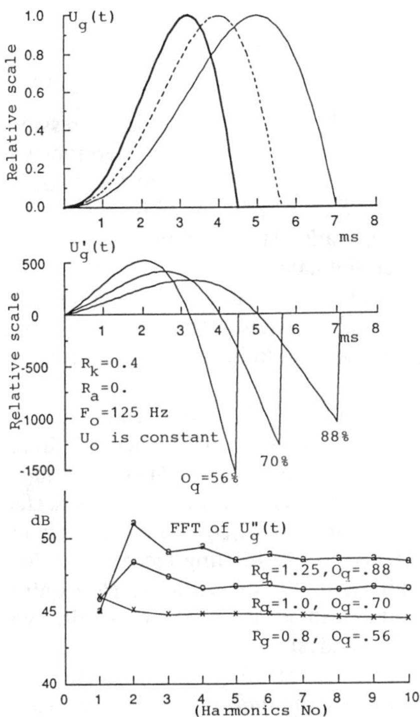

Fig. 4. Glottal flow (top), flow derivative (middle), and the normalized spectra sampled at harmonics (bottom) of the LF-model for three R_g values: $R_g = 0.8$, 1.0, and 1.25 (corresponding to open quotients of 88%, 70%, and 56%, respectively). The other model parameters are constant. $R_k = 0.4$, $F_0 = 125$ Hz, and $R_a = 0$. Note that the U_0 is adjusted to be the same amongst these three calculations.

spectrum analysis or afterwards in the frequency domain. The resulting spectrum is proportional to the source spectrum submitted to differentiation through the radiation transfer. This spectrum is further preemphasized with f/F_0, i.e., with the fundamental as a reference. Ideally with $T_a = 0$ this +12 dB/Oct preemphasized glottal flow would have a constant spectrum level at frequencies well above F0 or F1. At a distance of a cm from the speaker it is simply:

$$A_k' = \frac{E_e}{\pi^2} \times \frac{\rho}{4a} \tag{6}$$

Since a finite return phase will introduce an additional -6 dB/Oct role off above a cut-off frequency $F_a = 1/(2\pi T_a)$ one should as an initial step compensate it by an inverse operation.

F_a may vary from 60 Hz at a highly abducted phonation as in a voiced [h] up to 4000 Hz and is typically 2000 Hz for an ideal vowel. The reduction in formant amplitudes related to a low F_a constitutes a departure from the proportionality between E_e and formant amplitudes, see Figure 13 in Fant and Lin (1988).

A basic spectrum parameter is the ratio of the amplitude of the normalized source fundamental A_0 to its higher harmonics A_k' which comes out as:

$$\frac{A_0}{A_k'} = \frac{\pi k}{R_g} \times \frac{E_i}{E_e} = \pi^2 k F_0 \frac{U_0}{E_e} \tag{7}$$

By combining eqs. (7) and (4a) we have for $R_k < 0.4$:

$$\frac{A_0}{A_k'} = [2.5 \times \frac{R_k}{R_g} + 10 \times R_a] \times k \qquad (8)$$

Observe that an approximation $k = 1$ is valid for $R_g < 1.1$ only. These expressions show that the spectral balance of the source fundamental versus its higher harmonics is more closely related to the direct flow parameters U_0/E_e or E_i/E_e than to R_k alone. At constant R_k and U_0 an increase of R_g or a decrease of R_a (i.e., of T_a or an increase in F_a) will increase E_e and A_k' and thus decrease the A_0/A_k' ratio. The remaining parameter to be determined is R_g, which can be derived by spectral matching of the fundamental versus the second harmonic of the normalized source flow or more directly from a time domain analysis, e.g., from an E_e/E_i measure, eq. (7). Table 1 shows the amplitudes of the fundamental A_0 and of the second harmonic A_2 with respect to the limiting level A_k' of the normalized source spectrum.

For analysis purposes one could substitute E_e or U_0 for R_k. E_e/E_i is directly apparent as the peak ratio in the derivative flow. However, E_i is often obscured by acoustic interaction which also may affect an estimate of T_p and thus of R_g. U_0 appears to be a more robust measure and has the advantage of a relative stability as a carrier in connected speech and a simple relation to A_0. The envelope of $U_0(t)$ and $E_e(t)$ within an utterance can be easily traced from preprogrammed continuous inverse filtering records with low accuracy demands. For voices with relatively high A_0/A_k' the extraction of U_0 requires simple integration only (Fant, 1961a; 1979a). It might also be an advantage to write synthesis rule with respect to the temporal variation of A_0 and A_k'.

It is of interest to note that there also exists a relative stability of U_0/E_e. This parameter has the dimension of time. It is the projection on the time-axis of the tangent to the glottal flow at closure drawn from the level of U_0, see eq. (4) and Figure 1. It was originally adopted by Sundberg and Gauffin (1979) and was referred to as "closing time" with the notation S_c. It is of the order of 0.5 - 1.5 ms, and typically 1 ms for both male and female voices (Fant and Lin, 1988). Females have about 4-6 dB smaller U_0 and E_e than of men but because of the higher F0 the difference in the spectrum levels is less. Formant amplitudes are proportional to both E_e and F0. The often higher A_0/A_k' of female than of men is related to lower R_g and higher R_a and occasionally higher R_k, see eq. (8), which also implies greater O_q. Figure 4 exemplifies this relation in the case of varying R_g. However, at a constant (U_0/E_e) the A_0/A_k' ratio is directly proportional to F0, see eq. (7). This is a less complicated relation. Because of the relative closeness of F0 to F1 the A_0 attains an additional boost in the female vowel spectrum, see further Fant and Lin (1988).

CONCLUSIONS

Acoustic and aerodynamic-mechanical interaction and subglottal coupling effects have been briefly discussed. It remains to verify to what extent a linear synthesis scheme preserving a best spectral match may suffice for highest demands on synthesis quality. A knowledge of interaction effects is needed for an understanding of sometimes large deviations from ideal waveforms in inverse filtering.

The covariation of the LF parameters in connected speech is complex. As noted by Gobl (1988), and Gobl and Karlsson (1991), E_e varies inversely with R_k and R_a which increase in an abduction gesture. Increased E_e also follows increased R_g as in a pressed voice. The carrier nature of U_0 as a rather stable parameter increasing with subglottal pressure and decreasing with supraglottal constriction, should be made use of as reference to support a more basic and systematic description of parameter inter-relations as implied by our analytical survey, eqs. (2-7) which also indicate the spectral correlates. A substantial part of our presentation is devoted to frequency-time relations in production theory, recently derived by Fant (1988) and Fant and Lin (1988). A frequency domain derivation of glottal flow parameters has the benefit of preserving a resynthesis spectral check. The very direct relation between U_0 and A_0 and between E_e and spectral levels in the formant domain suggests the use of a parameter U_0/E_e, the "closing time" substituting or supplementing the R_k parameter as a more complete and direct spectrum shape correlate. The finite return phase represented by the return time T_a or $F_a = 1/(2\pi T_a)$ is besides U_0/E_e or the corresponding A_0/A_k' the most important parameter, essential for describing abduction-adduction gestures in connected speech. The spectral consequence of the T_a parameter has been incorporated by Blomberg (1989) in an adaptive scheme for speech recognition.

It remains to test in practice the relative benefit of the alternative parameter sets that we have proposed and to test the feasibility of frequency domain inverse filtering. The purpose of deriving glottal flow parameters from their frequency domain correlates is to allow voice source analysis from ordinary tape recordings without precautions of preserving a HiFi low frequency response and to guarantee a correct spectrum match. A combination of time domain and frequency domain methods may be optimal.

Programs have been written that allow for a translation from alternative parameter sets to the conventional E_e, R_k, R_g, and R_a parameters and vice versa and also the transformation to generative synthesis parameters (Lin, 1990).

REFERENCES

Note: STL-QPSR is an abbreviation of Speech Transmission Laboratory Quarterly Progress and Status Report. Department of Speech Communication and Music Acoustics, Royal Institute of Technology (KTH), Stockholm

Ananthapadmanabha, T.V. and Fant, G. (1982). Calculation of true glottal flow and its components. *Speech Comm.*, 1:167-184.

Ananthapadmanabha, T.V. (1984). Acoustic analysis of voice source dynamics. *STL-QPSR*, 2-3:1-24.

Bickley, C.A. and Stevens, K.N. (1986). Effects of a vocal tract constriction on the glottal source: Experimental and modelling studies. *J. Phonetics*, 14:373-382.

Blomberg, M. (1989). Voice source adaptation of synthetic phoneme spectra in speech recognition. In: *Proc. European Conf. on Speech Communication and Technology, EUROSPEECH 89*, Vol. 2, pp. 621-614.

Briess, B. and Fant, G. (1962). Studies of voice pathology by means of inverse filtering. *STL-QPSR*, 1:6.

Carlson, R., Fant, G., Gobl, C., Granström, B., Karlsson, I., and Lin, Q. (1989). Voice source rules for text-to-speech synthesis. *Proc. ICASSP 1989*, pp. 223-236.

Cederlund, C., Krokstad, A., and Kringelbotn, M. (1960). Voice source studies. *STL-QPSR*, 1:1-2.

Cederlund, C. and Mártony, J. (1960). Voice source studies. *STL-QPSR*, 2:8.

Fant, G. (1961a). The acoustics of speech. In: *Proc. of the 3rd Intern. Congr. Acoustics*,, Elsevier, Stuttgart, 1959, pp. 187-201.

Fant, G. (1961b). A new anti-resonance circuit for inverse filtering. *STL-QPSR, 4:1-6.*

Fant, G. (1979a). Glottal source and excitation analysis. *STL-QPSR*, 1:85-107.

Fant, G. (1979b). Voice source analysis - a progress report. *STL-QPSR*, 3-4:31-54.

Fant, G. (1980). Voice source dynamics. *STL-QPSR*, 2-3:17-37.
Fant, G. (1982a). Preliminaries to analysis of the human voice source. *STL-QPSR*, 4:1-27.
Fant, G. (1982b). The voice source acoustic modeling. *STL-QPSR* , 4:28-48.
Fant, G. (1986). Glottal flow: Models and interaction, *J. Phonetics*, 14:393-399.
Fant, G. (1987). Interactive phenomena in speech production. Proc. XIth Intern. Congr. Phonetics Sci., Vol. 3, pp. 376-381, Tallin, Aug., 1987.
Fant, G. (1988). Glottal flow parameters from the frequency domain. Paper presented at 2nd Symp. on Advanced Man-Machine Interface through Spoken Language, Hawaii, Nov., 1988.
Fant, G. and Ananthapadmanabha, T.V. (1982). Truncation and superposition. *STL-QPSR*, 2-3:1-17.
Fant, G. and Lin, Q. (1987). Glottal source - vocal tract acoustic interaction. *STL-QPSR*, 1:13-27.
Fant, G. and Lin, Q. (1988). Frequency domain interpretation and derivation of glottal flow parameters. *STL-QPSR*, 2-3:1-21.
Fant, G. and Mártony, J. (1963). Formant amplitude measurements. *STL-QPSR*, 1:1-5.
Fant, G. and Sonesson, B. (1966). Indirect studies of glottal cycles by synchronous inverse filtering and photo-electrical glottography. *STL-QPSR*, 4:1-3.
Fant, G., Liljencrants, J., and Lin, Q. (1985a). A four-parameter model of glottal flow. *STL-QPSR*, 4:1-13.
Fant, G., Lin, Q., and Gobl, C. (1985b). Notes on glottal flow interaction. *STL-QPSR*, 2-3:21-45.
Fant, G., Ishizaka, K., Lindqvist-Gauffin, J., and Sundberg, J. (1972). Subglottal formants. *STL-QPSR*, 1:1-12.
Fant, G., Ondrácková, J., Lindqvist-Gauffin, J., and Sonesson, B. (1966). Electrical glottography. *STL-QPSR*, 4:15-21.
Gauffin, J. and Sundberg, J. (1980). Data on the glottal voice source behaviour in vowel production. *STL-QPSR*, 2-3:61-70.
Gobl, C. (1988). Voice source dynamics in connected Speech, *STL-QPSR*, 1:123-159.
Gobl, C. and Ní Chasaide, A. (1988). The effects of adjacent voiced/voiceless consonants on the vowel voice source: a cross language study. *STL-QPSR*, 2-3:23-59.
Gobl, C. and Karlsson, I. (1989). Male and female voice source dynamics. In: *Vocal Fold Physiology: Acoustic, Perceptual, and Physiological Aspects of Voice Mechanisms*, edited by J. Gauffin and B. Hammarberg (this volume).
Karlsson, I. (1988). Glottal wave form parameters for different speaker types. In: Proc. of SPEECH 88, 7th FASE Symp., Edinburgh, pp. 225-231.
Klatt, D.K. and Klatt, L.C. (1990). Analysis, synthesis, and perception of voice quality variations among female and male talkers. *J. Acoust. Soc. Am.*, 87:820-857.
Lin, Q. (1987). Nonlinear interaction in voice production. *STL-QPSR*, 1:1-12.
Lin, Q. (1990). *Speech Production Theory and Articulatory Speech Synthesis*. Doctoral thesis, Royal Inst. of Technology, Stockholm.
Lindqvist-Gauffin, J. (1963). Inverse filtering equipment. *STL-QPSR*, 1:13.
Lindqvist-Gauffin, J. (1964). Inverse filtering - Instrumentation and techniques. *STL-QPSR*, 4:1-4.
Lindqvist-Gauffin, J. (1965). Studies of the voice source by means of inverse filtering. *STL-QPSR*, 2:8-13.
Lindqvist-Gauffin, J. (1970). The voice source studied by means of inverse filtering. *STL-QPSR*, 2:3-9.
Mártony, J. (1961). Studies of the voice source. *STL-QPSR*, 4:9.
Mártony, J. (1964). On the vowel source spectrum. *STL-QPSR*, 1:3-4.
Mártony, J. (1965). Studies of the voice source. *STL-QPSR*, 1:4-9.
Miller, R.L. (1959). Nature of the vocal cord wave. *J. Acoust. Soc. Am.*, 31:667-679.
Nord, L., Ananthapadmanabha, T.V., and Fant, G. (1984). Signal analysis and perceptual tests of vowel responses with an interactive source filter model. *STL-QPSR*, 2-3:25-52.
Rothenberg, M. (1981). An interactive model for the voice source. *STL-QPSR*, 4:1-17.
Rothenberg, M. (1985). Cosi fan tutte and what it means. Draft for discussion presented at the 4th Int. Conf. on Vocal Fold Physiology, Yale University, New Haven, CT.
Sundberg, J. and Gauffin, J. (1979). Wave form and spectrum of the glottal voice source. In: *Frontiers of Speech Communication*, edited by B. Lindblom and S. Öhman, pp. 301-322. Academic Press, London.

8

Simultaneous Modelling of EGG, PGG, and Glottal Flow

Bert Cranen

Dept. of Language and Speech (Phonetics section), Nijmegen University, NL-6500 HD Nijmegen, The Netherlands

It is well known that the way in which the kinetic energy of the glottal air flow is transformed into sound strongly depends on the details of how the geometry of the glottis changes with time. For a long time it has been thought that projected glottal area (as measured by means of photoglottography) is an adequate descriptor for glottal geometry as far as the acoustic voice source is concerned. Since Ishizaka and Flanagan (1972), however, indications have accumulated that various other details of the three-dimensional glottal shape contribute to how a voice will actually sound. Ishizaka and Flanagan have derived a formula which relates glottal flow to the geometry of the glottis in a two-mass model. Although the glottis in a two-mass model is highly stylized, the formula is also applicable to physiologically more realistic geometries as long as the basic assumptions of its derivation are not violated (no separation of the flow from the walls within the glottis and consequently no other energy loss than viscous loss at the walls of the glottal duct). For our purposes it is important to note that the results of Ishizaka and Flanagan can be used to show that the projected glottal area does not capture all aspects of glottal geometry that are essential for understanding the aerodynamics and acoustics of phonation, but that a hypothetical area function that we will call the "effective glottal area" does. Under the assumption that the inertia of the air and the viscous losses within the glottis can be neglected, the effective glottal area is defined as (Cranen and Boves, 1987):

$$Ag \approx \sqrt{\frac{1.37\, A_{g1}^2\, A_{g2}^2}{0.37\, A_{g1}^2 + A_{g2}^2}} \qquad (1)$$

where A_{g1} is the area of the glottal inlet, and A_{g2} the area of the glottal outlet.

The effective glottal area allows one to think of a time-varying glottis for which the upper and lower margins move out of phase as equivalent to a time-varying glottis which has a uniform cross-section in the direction of flow throughout the entire glottal cycle. The effective glottal area concept seems to comprise those aspects of glottal geometry that are most important from an aerodynamic/acoustic point of view. To validate this idea experimentally, however, simultaneous measurements of glottal geometry and glottal flow will have to be carried out.

Unfortunately, glottal geometry cannot be measured directly, at least not during normal speech production, and the measurements that can be obtained, like EGG, PGG and flow, are at best indirect indicators. This makes the estimation of glottal geometry from measurable signals in an essential way dependent on a theory about the relation between the phenomena. It is our goal to design a computer model capable of estimating glottal geometry during speech from EGG, flow, and perhaps also PGG. Eventually, we expect to make the step from the estimation of glottal geometry to an improved description and understanding of aerodynamics and acoustics of phonation.

STATEMENT OF THE PROBLEM

At first glance the model proposed by Titze (1984) seems to fulfil all our requirements. It allows the simulation of EGG and PGG (i.e., projected glottal area); with a minor extension the model also allows simulation of effective glottal area.

In Figure 1, simulated PGG, EGG and effective glottal area waveforms are shown for two different settings of the model. The figure serves to illustrate how one can run into trouble if one demands that not only PGG and EGG, but also effective glottal area simulations show characteristics similar to real observations for one setting of the model.

Figure 1a relates to a pre-phonatory setting where the folds are well adducted and where the glottis has a strongly convergent shape ($A_{g1} \gg A_{g2}$). Figure 1b shows the results of a simulation where the folds are slightly abducted and the glottis has a more uniform cross-sectional area (A_{g1} and A_{g2} are of the same order of magnitude). In both simulations it was assumed that the lower and upper margins make sinusoidal excursions with an amplitude which is largest in the middle of the folds and which decreases sinusoidally towards the anterior and posterior boundaries (cf., Titze (1984). The amplitude of the vibrations of upper and lower margin were set to identical values. The resulting glottal areas (A_{g1} and A_{g2}) are denoted by dotted lines in the upper panels of Figure 1a and 1b. The solid line in the upper panels reflect the minimum of the corresponding A_{g1} and A_{g2} waveforms, i.e., the projected glottal areas. Note that the solid lines always obscure part of the dotted lines. In the second and third panels, the simulated EGG's (i.e., contact areas) and the derivatives are shown.

Due to the convergent shape of the glottis the PGG waveform in Figure 1a is identical to A_{g2} and thus quite symmetrical while the EGG and d/dt(EGG) waveforms in Figure 1a show a marked asymmetry between the way in which the contact area develops during opening and closing. Similar phenomena can be observed in real PGG and EGG recordings, and one might be inclined to conclude that the corresponding pre-phonatory setting is typical for normal phonation. However, with the pre-phonatory settings which are necessary to obtain believable PGG and EGG waveforms, it appears impossible to obtain effective glottal areas which show the same characteristics as those which we think to see in real recordings. According to our experience glottal flow pulses (and consequently effective glottal areas) for a male voice during normal speech production are often characterized by a closure slope that can be divided into two separate regions very much as in the lower panel of Figure 2. In our interpretation, such a waveform signals a combination of glottal leakage and vertical phasing, and a pre-phonatory glottal shape which is almost uniform. Consequently, for effective glottal areas like that in the lower part of Figure 2 a much more uniform and abducted pre-phonatory setting is required. However, with such a pre-phonatory setting, the model predicts that EGG

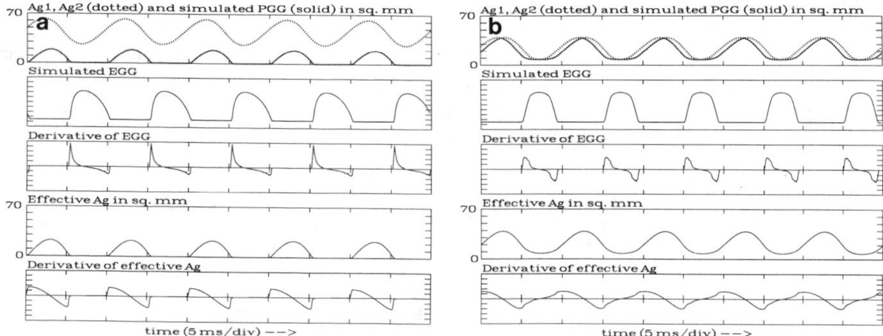

Fig. 1. From top to bottom: simulation of projected glottal area, EGG, derivative of EGG, effective glottal area, and derivative of effective glottal area by means of the model of Titze for two different settings of the model. Using the same terminology as in Titze (1984) where ξ_{01} and ξ_{02} denote the pre-phonatory displacements of the lower and upper margins of the folds at the level of the vocal processes and where ξ_m denotes the common vibratory amplitude, the settings of the model were in (**a**) Phasing quotient Q_p = 1/12 (equivalent to vertical phasing = 30 degrees); Shape quotient $Q_s = (\xi_{01} - \xi_{02})/\xi_m$ = 3; Abduction quotient ($Q_a = \xi_{02}/\xi_m$) = 0.1 and in (**b**) Phasing quotient (Q_p) = 1/12; Shape quotient (Q_s) = 1; Abduction quotient (Q_a) = 1.5.

waveforms become almost symmetrical as in Figure 1b; also, the open glottis interval becomes larger. More extensive simulations in which the parameters of the model were systematically varied (cf., Cranen, 1988) seemed to suggest that the requirement of both effective glottal area and EGG being simulated in a realistic way leads to contradictory demands for the model.

Every theory about the relation between EGG, PGG, glottal flow and glottal geometry will have a relatively large number of parameters. An important requirement for any modeling approach is that the number of parameters used must not be so large that they remain undetermined by the measurements. Therefore, the maximum amount of information present in PGG, EGG and glottal flow should be used. The question arises, however, whether it is possible to specify beforehand what signal characteristics represent "real" information. From many details in the measured waveforms it is not clear what they represent in terms of glottal geometry changes; it even cannot be excluded that some of these details are artefacts of the measurement method. Moreover, due to the non-linear nature of the system it is quite possible that small changes in glottal geometry have appreciable effects on recorded glottal waveforms. "Blindly" modeling all details in measured waveforms by minimizing some mathematically convenient cost function makes one run the risk of emphasizing aspects of waveforms which are not relevant for the problem under consideration, or even worse, of ending up with seemingly conflicting requirements for the model.

In this paper we hypothesize that a partial answer can be found by considering the coincidence of waveform events. We think that by looking at waveforms of PGG, EGG and glottal flow, as well as their derivatives, "events" can be defined that may or may not have a relation with a (sudden) change in glottal geometry. If the event detected in one signal coincides with an event in an other signal, the chance that the event reflects an important change in glottal geometry becomes larger. The moments of coinciding events can then be used as reference points in a simulation.

TIMING INFORMATION IN EGG, PGG AND GLOTTAL FLOW ESTIMATES

The interpretation of PGG, EGG and glottal flow waveforms has been extensively discussed in the literature and there is little that we could add that is not already known by considering these signals separately. We think, however, that the three signals in combination have an added value, especially if their first derivatives are also taken into account since the latter signals give additional information about the speed with which the glottal geometry changes. Especially interesting are the timing relations that can be found by considering the glottal flow as a skewed version of the "effective glottal area". In order to define our interpretation framework, let us first make a short inventory of what we consider the most important knowledge about the separate waveforms of PGG, EGG, and glottal flow.

It is well known that the PGG cannot be absolutely calibrated in terms of glottal area. Furthermore, the light picked up by the photo-sensor will not only change due to the time-varying glottal slit, but will probably also be slightly modulated when the glottis is closed and the contact area and medial compression change. This even makes an approach where PGG is interpreted as a normalized version of projected glottal area [like we did when applying Titze's model (cf., Figure 1)] somewhat uncertain. Information that we consider relatively robust and that can be extracted fairly easily from the PGG and its derivative, are the moments of glottal closure, glottal opening and maximum projected glottal area.

The EGG waveform is not interpretable in absolute terms either. In a situation where the electrodes have a fixed position with respect to the vocal folds, the relation between the normalized ac-part of the EGG-signal and vocal fold contact area seems to be linear in a first approximation (Scherer et al., 1988). On the other hand, it is also known that various details in the waveform are dependent on the placement of the electrodes, vertical movement of the larynx, fat tissue composition, etc. It is not clear how these factors will affect the relation between vocal fold contact area and EGG, which in our simulations we have assumed to be

$$EGG(t) = \frac{K_1}{K_2 + A_c(t)} \tag{2}$$

where K_1 and K_2 denote constants, A_c denotes contact area and t denotes time, cf,. Childers et al. (1986).

Although various researchers have investigated the relation between EGG waveform and changes in the glottal geometry, their findings cannot easily be incorporated in models. This is not strange if one realizes that one may barely expect to find a unique relation between EGG and glottal geometry: Since the vocal folds may vibrate very differently in various situations the contact area is a very complex function of vertical phasing, horizontal phasing, abduction, etc. As a consequence, certain details may be present in some EGG recordings and not in others, but it could also occur that some details have a different meaning dependent on the specific vibration mode.

Extrema in the first derivative have been proved to be relatively reliable indicators for moments of glottal opening and closure (Childers and Krishnamurty, 1985). Examination of our own recordings with respect to the coincidence between the (automatically detected) moments of glottal opening and closure defined by means of the PGG and its derivative on the one hand, and the moments defined by means of the derivative of the EGG on the other have confirmed this finding.

Since glottal flow cannot be measured directly, various indirect methods have been proposed in the literature, each with their own advantages and disadvantages. Whatever method is used, it appears that always some sort of inverse filtering is involved. In this paper we will assume that the glottal flow (U_g) can be described by the following formula:

$$U_g = A_g \sqrt{\frac{2\,P_{tr}}{k\,\rho}} \tag{3}$$

where A_g denotes the "effective glottal area" [cf., Eq. (1)], P_{tr} denotes transglottal pressure, k is a constant, and ρ the mass density of the air.

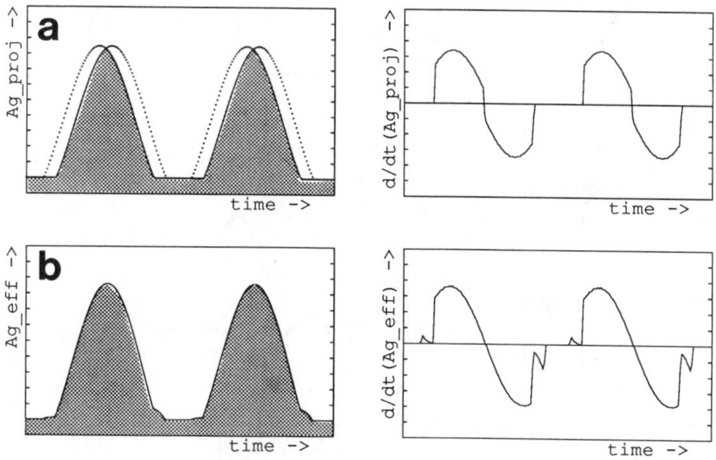

Fig. 2. If it is assumed that the areas of the glottal inlet and outlet vary sinusoidally around an offset value during the interval the folds have not collided and that the pre-phonatory shape is uniform, the projected glottal area (shaded area in **a**) is different from the effective glottal area (shaded area in **b**). Note that the latter is constant only if A_{g1} and A_{g2} are both constant and that the moments where upper and lower margins of the folds touch can be easily detected from the derivative of the effective glottal area (bottom panel in **b**).

The fact that we use the *effective glottal area* makes our way of interpreting glottal flow waveforms slightly different from the approaches normally encountered in the literature. From Eq. (3) it can be inferred that the glottal flow waveform has basically the same shape - and consequently carries basically the same information - as the effective glottal area. Generally, the major difference will be that the glottal flow will be skewed to the right and may have some formant ripple superimposed (due to the transglottal pressure term). As a consequence, it must be expected that "vertical phasing" in combination with glottal leakage causes a clearly observable effect in the glottal flow. The effect to be expected is illustrated in Figure 2, where the effective glottal area is sketched for a situation where A_{g1} and A_{g2} are both sinusoidal, and where a glottal leak is present. Note that all four moments where either the lower or upper margins of the vocal folds come into contact or separate can be detected from the effective glottal area

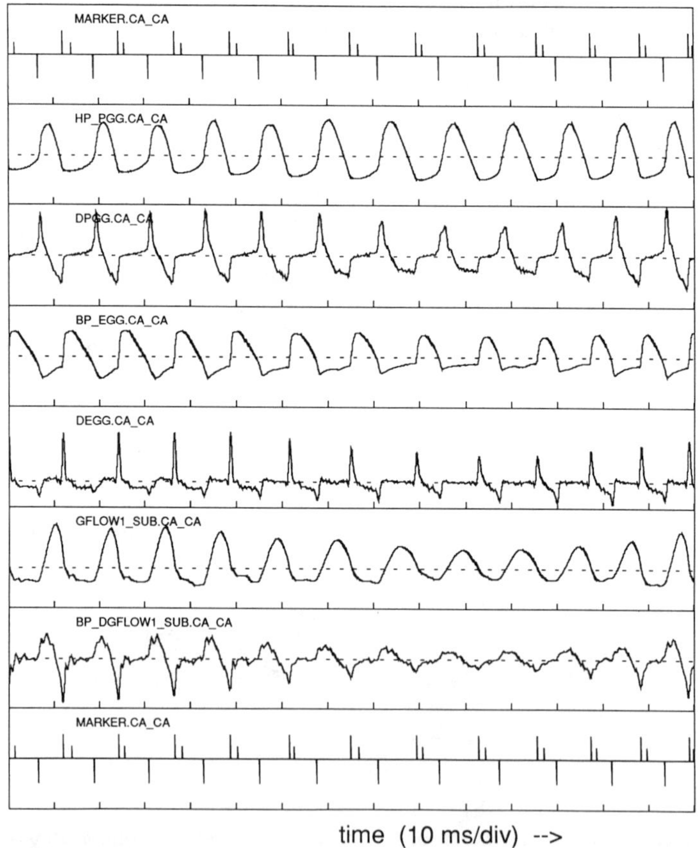

Fig. 3. 150 ms segment of an /aza/ transition. The simultaneous recordings are taken from the utterance /zaza/ spoken by a Dutch male speaker (LB). From top to bottom are shown: markers derived from the EGG (see text), PGG, derivative of the PGG, EGG, derivative of the EGG, glottal flow estimate, derivative of the glottal flow estimate, same marker as in the top panel to facilitate the alignment of a ruler.

function. Thus, compared to the projected glottal area, the effective glottal area function contains much more information about vocal fold motion in the direction of flow. In practice the sudden changes in the derivative of the effective glottal area (and the glottal flow) will not be that prominent, since the areas of the inlet and outlet of the glottis change more gradually (cf., Figures 1 and 3).

In Figure 3 an example is shown of a set of simultaneously recorded real signals of a segment from the utterance /zaza/. Identical marker signals derived from the EGG are shown in the top and bottom panels. The largest positive spikes in the marker signal denote the moments where the first derivative of the EGG shows a maximum. The negative spikes denote the minima in the derivative of the EGG. The smaller positive spikes denote the maxima of the EGG itself. The other signals denote (from top to bottom) PGG, first derivative of PGG, EGG, first derivative of EGG, glottal flow estimate [derived from subglottal pressure gradient (cf., Cranen and Boves 1988) and first derivative of glottal flow estimate.

It can clearly be seen that the moments derived from the first derivative of the EGG coincide with events in other waveforms like PGG, first derivative of PGG, glottal flow and first derivative of glottal flow. These events correspond to the closing and the opening of the glottis, in the way that is testified in the literature. For this given set of signals, however, there are additional events that can be discerned and interpreted. From Eq. (1) it can be inferred that the effective glottal area becomes constant only during part of the glottal cycle if (1) the flow is forced to zero, or if (2) the glottal configuration is constant over the entire depth.

Note that the duration of this interval is not necessarily equal to the closed glottis interval as detected by the EGG (or PGG). This will be the case only if (1) there is no vertical phase difference, or if the pre-phonatory configuration is either highly convergent ($A_{g1} \ll A_{g2}$), or (2) highly divergent ($A_{g1} \gg A_{g2}$), since then the waveform of the effective glottal area equals either A_{g1} or A_{g2}.

From observation of the glottal flow waveform it seems warranted to conclude that for this specific voice there was a glottal leak in combination with vertical phasing. The closure slope of the glottal flow pulse can be clearly divided into two parts, the second part being easily recognized as due to vertical phasing (cf., Figure 2).

If we are willing to assume that in this speaker's voice the horizontal phasing is negligible (i.e., the folds do not move like a zipper that is pulled close from anterior to posterior) the contact area between the moments at which the folds first touch and the moment when the glottis re-opens is completely determined by vertical phasing. This, then, would mean that the interval between the maximum in the derivative of the EGG and the maximum of the EGG proper corresponds to the interval in Figure 2 where the effective glottal area approaches its minimum after the "closure" of the glottis when A_{g1} reaches its minimum. Closer examination of Figure 3 reveals that the interval during which contact area increases coincides quite nicely with the interval in which glottal flow gradually approaches its minimum value after the moment where the flow derivative reached its minimum. This appears to hold not only for the steady vowel part during /a/, but also during the transition to the consonant /z/.

We have seen similar patterns of EGG (PGG) and flow in a number of other talkers. Moreover, we have been able to follow the evolution of EGG (PGG) and flow in other VCV and CVCV utterances, where the abduction coefficient reaches a peak in the consonant, causing an increase of the duty cycle of the glottal flow function, a more symmetrical EGG, and a less pronounced presence of the second part of the closure slope of the flow function, due to the increasing leak opening. More quantitative investigations of the timing relations described above between EGG and glottal flow estimates are underway.

SUMMARY AND CONCLUSION

In this and previous studies (e.g., Cranen and Boves, 1987), we have argued that projected glottal area is not sufficient to predict glottal flow, and that phenomena like vertical phasing and glottal leakage have to be taken into account properly when all details in the glottal flow waveform are to be understood. Therefore, we believe that a comprehensive explanatory model of the glottal geometry should allow one to simulate both projected glottal area and effective glottal area simultaneously (preferably with their derivatives since it often allows a better definition of "events") as well as the EGG (and its derivative). A model will be more convincing if it succeeds in tracking (or predicting) glottal parameter tracks in dynamic situations. In VCV-type utterances the glottal settings vary dynamically. Therefore, these types of waveforms are very valuable if it comes to "prove" that a given model is adequate. In many of our recordings we were able to show a remarkable coincidence of moments defined by means of the EGG waveforms (and its derivative) on the one hand, and of moments defined by means of the effective glottal area on the other. We think that it is worthwhile to investigate these phenomena in more detail and try to simulate them since they impose a number of extra restrictions on the choice of the model parameters. The more cues that can be simulated without conflicting demands for the model, the higher becomes the probability that the model is correct.

REFERENCES

Childers, D.G. and Krishnamurthy, A.K. (1985). A critical review of electroglottography. *CRC Crit. Rev. Biomed. Eng.*, 12:131-161.

Childers, D.G., Hicks, D.M., Moore, G.P., and Alsaka, Y.A. (1986). A model for vocal fold vibratory motion, contact area, and the electroglottogram. *J. Acoust. Soc. Am.*, 80:1309-1320.

Cranen, B. (1988). Simultaneous modeling of EGG, PGG and glottal flow. *J. Acoust. Soc. Am.*, 84:S82.

Cranen, B. and Boves, L. (1987). On subglottal formant analysis. *J. Acoust. Soc. Am.*, 81:734-746.

Cranen, B. and Boves, L. (1988). On the measurement of glottal flow. *J. Acoust. Soc. Am.*, 84:888-900.

Ishizaka, K and Flanagan, J.L. (1972). Synthesis of voiced sounds from a two-mass model of the vocal cords. *Bell Syst. Tech. J.*, 51:1233-1268.

Scherer, R.C., Druker, D.G., and Titze, I.R. (1988). Electroglottography and direct measurement of vocal fold contact area. In: *Vocal Physiology: Voice Production, Mechanisms and Functions*, edited by O. Fujimura, pp. 279-291. Raven Press, New York.

Titze, I.R. (1984). Parameterization of the glottal area, glottal flow, and vocal fold contact area. *J. Acoust. Soc. Am.*, 75:570-580.

9

Phonation from a Continuum Mechanics Point of View

Richard S. McGowan

Haskins Laboratories , 270 Crown Street, New Haven CT 06511, USA

Some aspects of the continuum mechanics of phonation are described here. Why should we be interested in mechanics, either fluid or solid? Further, why should we be interested in continuum mechanics? Consider the two-mass model as an example of a mechanical model in regards to the first question. This is a mechanical model because the input and output parameters are mechanical parameters and physical laws are used to relate them. The two-mass model illustrates the mechanically important energy flow and stability properties. Other kinds of models, perhaps of the vocal tract or of the larynx itself, are important in other contexts to tell us that a model is possible in complicated situations. For instance, it may be too complicated to explain the control of the vocal tract, or even the larynx, using a physically based model. Here, more abstract control models provide "existence proofs" for lawful behaviour.

The continuum approach to mechanics should be pursued because it can bring us closer to physically measurable quantities than can lumped-element models. Continuum mechanics treats materials, like air, as though their parameters, such as density and velocity, vary continuously in space. The smallest spatial scale studied is much larger than the molecular scale. For instance, the Young's modulus of the epithelium can be measured (Titze and Durham, 1987) and predictions made based on a continuum model, as in certain numerical simulations. It is more difficult to relate the physically measurable quantities to a lumped-element model, like the two-mass model.

Following energy flow and being aware of stability properties in the larynx tells us the nature of the sound and the conditions under which sound is produced. We want to know under what conditions the folds will oscillate, or the instability of the open folds under the influence of air flow. When the folds are vibrating, we want to know how much energy is being absorbed by the folds, and how much of the energy that is left in the air will actually contribute to acoustic output. (Some of the energy travelling through the solid or travelling in the air in a nonacoustic mode can later be radiated as sound.) A knowledge of the instability of the air motion itself will tell us how much energy of air motion becomes predominantly nonacoustic turbulent energy. In the first part of this paper, the issues of energy balance and stability in air will be discussed, supposing that the folds are given sufficient energy to oscillate. The mechanics of the mucousal wave will be considered in the second part of the paper. Again, stability and energy balance are the central issues.

AIR MOVEMENT DURING PHONATION

During phonation the air below the glottis and in the lungs has potential energy. When the folds open, a bit of air leaks out so that some of the potential energy is released as the kinetic energy of air motion. If we consider only the possibility of acoustic motion, then the velocity of air at the glottis at time t will be signaled at the mouth at time $t + l/c$, where l is the length of the vocal tract and c is the speed of sound. Note that it is not the particles of air that leave the glottis at time t that are sensed at the mouth at time $t + l/c$, but rather the events are transmitted down the tube by wave action: bits of air pushing neighbouring bits of air. To conserve mass, there must also be a net change in the density of air as the signal travels down the tube, so that the wave is compressive travelling down the tube. (A rarefaction wave is sent travelling toward the lungs.) The magnitude of the signal that actually reaches the mouth will depend on the waves reflected back toward the glottis. For instance, the signal at the mouth depends on the relative quantity of the potential energy in the lungs compared to the energy of the reflected wave (i.e., on whether the air leaking from the glottis depends greatly on the reflected wave: source-tract interaction.)

However, this is not what happens in the real vocal tract situation. The acoustic equations that describe the situation above are only an approximation to the continuum mechanics of the air in the vocal tract. These equations do not take into account things like rotational motion of the air that can result from the viscous shear stress in the air. This rotational motion does not allow us to make the acoustic approximation right away. The continuum mechanics must be considered in its detail.

Viscous shear stress results in a frictional force. Shear stress results when layers of air move by one another at different velocities. The frictional force acts opposite to the direction of motion. So, if the flow is in one direction, and the velocity is changing only in a perpendicular direction (planar flow), then the velocity, at any time, can be plotted as a function of position in that perpendicular direction. The magnitude of the frictional force opposing the motion is proportional to the curvature of the resulting curve. Because of the shear stress, there is a net torque on any small volume of air and rotational air motion will result.

There can be a great deal of this frictional force in the glottis because the air speed must increase from zero at the epithelium to perhaps as high as 5000 cm/sec in a few millimetres at the center of the glottis. This frictional force can set air into rotational motion, which can be convected into the vocal tract. Further, there is air in the vocal tract near the glottal exit that is not travelling at nearly the speeds of the air in the jet exiting from the glottis, leading to large gradients of velocity and the production of more rotational motion. The rotational air motion is not a part of the acoustic motion of the air, although it is also unsteady. There are other arguments to show the existence of rotational motion of air near the glottis based on the conservation of mass and momentum (McGowan, 1988).

Beyond the loss of energy, the rotational motion would appear to have little consequence to the acoustic output of speech. Indeed, in the first approximation, the propagation of sound is decoupled from the rotational motion (Chu and Kovaszany, 1957). But there is an important consequence, because the unsteady rotational motion can act as a source of sound, particularly when it interacts with solids like the vocal folds. I hope that this provides an example of why we should be concerned about energy balance considerations that can be uncovered using continuum mechanics. Stability of motion is also of concern here. If the rotational air motion is turbulent to some degree, the sound sources due to rotational motion will be noisy. The issue of stability of the oscillating phonatory jet should be addressed experimentally.

MECHANICS OF THE MUCOUSAL WAVE

In this section of the paper I will describe a continuum mechanics approach to the mucousal wave of the vocal folds. This analysis will allow us to consider the growth of the mucousal wave based on the mechanical properties of the biological materials and other clinically important materials. The continuum approach gives a more straightforward mapping from the real larynges to the model than does the lumped element approach. However, the lumped element approach, as exemplified by the two-mass model, can tell us much about the proper approximations to include in the simplest continuum model.

The first hint that the two-mass model gives is that only pressure stress, and not viscous shear stress, need be considered in relation to the force balance on the solid surface. (Viscous shear stress is considered in the calculation of flow resistance only, and as has just been demonstrated, has important consequences in the motion of the air). Another hint is that only the dynamics of the surface of the folds in a direction normal to the mid-line of the glottis need be considered. The forces of air on the solids in the direction of the vocal tract axis are of no consequence as far as the motion of the masses is concerned. (Recall that only the simplest model is being considered.) Therefore, the particular geometric feature of the folds jutting toward the centerline in relation to the solid boundaries of the trachea and pharynx has constriction of flow as its only mechanically salient feature. This constriction results in high air speeds in the glottal region and a resistance to flow caused by the formation of rotational fluid motion at the entrance and exit of the glottis.

All these simplifications will be made here, along with the further restriction that the initial steady air velocity be the same throughout the air channel, although the effects of flow resistance due to rotational air motion at the entrance and exit to the glottis will have to be included. That is, the effect of the glottis here is to obstruct the flow and not to speed it up. This makes the problem tractable, while still illustrating the basic wave growth mechanism. More sophisticated analytical techniques are needed to include this spatial variation in the initial steady air velocity.

To begin the continuum model, Hirano's description of the vocal folds is abstracted for the model layered structure (Hirano, 1981). There is a layer of air flowing with velocity U over a thin, elastic, stiff epithelium, a fluid Reinke's space, and a ligament-muscle impedance boundary. The epithelium is supposed to lie in the $z = 0$ plane and the air flows in the x-direction. The y-direction will be the breadth dimension in this essentially two-dimensional picture. (The $z = 0$ plane will be called the horizontal plane and the z-direction is the vertical direction).

The sequence of steps in this analysis is as follows. The equation of motion for the epithelium will be stated. It is supposed that a spatially sinusoidal perturbation is applied to this layered structure in the x-direction, which will produce pressure perturbations in the air and Reinke's space and vertical position changes in the epithelium. The spatial variations will be related to the time variations through a complex number called wave speed, c. The question to be answered is: Do these perturbations grow or decay in time? The answer to this question will depend on where in the complex plane c lies. If the perturbations grow in time, then the structure is linearly unstable to the particular sinusoidal perturbation and a wave will be presumed to result.

The equation of motion for the model epithelium for small perturbations from the plane $z = 0$ is (Miles, 1956)

$$m\frac{\partial^2\zeta}{\partial t^2} - T\frac{\partial^2\zeta}{\partial x^2} + D\frac{\partial^4\zeta}{\partial x^4} = -\Delta p \tag{1}$$

where ζ is the elevation above $z = 0$, m the mass/area, T the tension/breadth, D the bending stiffness/breadth, $\Delta p = p_a|_{z=0} - p|_{z=0}$, p_a the perturbation air pressure and p the perturbation Reinke's space pressure.

As the air pressure increases relative to the pressure in Reinke's space, the epithelial surface tends to move in the direction of Reinke's space. It is restrained from moving too far by the tension and bending stiffness. Bending stiffness will be neglected for now, as it can be included in a later analysis without much work. The dynamics of the epithelium are described by

$$\frac{\partial^2\zeta}{\partial t^2} - \frac{T}{m}\frac{\partial^2\zeta}{\partial x^2} = -\frac{\Delta p}{m} \tag{2}$$

This appears to be a forced wave equation with the restoring force proportional to the curvature of the epithelium. The stronger the constant of proportionality, that is, the larger T/m, the faster the wave travels, because the wave speed equals the square root of this quantity. Recall that quantities that obey the unforced wave equation travel without change of shape.

The apparent forcing is provided by the difference in the air and Reinke's space pressure at the epithelium. However, it turns out that this difference in pressure is a function of the surface elevation, ζ, so that the differential equation is really an unforced, homogeneous equation. One might want to think of this as a system with very strong feedback. After finding the pressure difference in terms of the elevation, ζ, it will be seen that the equation is no longer the simple wave equation, but a slightly more complicated equation allowing for wave-like behaviour, but where surface shapes can change over time. In fact, some solution shapes may grow in amplitude, so that these shapes can be expected to become visible from very small initial perturbations. These shapes are linearly unstable.

Recall that sinusoidal perturbations are to be considered. First, it is supposed that all quantities can be Fourier decomposed in space and time, so we write

$$f = \tilde{f}e^{ik(ct-x)}, \quad \tilde{f} = \tilde{f}(z) \tag{3}$$

for all dependent variables, where the real part of the above expression is taken. k is a real number known as the wave number and equals $2\pi/\lambda$, where λ= wavelength. By making this substitution, the stability of the surface to sinusoidal perturbations will be studied. c is the wave speed, which may be complex. The real part of c times the wavenumber gives the circular frequency. If c has a negative imaginary part, there is growth in time. One of the goals here is to find the value of c by substituting equation (3) into the equation of motion, equation (2). Before this can be done, the pressure difference, Δp, must be written in terms of the elevation, ζ. That is, the feedback must be found explicitly.

The expressions for air pressure and Reinke's space pressure depend on the governing equations and the boundary conditions at the mid-line of the air channel and at the ligament-muscle boundary. It can be shown that (McGowan, 1989)

$$\tilde{p}_a|_{z=0} = \frac{\rho_a}{k\tanh(kh_0)}\left\{\frac{\partial^2\tilde{\zeta}}{\partial t^2} + 2U\frac{\partial^2\tilde{\zeta}}{\partial t\,\partial x} + U^2\frac{\partial^2\tilde{\zeta}}{\partial x^2}\right\} \tag{4}$$

where h_0 is the half-width of the air channel and ρ_a is the density of air. Note that for kh_0 small, or surface wavelength much greater than channel half-width, $\tanh(kh_0)$ is small and the effect of the air on the epithelium is greatly enhanced over the situation where the flow is not channelled. For instance, the Bernoulli effect, as represented by the final term in the above equation is enhanced. This will be seen to lead to a much greater likelihood for the growth of surface waves.

It turns out that if Reinke's space is shallow compared to the surface wavelength, then the epithelium senses the ligament-muscle boundary pretty much directly. If this boundary is modelled as a second-order, locally reacting surface with mass per unit area M, spring constant per unit area K, and damping per unit area R, then

$$\tilde{p}\,|_{z=0} = 0 = \frac{1}{kc}\{iR - [M(kc) - \frac{K}{kc}]\}\frac{\partial^2\tilde{\zeta}}{\partial t^2} \tag{5}$$

Using equations (4) and (5), we can rewrite equation (2):

$$\mu\frac{\partial^2\tilde{\zeta}}{\partial t^2} + \frac{R}{m}\frac{\partial\tilde{\zeta}}{\partial t} + \frac{T}{m}\frac{\partial^2\tilde{\zeta}}{\partial x^2} + \left[\frac{K}{m} - \frac{\rho_a U^2}{mh_0}\right]\tilde{\zeta} = 0 \tag{6}$$

where $\mu = (1 + M/m)$. Here, the first and second terms in curly brackets of equation (4) have been neglected. Equation (6) still describes a type of wave propagation with damping provided by the ligament-muscle boundary and with an altered restoring force. The damping will tend to decrease the amplitude of any disturbance. The restoring force is altered by the presence of the flow and the underlying ligament-muscle tension, as shown by the factor in the square brackets. This alteration makes the wave dispersive. A dispersive wave is one whose wave speed depends upon wavelength, and this is one reason shapes do not propagate without change.

A nondispersive wave results when equation (2) is taken without forcing. To see this the substitution

$$\zeta = \tilde{\zeta}e^{ik(ct - x)} \tag{7}$$

is made into equation (2) without the forcing term. The following constant wave speed is obtained:

$$c = \sqrt{\frac{T}{m}} \tag{8}$$

The result is that shapes propagate without change in this simpler situation. If, on the other hand, the same substitution is made into equation (6), neglecting damping, the following is derived for the wave speed

$$c = \sqrt{\frac{T}{m} + \frac{1}{k^2}\left(\frac{K}{m} - \frac{\rho_a}{mh_0}U^2\right)} = \sqrt{\frac{T}{m} + \left(\frac{\lambda}{2\pi}\right)^2\left(\frac{K}{m} - \frac{\rho_a}{mh_0}U^2\right)} \tag{9}$$

The wave speed depends on the flow velocity, as well as wavelength.

The instability leading to the formation of the mucousal wave has yet to be considered. First, a little background on this kind of problem will be discussed. When air flows over water, waves can sometimes result. When air flows over water the Bernoulli effect makes the air pressure over the surface less than it otherwise would be. In fact, for air speeds high enough the Bernoulli effect will overcome the restoring forces of surface tension and gravity near the surface, and the water is literally sucked into the air. This is known as a Kelvin-Helmholtz instability, and it is an instability of the static type, where the elevation grows exponentially without oscillation. In this situation, the wave speed, c, is purely imaginary. This type of instability does not depend on the damping in the system, because the effective spring constant changes sign and pushes the mass away from the former equilibrium. It was found, however, that the wind velocities necessary to initiate waves with this mechanism are much higher than those that are observed (Miles, 1959).

Another mechanism was sought that would simply overcome any natural damping in the water, rather than counteracting the surface tension and gravitational forces completely. One such mechanism was proposed by H. Jeffreys in a 1925 paper, and is referred to here as the sheltering hypothesis (Jeffreys, 1925). He proposed that the pressure of the air at the water surface on the windward side of a wave crest is greater than on the leeward side. However, if the airflow contains no vorticity, that is, if the air motion is irrotational this can not be the case. So, Jeffreys proposed that flow separation occurs on the wave crests and that vorticity is shed into the air. This sheet of vorticity divides the windward and leeward sides into regions where the pressure heads, $p_T = p_S + \rho_a U^2/2$, are different. While the velocity of the air at the water surface is zero everywhere, the static pressures, p_S, are different on the two sides of the crest because the pressure heads, p_T, are different. Mathematically, Jeffreys added a term to the equation of motion for surface waves on water that gives a force in phase with the surface velocity, so that work is done by air on the water for waves travelling in the direction of the wind. If the amount of work done is large enough to overcome damping, this leads to what is known as a dynamic instability, where exponentially growing oscillations occur.

As can be seen from equations (6) and (9) it is possible to attain static instability for the epithelium in the case that the air speed is high enough and the surface wavelength long enough to diminish the importance of the tension force of the epithelium. Static instability will also be more likely to occur if T and K are made small, say, by relaxing the cricothyroid muscle, and by making the air channel narrower. If the linear analysis applies to different operating points along the closing phase of the glottal cycle, then the percentage of closing phase spent near or at static instability will help to determine voice type. Creaky voice may be distinguished from chest voice in the amount of the glottal cycle spent near static instability. In fact, a small change in the parameters used by Ishizaka and Matsudaira in their linear stability analysis of the two-mass model would produce a static instability (Ishizaka and Matsudaira, 1972). However, as in the case of wind waves over water, another instability is usually operable, and it too depends on the loss of pressure head due to the formation of rotational air motion and separated flow.

The two-mass model illustrates this instability very nicely, so this analysis can be used to include the head-loss effect in the continuum model (Ishizaka and Matsudaira, 1972). The head-loss mechanism and the consequent resistance to flow depends on the elevations of the masses, providing another feedback. It was shown that the resulting pressure perturbations because of this dependence affected the lower masses (leftward in our coordinate system), but not, particularly, the upper masses. Further, it was found that the air pressure on the lower masses was higher than it otherwise would have been when the lower mass was away from the mid-line of the glottis and upper mass was raised toward the mid-line. This means that an extra term should be added to the differential equation. Instead of saying that the head-loss affects the lower masses, it will be said that it affects a region weighted by the function $W(x)$, which is substantially non-zero and positive only for $-a < x < 0$. And, instead of saying that the effect's magnitude depends on the elevations of the masses, it will be said to depend on the weighted sum of elevations, so the following term should be included in the differential equation (6),

$$\frac{\rho_a U^2}{m h_0} W(x) \int_{-\infty}^{\infty} \Gamma(x') \zeta(x') dx' \tag{10}$$

where $\Gamma(x)$ is positive for $-a < x < 0$ and negative for $0 < x < a$ and substantially zero otherwise. Just as in the case of Jeffreys' sheltering hypothesis, it can be shown that this term produces a force in phase with the surface velocity over a complete cycle for certain kinds of disturbances, meaning that energy will be input into the epithelium. When enough energy is input to overcome the damping, dynamic instability results. Suppose :

$$W(x) = \begin{cases} 1 \text{ for } -a < x < 0 \\ 0 \quad otherwise \end{cases} \qquad \Gamma(x) = \begin{cases} -\sin\left(\frac{2\pi}{2a} x\right) \text{ for } -a < x < a \\ 0 \quad otherwise \end{cases} \tag{11}$$

and make the problem periodic in space by giving W and Γ periodic extensions of period $4a$. Then the problem can be solved by writing ζ in a Fourier series in space, so that each Fourier coefficient is a function of time. Assuming that only the forward going wave of wavelength $4a$ is present, the following differential equation for that coefficient can be derived:

$$\frac{d^2\overline{\zeta_1}}{dt^2} + \frac{R}{m\mu}\frac{d\overline{\zeta_1}}{dt} + \left[\frac{T}{m\mu}k_1^2 + \left(\frac{K}{m\mu} - \frac{\mu_B}{\mu}\right)\right]\overline{\zeta_1} = \frac{\mu_B}{\mu}\frac{8}{3}(1 - i)\overline{\zeta_1} \tag{12}$$

where $k_1 = \frac{2\pi}{4a}$, $\mu_B = \frac{\rho_a U^2}{m h_0}$ and $\overline{\zeta^1}$ = Fourier coefficient for wavelength $4a$ traveling in the $+x$ direction.

Note there is a forcing $\pi/2$ out of phase with the restoring force, called here the out-of-phase forcing. This is provided by the extra term added to the differential equation, and is analogous, although not completely equivalent to the sheltering term used by Jeffreys. The Routh-Hurwitz criterion gives the following inequality for instability

$$\left(\frac{8}{3}\frac{\mu_B}{\mu}\right)^2-\left(\frac{R}{m\mu}\right)^2\left[\frac{T}{m\mu}k_1^2+\left(\frac{K}{m\mu}-\frac{11}{3}\frac{\mu_B}{\mu}\right)\right]>0 \qquad (13)$$

The square of the out-of-phase forcing providing the first term in the inequality must be large compared to latter term, which is the square product of damping and effective natural frequency. The natural frequency appears here because the rate of dissipation over a cycle depends on this frequency. Not only does the added head-loss term help to create the instability by increasing the magnitude of the out-of-phase forcing, but it also decreases the natural frequency, and, thus the efficacy of damping.

When the tension T is increased by either tensing the cricothyroid, or a lessening of K, the tension for shorter wavelengths increases. So, it may turn out that there is not sufficient air velocity to create a dynamic instability at the wavelength $4a$, but only at longer wavelengths. However, the instability mechanism depends critically on the relative phase of the epithelial surface at $x = -a$ compared to $x = a$. If the wavelength gets too long then this mechanism will no longer work. So, it appears there must be a critical tension, T, where instability will no longer ensue, at least with this head-loss mechanism. Then such influences as inertial loading or stall flutter must be relied on for instability when phase differences are no longer possible. This is the regime of falsetto voice.

ACKNOWLEDGEMENTS

This work was supported by NIH grants NS-13870, HD-1994, and NS-13617 to Haskins Laboratories.

REFERENCES

Chu, B. -T. and Kovaszany, L. S. G. (1957). Non-linear interactions in a viscous, heat- conducting, compressible gas. *J. Fluid Mech.*, 3:494- 514.

Hirano, M. (1981). *The Clinical Examination of Voice*. Springer-Verlag, Vienna.

Ishizaka, K. and Matsudaira, M. (1972). Fluid Mechanical Considerations of Vocal Cord Vibration, *SCRL monograph* #8. (Speech Communications Research Laboratory Inc., Santa Barbara, Calif).

Jeffreys, H. (1925). On the formation of water waves by wind. *Proc. Royal Soc. London* 107:189-206.

McGowan, R. S. (1988). An aeroacoustic approach to phonation. *J. Acoust. Soc. Am.* 88:696- 704.

McGowan, R.S. (1989). Growth of surface waves with application to the mucosal wave of the vocal folds. *Haskins Laboratories Status Report on Speech Research*, SR 97/98:41-50.

Miles, J. W. (1956). On the aerodynamic instability of thin panels. *J. Aeronautical Sciences* 23:771-780.

Miles, J. W. (1959). On the generation of surface waves by shear flow: Part 3. Kelvin-Helmholtz instability. *J. Fluid Mech.*, 6:583-598.

Titze, I. R. and Durham, P. L. (1987). Passive mechanisms influencing fundamental frequency control. In: *Laryngeal Function in Phonation and Respiration*, edited by T. Baer, C. Sasaki, and K. Harris, pp. 304-319. College-Hill Press, Boston.

10

An Investigation Into the Acoustics and Aerodynamics of the Larynx

Christine H. Shadle, Anna M. Barney, and David W. Thomas

Department of Electronics and Computer Science, University of Southampton, Southampton SO9 5NH, England

Studying the mechanism of sound generation at the vocal folds is difficult because it involves the interaction of acoustic, aerodynamic and mechanical systems, and because the folds are small, delicate, and fairly inaccessible. A variety of techniques have been employed, including observation of excised larynges (Baer, 1981), measurements in mechanical models (Scherer, 1981; Scherer et al., 1983; Binh and Gauffin, 1983), and computer simulation (Titze and Talkin, 1979; Ishizaka and Flanagan, 1972; Fant et al., 1985). Nevertheless, many questions remain unanswered. We still do not completely understand, for instance, the effect of the supraglottal acoustic impedance on vibration of the vocal folds. And, since most of the mechanical models used were static, the accuracy of the quasi-static approximation in the flow equations has not been tested.

In the work reported here, we chose to study the aerodynamic effect of vocal fold vibration by visualizing the flow through a life-size dynamic model of the vocal folds. The most straightforward criterion for a quasi-static approximation is that the glottal area should change insignificantly during the time it takes for a disturbance to convect through the glottis. If parameter values typical for human speech are used, this criterion is satisfied for all conditions except for fundamental frequencies above about 300 Hz. A similar range of equivalent parameters is used in the model to be described here. Recent work by Chapman and Glendinning (1989) on a system having similar geometry used this approximation to solve for pressure and particle velocity in the tract. As we shall see, however, their solution is unlikely to apply in the region immediately downstream of the glottis. The utility of the model is thus more likely to be in the definition of the regions in which an acoustic as opposed to aerodynamic solution holds, than in directly testing the validity of the quasi-static approximation. The qualitative flow visualization results reported here represent the initial steps towards this end.

Flow visualization has been used before in studies of the vocal folds, in particular by Binh and Gauffin (1983). In this case the models were static, and were used mainly to show that the different shapes and cross-sectional areas assumed by the larynx during a phonatory cycle result in vastly different flow patterns: for example, a diverging glottis tends to cause flow separation; an abrupt glottal entry results in a vena contracta within the glottis. Such patterns can affect the pressure and velocity distributions throughout the laryngeal region, and thus are important for any theoretical models of vocal fold vi-

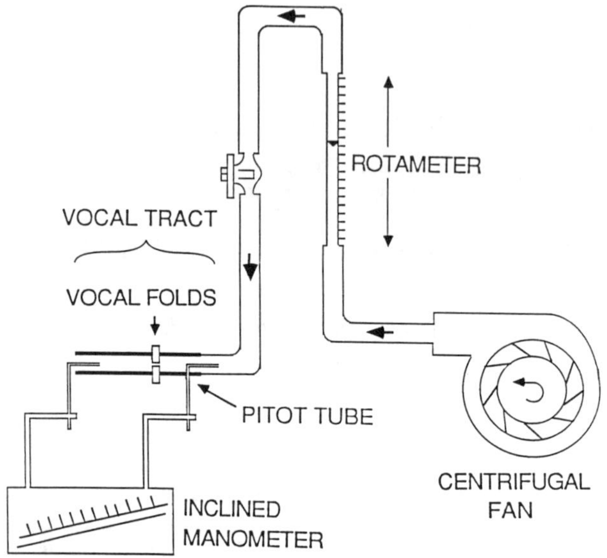

Fig. 1. (a) Diagram of static pressure-flow measurement setup, showing the placement of pitot tubes on either side of the stationary "vocal folds" to measure the pressure drop, and the rotameter, to measure volume velocity.

bration. The assumption is, of course, that a quasi-static approximation to the motion of the vocal folds is accurate enough for modelling purposes.

Studies involving static models have more often been used to measure the pressure at various points throughout the glottis, providing the quantitative data needed for theoretical models directly. Results from different models can vary significantly, as demonstrated by Scherer et al. (1983): they present a detailed comparison of the four pressure-flow relationships found by three different studies for slightly different static models of the larynx (Wegel, 1930; van den Berg et al., 1957; Ishizaka and Matsudaira, 1972). Upon comparing the equations to their own data, Scherer et al. found that Wegel's equation provided the worst fit in all cases, whereas Ishizaka and Matsudaira's expression for laminar flow provided the best fit. The relatively poor fit of van den Berg's equation was explained by a later study of Binh and Gauffin (1983), using a scaled-up model of the larynx.

The model we will be concerned with here is dynamic, and is principally designed to enable flow visualization rather than detailed pressure measurements. Its shape is considerably less realistic than any of the static models mentioned above. Since it is clear that the shape of the model, particularly in the glottis, affects the static pressure-flow relationship, we measured that relationship when the model was not moving and compared it to the equations studied by Scherer et al. (1983). The purpose of the comparison was to quantify the effect of using an idealistic shape, and to establish a context enabling comparison of the dynamic and static results. At the same time, we measured the effect of some simple variations in the tract shape, and performed some preliminary flow visualization. All of these static results are presented in Part 1.

Part 2 presents the flow visualization results for the model when in motion. We are interested in the following questions: what patterns does the flow assume during a glottal cycle, and how are these related to F0 and volume velocity? Is a quasi-static ap-

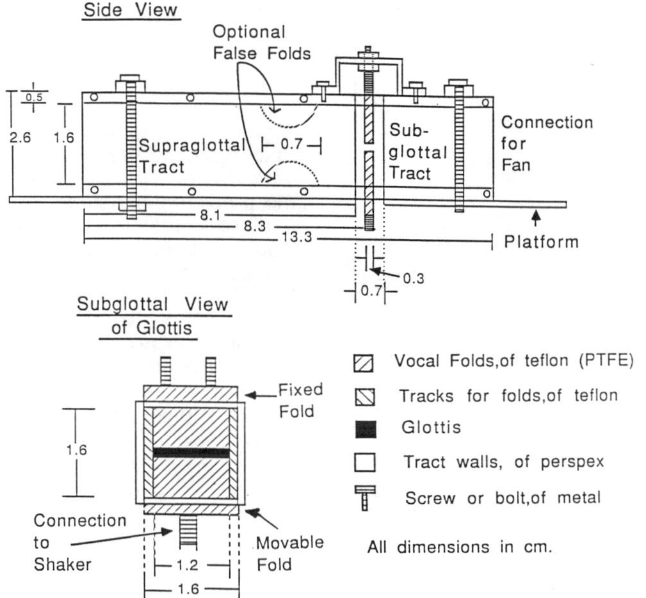

(b) Close-up cross-sectional views of the tract and "vocal folds" used in setups shown in Figure 1(a) and Figure 3.

proximation to laryngeal behaviour valid? Finally, can we observe any effect of acoustic loading?

PART 1: STATIC BEHAVIOUR OF THE MODEL

Method

A diagram of the apparatus used for the static flow measurements is shown in Figure 1. It consisted of a life-size "tract" of square cross-section made out of plexiglass, with shutters in the middle machined out of Teflon. The shutters, which formed the "vocal folds", ran along machined teflon tracks. The glottis thus had a rectangular profile, imitating a "one-mass" model. The tract was square in cross-section, rather than a more realistic circular cross-section, so that the flow could be observed without visual distortion. The dotted lines in Figure 1b indicate removable "false folds" made of plexiglass rod.

The air stream for the model was delivered by a centrifugal fan and regulated by a valve. The mean volume velocity was measured using a rotameter. Pressure was measured on both sides of the constriction by use of two pitot tubes attached to an inclined manometer. Subglottal pressure was found to be insensitive to location of the pressure tap as long as that was more than 3/4 D upstream of the glottis, where D = cross dimension = 1.6 cm. Downstream of the glottis, pressure recovery was complete within 4 to $5D$. The pressure taps were placed 1.6 cm upstream and 8.0 cm downstream of the glottis.

The model was life-size, with dimensions (shown on the figure) representative of an adult male. The pressure and flow were measured for four glottal areas (6, 12, 18, 24 mm^2) which correspond to the widths of 0.5, 1.0, 1.5 and 2.0 mm. These widths were checked by use of a feeler gauge.

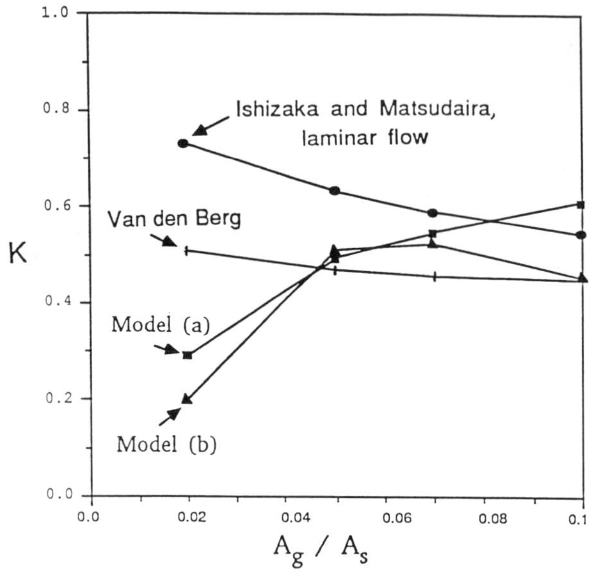

Fig. 2. *k* vs. the open-area ratio A_g/A_s, where *k* is the intercept of the line fit to the predicted/measured logarithmic pressure-flow relationships indicated. The curves shown are for Model **(a)** (with no tapering), Model **(b)** (with the Van den Berg profile), Van den Berg's equation and Ishizaka and Matsudaira's equation (given in Scherer et al., 1983).

Modelling clay was used to make the tract conform to the particular shape used by van den Berg, and therefore to check the effects of the abrupt change in area at the glottis.

Flow visualization was also performed for this static setup by removing the pitot tubes, and inserting a smoke probe upstream of the glottis. The smoke probe worked by burning oil at the tip of a probe. Only the original square tract cross-section was used for the flow visualization. Flow rates of 200 and 350 cm^3/sec and glottal areas of 6, 12, 18, 24 mm^2 were used, with and without the false folds. A halogen lamp was used as illumination.

Results

Pressure-flow characteristics for the basic, abrupt-entry tract (referred to as Model (a)) and for the tract formed to match van den Berg's model (Model (b)) were measured and compared to the equations discussed above. These comparisons are discussed in detail in Shadle et al. (1987). The principal points are obvious from Figure 2, a graph of *k* vs. the area ratio A_g/A_s. The coefficient *k*, which corresponds to the flow coefficient in the equation $\Delta P = k\,\rho U^2/A_g^{\,2}$, was obtained by fitting straight lines to the (logarithmic) pressure-flow characteristics; *k* is the intercept of each fitted line. A_g = the glottal area, and A_s = subglottal area, for each case. For the larger open-area ratios *k* tends to 0.5, as expected; at the area of 6 mm^2, an area not discussed by Scherer et al., none of the equations matches the data well. The discrepancies for the smallest area of 6 mm^2 may indicate that the assumption of Poiseuille flow within the glottis is inaccurate. For this small area, the predicted pressure drop within the glottis is an order of magnitude higher than the entry and exit losses, a condition not true of the other areas considered. Apart from this smallest area, models (a) and (b) fall within the predictions of the theories. We conclude that model (a) exhibits a pressure-flow characteristic comparable to static models having a more realistic shape.

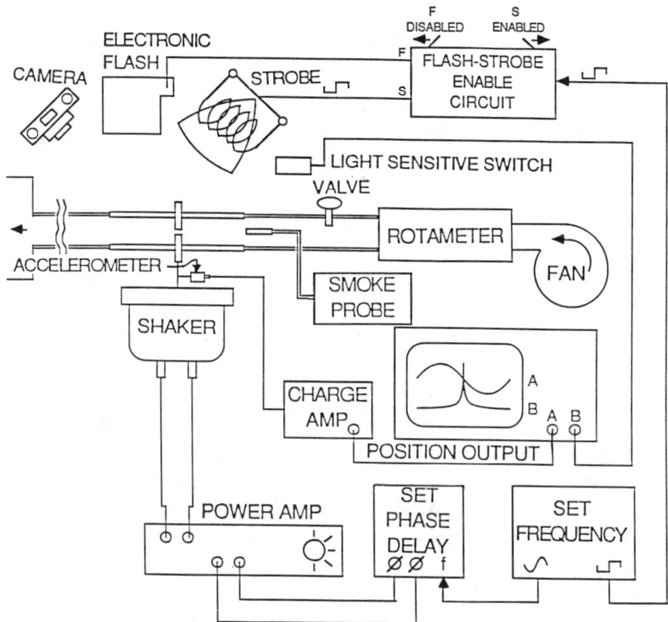

Fig. 3. Diagram of the dynamic flow visualization setup.

The flow visualization done for the static case was quite limited in scope, and will be covered only briefly. When the flow was visualized by inserting the smoke probe upstream of the glottis in the static setup, a jet was visible downstream of the vocal folds. Two principal observations were made concerning this jet. First, an off-center glottis caused the jet to veer towards the tract wall that was closer to the glottis. Second, when the "false folds" were inserted supraglottally, the jet straightened out, that is, the jet axis became parallel to the tract walls even for an off-center glottis.

PART 2: DYNAMIC BEHAVIOUR OF THE MODEL: FLOW VISUALIZATION

Method

The dynamic system (shown in Figure 3) is designed to answer the question, how does steady flow behave when it is interrupted periodically? Thus the setup is similar to that for the static experiments, but with one fold driven in simple harmonic motion by a mechanical shaker to which it is attached. The frequency and voltage selected on the two-phase oscillator that drives the shaker determine the frequency and amplitude of the vocal fold motion.

Only one fold could be moved in this mechanical design. In essence, the result is a model of a larynx with one paralysed vocal fold, with the important difference that pathological condition often results in incomplete glottal closure. Our model was capable of a completely closed glottis; in all diagrams shown here, that was the zero-phase condition.

A strobe, used to illuminate the model, was triggered by the same sinusoidal signal that controlled the shaker. A two-phase oscillator allowed control of the phase difference between the strobe and shaker. Photographs were taken by using an electronic flash triggered by the same strobe trigger signal, so that the film was exposed only during the time it took the flash to fire once. Thus the pictures did not incorporate any averaging, a technique which proved to give superior results. However, as a result the filming was done "blind", which resulted in a high wastage rate. Therefore at least three pictures were taken at each condition and phase angle.

The camera used was a Minolta SR-101T, a 35 mm single-lens-reflex. In order to achieve sufficient detail on the shots, a 13 mm extension tube was used with a 55 mm lens and haze filter. The camera was mounted on a tripod and operated by use of a shutter-release cable in order to mechanically isolate it from the rest of the heavily-vibrating system. Black and white Ilford HP5 film with film speed of 400 ASA was used exclusively.

The exact phase angle was determined by positioning a photodetector under the strobe lamp and mounting an accelerometer on the shaker, and comparing their outputs on an oscilloscope. Since the accelerometer was calibrated, the scope trace was also used to determine the peak-to-peak amplitude (i.e. the maximum vocal fold excursion distance) of the vocal fold motion. For the pictures shown here, the peak-to-peak amplitude was always 3 mm. The "mouth" of the tract exited into a 10 cm diameter flexible hose, which carried the acrid smoke away from the experimenter. In order to alter the supraglottal acoustic impedance, a long tube was attached between the tract and exit hose. This impedance tube was circular in cross-section, with an inner diameter of 2.8 cm, made of rigid PVC. Since the area of tract (2.6 cm^2) and impedance tube (6.2 cm^2) were of the same order of magnitude, and that of the exit hose (78.5 cm^2) was 10 times bigger, acoustically the exit hose was approximately like exiting into free space. The impedance tubes were designed to be one-quarter wavelength at the fundamental frequency so that a large acoustic impedance would be presented to the glottis of the model. Due to variation in the various interconnections, the final lengths from glottis to exit hose were approximately correct: for F0 = 80 Hz, the length with tube was 110 cm; for 100 Hz, the length with tube was 90 cm. The first formant frequencies were calculated to be 81 and 100 Hz respectively. The magnitude of the impedance was thus near, if not precisely at, its maximum value.

Results

Figure 4 is a diagram of the flow in the region downstream of the vocal folds. The figure, which captures essential details of the photographs, shows a sequence of phase angles for a fundamental frequency (F0) of 100 Hz, flow speed (*U*) of 350 cc/s, and two lengths of supraglottal tract, 19.5 and 90 cm. All possible combinations of two values of F0 (80, 100 Hz), of *U* (200, 350 cm^3/sec), and of tract length (19.5 cm, and the quarter-wavelength at the F0 value used) were photographed.

The most obvious feature shown by the figure is the development of the jet during a glottal cycle. In most cases, nothing can be seen at 45° or 90°. Here, for the without-load case (19.5 cm tract), a small jet appears perpendicular to the glottis at 135°. At successive phase angles the jet lengthens and widens, mixing with the surrounding air until the plume loses definition. The timing of the jet appearance is quite asymmetric with respect to the glottal area. Not only is the same pattern not observed for the same open area A_g at different phases (which is not surprising), but evidence of any jet activity at all is largely restricted to the latter half of the cycle. It is interesting to note, however, that the phase

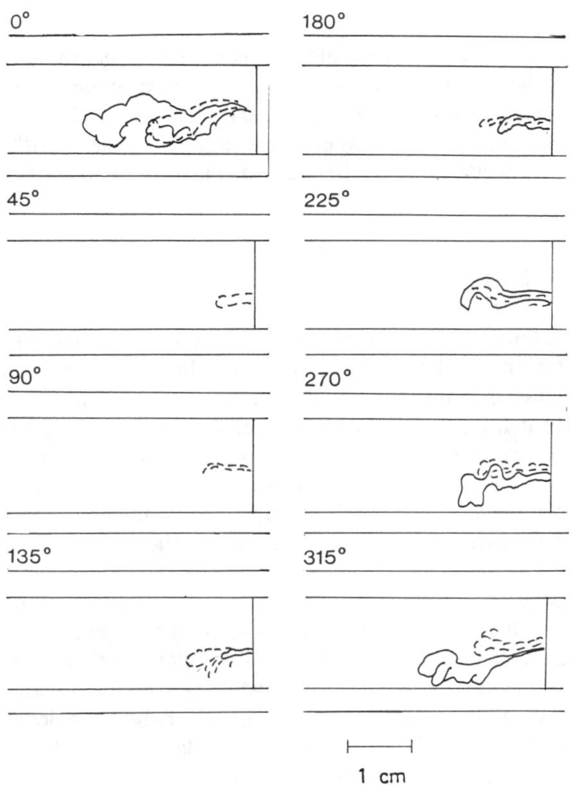

Fig. 4. Flow patterns shown diagrammatically in region downstream of vocal folds. Air flows from right to left. 0° is closed, 180° is maximum open. Solid lines are without impedance tube, dashed lines are with tube. F0 = 100 Hz, U = 350 cm^3/sec.

angle at which the jet first appears shifts earlier by about 45° when the quarter-wavelength tube is in place.

Various differences, such as more vortices visible in the developed jet, can be observed when comparing the cases with and without the quarter-wavelength tube in place, but for the most part they do not appear consistently enough or with a great enough magnitude to rule out the effect of variations due to the experimental method. It is worth noting, however, that when the jet is its maximum length, it generally tends towards the bottom rather than the top of the tract. Since the bottom shutter is the moving one, the center line of the glottis is effectively slightly below the center line of the tract. From the static flow visualization results, one would therefore predict that the jet would tend downwards; this prediction is borne out, even though in the dynamic case, the center line is constantly moving.

In order to compare all combinations of phase angle, U, F0, and acoustic load more easily, the total length of the jet visible in each photo was measured. Although it can be difficult to measure the ''edge'' of a smoke cloud, the results were reasonably consistent. First, the maximum length of the visible cloud occurred for the higher flow rate in the "without acoustic load" (i.e. tract length = 19.5 cm) cases, and the maximum length overall (3.4 cm) occurred when the higher F0 value was used, as well. These observations are as expected, since the jet is most visible against the background when it has mixed least with the surrounding air, and it will travel further while mixing if it is moving faster.

The difference between "with" and "without" acoustic load is not so easily predicted. For the without-load cases, visible jet length increases linearly with phase angle; for the with-load cases, the length increases for smaller phase angle, and then essentially levels off. Thus, even in this situation of forced excitation, where the oscillation of the "folds" is determined externally, the acoustic impedance of the tract affects the development of the jet significantly.

DISCUSSION

The quarter-wavelength tube is longer than the unaugmented tract tube, and hence the inertance of the supraglottal tract of the model should be increased. Increasing the inertance of the vocal tract has been shown in many simulations to increase the skewing of the glottal pulse, that is, to increase the delay between the glottal area function and the glottal volume velocity. The skewing does not increase linearly with the tract inertance, but it would predict that the air flows through the glottis later when the tract is longer (Fant, 1982). However, the situation is complicated when F0 is equal to the first tract resonance, since then previous glottal cycles can carry over, producing ripples in the glottal volume flow (Fant et al., 1985).

If we assume that the first appearance of the jet occurs when the volume flow has risen above some critical amplitude, then a shift of the first appearance of the jet earlier in the glottal cycle (as we observed) would indicate a skewing of the glottal volume flow earlier in the cycle (the opposite of the prediction). Clearly it would be useful to measure the particle velocity and sound pressure just downstream of the glottis, rather than deducing them from essentially qualitative data. But it is also possible that data measured at the glottis of a mechanical model may not directly correspond to simulated glottal flow variables; there may be an aerodynamic equivalent to the acoustic near- and far-field concepts.

Such a concept was outlined by Chapman and Glendinning (1990) in their theoretical analysis of a compressed-air loudspeaker, which was similar geometrically to the model discussed above but was used at sonic flow rates. They first derived a nonlinear pressure-velocity relationship at the glottis using the mean glottal area, and then by allowing the pressure, velocity and area to be time-varying, they arrived at a linear relationship for pressure and velocity in the duct. They noted that the linear solution is unlikely to apply within the mixing region near the glottis due to the nonuniformity of the flow there, but the values at the radiating "lip" end were confirmed experimentally (Glendinning et al., 1990).

In the model studied here, flows are subsonic. Preliminary derivations indicate that a similar method of solution will work, but the solution will be more complex. It is definitely of interest to us to determine the farthest-upstream point in the tract at which the acoustic solution is valid. Work is underway to make the detailed tract measurements necessary to establish this, but it seems likely to be of the same order as the distance over which the jet was distinctly visible in the flow visualization.

CONCLUSION

In conclusion, the vocal-tract and vocal-fold model described here, although lacking the tapering found in the real vocal tract, was shown to have static pressure-flow characteristics comparable to more realistic static models. The simpler shape made both static and dynamic flow visualization possible; we thus have a new tool for investigating the role of aerodynamic forces at the glottis. The dynamic flow visualization showed principally that there is a steady progression of jet formation and dispersion, confined largely to the latter half of the glottal cycle. Further, this progression occurs earlier in the cycle when F0 is approximately equal to the first resonance frequency of the tract. Finally, the region over which the jet was observed provides an initial estimate of the limit of validity of the theoretical solution.

ACKNOWLEDGMENTS

We would like to acknowledge P.J. Ashford, for his work in the initial stages of the project and his static flow data. We would also like to thank S.J. Elliott, P.A. Nelson, J. Gauffin, J. Liljencrants, G. Fant and Q-G. Lin for helpful discussions. This work was supported in part by the North Atlantic Treaty Organization under a Grant, and by the Acoustical Society of America under the Hunt Fellowship, both awarded in 1984 to C. Shadle, and by the Science and Engineering Research Council and IBM UK Scientific Centre under a CASE award.

REFERENCES

Baer, T. (1981). Observation of vocal fold vibration: measurement of excised larynges. In *Vocal Fold Physiology*, edited by K.N. Stevens and M. Hirano, pp. 119-135. Univ. Tokyo Press, Tokyo.

van den Berg, Jw. , Zantema, J.T., and Doornenbal, P. (1957). On the air resistance and the Bernoulli effect of the human larynx. *J. Acoust. Soc. Am.*, 29:626-631.

Binh, N. and Gauffin, J. (1983). Aerodynamic measurements in an enlarged static laryngeal model. *STL-QPSR* 2-3:36-60 (Dept. of Speech Communication and Music Acoustics, Royal Institute of Technology, Stockholm).

Chapman, C.J. and Glendinning, A.G. (1990). A Theoretical Analysis of a Compressed Air Loudspeaker. *J. Sound Vib.*, 138:493-500

Fant, G. (1982). Preliminaries to analysis of the human voice source. *STL-QPSR* 4:1-27 (Dept. of Speech Communication and Music Acoustics, Royal Institute of Technology, Stockholm).

Fant, G., Lin, Q.-G., and Gobl, C. (1985). Notes on glottal flow interaction. *STL-QPSR* 2-3:21-45 (Dept. of Speech Communication and Music Acoustics, Royal Institute of Technology, Stockholm).

Glendinning, A.G., Nelson, P.A., and Elliott, S.J. (1990). Experiments on a Compressed Air Loudspeaker. *J. Sound Vib.*, 138:479-492.

Ishizaka, K. and Flanagan, J. (1972). Synthesis of voiced sounds from a two-mass model of the vocal cords. *Bell Syst. Tech. J.*, 51:1233-1268.

Ishizaka, K. and Matsudaira, M. (1972). Fluid mechanical considerations of vocal cord vibration. *SCRL Monograph* No. 8, April.

Scherer, R.C. (1981). *Laryngeal fluid mechanics: Steady flow considerations using static models.* Ph.D. thesis, University of Iowa, Iowa City, IA.

Scherer, R.C., Titze, I.R., and Curtis, J.F. (1983). Pressure-flow relationships in two models of the larynx having rectangular glottal shapes. *J. Acoust. Soc. Am.*, 73:668-676.

Shadle, C.H., Elliott, S.J., and Nelson, P.A. (1987.) Visualization of the air flowing through a dynamic model of the vocal folds. *ISVR Technical Report* 154, (University of Southampton).

Titze, I.R. and Talkin, D.T. (1979). A theoretical study of the effects of various laryngeal configurations on the acoustics of phonation. *J. Acoust. Soc. Am.*, 66:60-74.

Wegel, R.L. (1930). Theory of vibration of the larynx. *Bell Syst. Tech. J.*, 9:207-227.

11

Generalized Translaryngeal Pressure Coefficient for a Wide Range of Laryngeal Configurations

Ronald C. Scherer and *Chwen-Geng Guo

*The Wendell Johnson Speech and Hearing Center, The University of Iowa, Iowa City, Iowa 52242, USA, *The Recording and Research Center, The Denver Center for the Performing Arts, 1245 Champa Street, Denver, Colorado 80204, USA*

The quality of voiced speech is dependent upon the volume velocity signal produced at the exit of the larynx. The pressure drop across the larynx drives air through the glottis, and is therefore a primary aspect of the creation of the volume velocity signal and laryngeal mechanics in general. A sufficiently complete description of translaryngeal pressure-flow information is necessary for both modelling and an adequate understanding of laryngeal function.

The configuration of the glottis continuously changes during phonation (e.g., Hirano, 1977). The glottis dynamically varies in the angle between the vocal folds, glottal shape, and diameter. The shape can change from a convergence during the first part of the glottal cycle when the airflow begins to pass through the glottis, to a divergence during glottal closure. Laryngeal flow resistance depends upon pressure loss created by viscosity, and should be especially sensitive to the closeness of the two vocal folds and to the angle of divergence.

A number of earlier reports have studied flow resistance within static larynx models (Wegel, 1930; van den Berg et al., 1957; Ishizaka & Matsudaira, 1972; Scherer, 1981; Gauffin et al., 1983; Scherer & Titze, 1982, 1983; Scherer, 1983; Scherer et al., 1983a, b; Gauffin & Liljencrants, 1988). The most complete modelling of laryngeal shape was performed by Binh and Gauffin (1983) who used a variety of convergence and divergence configurations. Their model, however, incorporated a quasi-stairstep change in glottal diameter from the inferior to superior glottal ends. In all steady flow modelling, as in the present study, the quasi-steady flow approximation to glottal flow has been adopted (Flanagan, 1958).

The translaryngeal pressure can be expressed as the translaryngeal pressure coefficient. This term is defined as the translaryngeal pressure drop divided by the dynamic pressure estimated at the minimal glottal cross sectional area. The dynamic pressure is defined as one-half times the density of air times the squared velocity of air flowing through the minimal glottal location. The velocity is usually taken as the volume flow divided by the cross sectional area. The importance of this term and other pressure drop terms throughout the larynx is reflected in many studies of modelled laryngeal

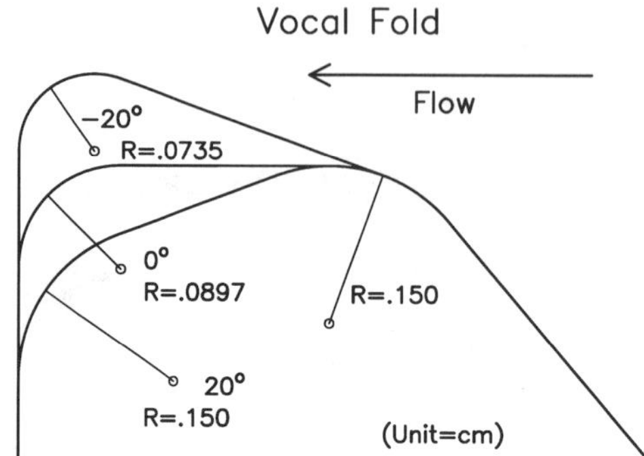

Fig. 1. Outline of the vocal fold shapes for half of -20 degree (glottal convergence), 0 degree (uniform glottis), and +20 degrees (glottal divergence). Distances are in cm corresponding to the life-size equivalent vocal folds

function (e.g., Ishizaka & Flanagan, 1972; Titze, 1973, 1974, 1986, 1988; Titze & Talkin, 1979; Ishizaka, 1981, 1985; Ananthapadmanabha & Fant, 1982; Ananthapadmanabha & Gauffin, 1985; Cranen & Boves, 1987; Guerin, 1985; Koizumi et al., 1987). The results from the present study should help make these types of models more realistic from the laryngeal aerodynamics point of view.

METHODS

The larynx models created for this project are collectively referred to as model M5. They were larger than normal (prototype) size by a factor of 7.5. This size was chosen in order to provide relatively small but measurable glottal diameters.

Model M5 consisted of a rectangular airway within which were placed sets of vocal fold pieces which were attached firmly to the model airway sides by screws. Each vocal fold was precisely milled by a digital mill. Typical shapes for one of the vocal folds in the model are shown in Figure 1. The prototype glottal thickness was 0.3 cm with glottal length of 1.2 cm. The vocal fold glottal surface was flat. The radius of curvature for the lower margin was 0.15 cm. The radii for the upper glottal margin were determined by the expression $R_u = R_o/(1\text{-}\sin[b/2])$, where R_u is the radius of the upper margin, R_o is the radius of the upper margin when the vocal folds form a uniform duct (0.0987 cm), and b is the included glottal angle which ranged between 40 degrees divergence to 40 degrees convergence. The authors believe that this specification created a realistic vocal fold contour.

Figure 2 is a schematic of the airway with vocal folds inside. The box, vocal fold pieces, and entry convergence upstream of the trachea were made out of plexiglas. The sections of the airway upstream and downstream of the vocal folds were both rectangular, with a lateral (prototype equivalent) width of 2 cm when the maximum glottal diameter (0.32 cm) was used, and an anterior-posterior dimension of 1.2 cm.

Pressure taps were located (an equivalent prototype length of) 0.16 cm upstream of the start of the vocal fold piece, and 3.1 cm downstream of the vocal folds. The translaryngeal pressure drop was measured by Validyne pressure transducers (Mp45, DP103). The airflow was created by suction downstream of the model. A pneumotach

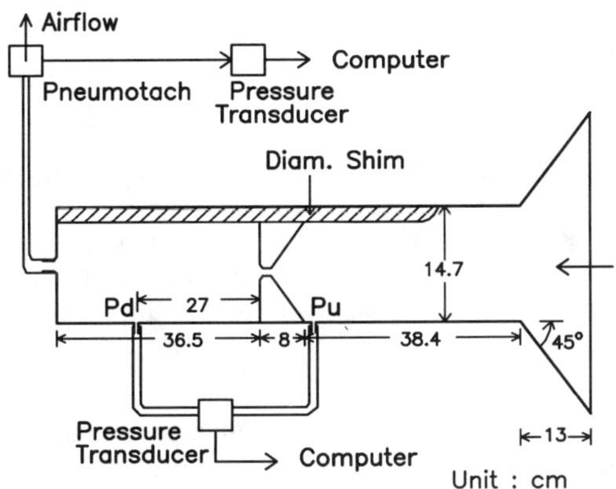

Fig. 2. Schematic of the experimental set-up

system (Hans Rudolph 3719, 4813) within the downstream section was used to measure the airflow.

After a chosen vocal fold configuration was set in the airway box, and the glottal diameter measured, a sequence of airflows was drawn through the box. For the 63 configuration cases (9 angles times 7 diameters), a total of 2295 pressure-flow values were obtained. Each pressure and flow measurement was recorded by computer interface. The inaccuracy of both pressure and flow measurement was a maximum of approximately ± 4% from all sources (multiple transducers, multiple calibration devices, and repeatability over time). Glottal diameter was directly measured with feeler gauges and separators, with a typical error of approximately 1.25%. The pressure coefficient had an error of approximately 5.5%, and Reynolds number (4 times flow divided by the perimeter times viscosity) of approximately 3.5% (Taylor, 1982).

RESULTS

The data in nondimensional form (pressure coefficient P^* versus Reynolds number Re) were graphed, and a curve of the form

$$P^* = \frac{A_1}{\mathrm{Re}} + A_2 \tag{1}$$

where A_1 and A_2 are coefficients, was fit to the data by eye such that the fit was best between 1 and 50 cm H_2O. The A_1 term corresponds to the laminar dependence at low flows and the A_2 term emphasizes the turbulent dependence at high flows. Values for the A_1 and A_2 coefficients were obtained for each of the 63 cases. The P^* equation can be converted into a quadratic equation (through the origin) relating dimensional pressure and flow values.

The pressure coefficient values are typically relatively very high for the smallest diameter. The highest range was found for the uniform glottis for a diameter of 0.00424 cm. The pressure coefficient ranged between approximately 150 to 4.6 between 1 and 100 cm H_2O, respectively. The accuracy of transducer function was verified for these high values. Much of the pressure coefficient value for small diameters (and especially for the uniform duct) comes most likely from the viscous loss within the glottis. It is also noted that the pressure coefficient tends to lie below 1.0 for larger diameters and larger pressures. This implies that near maximum glottal opening, modelled flow may reach higher values than previously estimated.

In Table 1 the pressure coefficient values are given for each of the approximate diameter values and at translaryngeal pressure values of 5, 10, and 15 cm H_2O. The pressure coefficient was averaged across all angles. The standard deviation values suggest the increasing range of the pressure coefficient values across angles as diameter decreases. For the smallest diameter, the indication of relatively high values again is suggested.

General Equation

The pressure coefficient equation (1) has coefficients A_1 and A_2 that are functions of angle and aspect ratio, where aspect ratio *(R_a)* is defined as the anterior-posterior glottal length divided by glottal diameter:

For A_1 the following equations were derived:

Case 1. If $R_a \leq 10^{10}$, then $A_1 = A_{11} - A_{12}\log R_a + A_{13}\log^2 R_a$ (2)

$$\text{where} \quad A_{11}, A_{12}, A_{13}, \begin{cases} \dfrac{C_1}{x^2 + C_2} + C_3 & x \leq 0 \\ \dfrac{C_4}{x^2 + C_5} + C_6 x + C_7 & x \geq 0 \end{cases} \tag{3}$$

and x is the angle in degrees, and the values of C_i are given by:

	C_1	C_2	C_3	C_4	C_5	C_6	C_7
A_{11}	11609.88	25.33	103.953	2155.70	7.143	3.32	260.506
A_{12}	2858.96	3.90	91.632	524.24	1.03	1.77	315.728
A_{13}	607.60	1.413	50.003	692.00	2.141	-0.806	156.797

$$\text{Case 2. If } R_a > 10^{10}, \text{ then} \begin{cases} A_1 = 5000 & \text{for } x < 0 \text{ (Convergent)} \\ A_1 = 15000 & \text{for } x \geq 0 \text{ (Divergent)} \end{cases} \tag{4}$$

For A_2 the following equations were derived:

Case 1. If $R_a \leq 1000$, then $A_2 = A_{21} - A_{22}\log R_a + A_{23}\log^2 R_a$ (4)

where $A_{21}, A_{22}, A_{23} = C_0 + C_1 x + C_2 x^2 + C_3 x^3 + C_4 x^4$, (5)

and x is the angle in degrees, and the values of C_i are given by:

	C_0	C_1	C_2	C_3	C_4
A21	0.786	0.00298	0.00130	-0.00000414	-0.000000693
A22	-0.333	0.0106	0.00189	-0.00000876	-0.000001041
A23	-0.151	0.00344	0.000638	-0.00000229	-0.000000362

Case 2. If $R_a > 1000$ then $A_2 = 0.7$

Table 1: *Pressure coefficient values at translaryngeal pressure values of 5, 10 and 15 cm H_2O averaged over the angles -40, -20, -10, -5, 0, 5, 10, 20, and 40 degrees.*

Diameter	5 cm H_2O		10 cm H_2O		15 cm H_2O	
cm	M	S.D.	M	S.D.	M	S.D.
0.32	1.03	0.0783	-	-	-	-
0.16	1.01	0.135	1.02	0.0716	-	-
0.08	1.05	0.135	0.984	0.775	0.985	0.065
0.04	1.05	0.146	0.961	0.123	0.948	0.110
0.02	1.30	0.424	1.20	0.309	1.15	0.264
0.01	2.89	4.10	1.98	2.06	1.71	1.45
0.005	11.7	25.6	6.54	13.0	4.49	8.48

Graphical examination of the general equation for diameters less than 0.005 cm (the smallest diameter empirically tested) showed smooth curves with reasonable extensions to small diameters. In the important range of 1 to 50 cm H_2O, the average difference of prediction from data was 6.98% (S.D. = 6.44%). The average percentage difference between data and prediction for all the data, ranging from approximately 0.01 cm H_2O to 390 cm H_2O, was 7.99% (S.D. = 8.00%).

DISCUSSION

The data and general equation indicate that the flow resistance for a uniform glottis at any specific diameter is relatively large compared to non-zero glottal angles. For small diameters, the difference beyond ± 10 degrees can be nearly an order of magnitude. It is reasonable to assume that for angles close to zero, viscosity takes on a relatively important role within the glottal duct and accounts for much of the flow resistance. As diameter decreases, results suggest that the relative difference between resistance for divergence and convergence at the same angles becomes more pronounced, with greater resistance for the diverging angle. This may be due to the relatively greater turbulence expected as the flow separates from the diverging sides of the glottis. Greater resistance for the diverging case for small diameters may also be due to greater viscous resistance at the minimal glottal diameter location because the radius of curvature for the entrance for diverging shapes is larger than the exit radius for converging shapes.

It is additionally noted with some interest that for diameters greater than about 0.01 cm, the resistance for converging glottal angles is slightly greater than for diverging angles of the same value (except near zero degrees). For example, for a diameter of 0.04 cm and angles of -10 and +10 degrees, the resistance for convergence is 7% greater than the resistance for divergence. We speculate for this case of 10 degrees and 0.04 cm diameter that the diameter is sufficiently small that flow separation does not take place (appreciably) on the glottal walls (Kline, 1959), creating a significant pressure recovery within the glottis. Furthermore, the flow at the exit of the convergence may create a vena contracta that accentuates pressure losses. These findings are in apparent opposition to those of Gauffin and Liljencrants (1988) and Binh and Gauffin (1983). Further comparison of data from this study to the findings of earlier studies will made in an expanded report.

CONCLUSION

The fluid mechanics of the larynx is an important aspect of a complete theory of phonation. The airflow through the glottis is dependent on the translaryngeal pressure and glottal configuration. This study of laryngeal pressure-flow relationships was motivated by the need for completeness in specifying these relationships.

This study examined the translaryngeal pressure-flow relationship within a model (M5) of the larynx. Steady flows were used within 63 configurations of the glottis (9 angles, 7 diameters).

The general equation obtained in this study holds for all data within the translaryngeal pressure range of 1 to 50 cm H_20 within approximately 7%. The general equation was modelled within the 40 degree convergence to 40 degree divergence range. The model results were extended to diameter values less than 0.005 cm (it is recognized that this extension needs to be validated).

The translaryngeal pressure coefficient can be used as a concise expression of the overall pressure-flow relationship across the glottis. The coefficient value is not constant. It can range below 1 and above 50. The value is relatively very high for a uniform glottal duct of small diameter.

The primary effect of using the variable pressure coefficient values found in this study instead of a constant value would be to increase the flow resistance near glottal closure as well as increase the peak flows near maximum glottal opening. These effects would potentially provide greater flow gradients during flow reduction before glottal closure. The acoustic and functional consequences need to be explored.

ACKNOWLEDGEMENTS

We would like to thank John Dyson and his staff of the Medical Instrument Shop of the University of Iowa for building the larynx models. We also thank Anita Kress for early programming and Deborah Garrison for manuscript typing. This study was supported by the National Institutes of Health, grant number R01-NS16320, and by the Bonfils Foundation.

REFERENCES

Ananthapadmanabha, T.V. and Fant, G. (1982). Calculation of the true glottal flow and its components. *STL-QPSR* 1:1-30. (Dept. of Speech Communication and Music Acoustics, Royal Institute of Technology, Stockholm).

Ananthapadmanabha, T.V. and Gauffin, J. (1985). Some results on the acoustic and aerodynamic factors in phonation. In: *Vocal Fold Physiology: Biomechanics, Acoustics and Phonatory Control*, edited by I.R. Titze and R.C. Scherer, pp. 402-413. The Denver Center for the Performing Arts, Denver.

Berg, J.W. van den, Zantema, J.T. and Doornenbal, P. Jr. (1957). On the air resistance and the Bernoulli effect of the human larynx. *J. Acoust. Soc. Am.* 29:626-631.

Binh, N. and Gauffin, J. (1983). Aerodynamic measurements in an enlarged static laryngeal model. *STL-QPSR* 2-3:36-60. (Dept. of Speech Communication and Music Acoustics, Royal Institute of Technology, Stockholm).

Cranen, B. and Boves, L. (1987). The acoustic impedance of the glottis - Modeling and measurements. In: *Laryngeal Function in Phonation and Respiration*, edited by T. Baer, C. Sasaki and K. Harris, pp. 203-218. Little, Brown and Company (Inc.), Boston.

Flanagan, J.L. (1958). Some properties of the glottal sound source. *J. Speech Hear. Res.* 1:99-116.

Gauffin, J., Binh, N., Ananthapadmanabha, T.V., and Fant, G. (1983). Glottal geometry and volume velocity waveform. In: *Vocal Fold Physiology: Contemporary Research and Clinical Issues*, edited by D.M. Bless and J.H. Abbs, pp. 194-201. College-Hill Press, San Diego

Gauffin, J. and Liljencrants, J. (1988). The role of convective acceleration in glottal aerodynamics. In: *Vocal Physiology: Voice Production, Mechanisms and Functions*, edited by O. Fujimura. Raven Press, New York.

Guerin, B. (1985). Effects of the source-tract interaction using vocal fold models. In: *Vocal Fold Physiology: Biomechanics, Acoustics and Phonatory Control*, edited by I.R. Titze and R.C. Scherer, pp. 482-499. The Denver Center for the Performing Arts, Denver.

Hirano, M. (1977). Structure and vibratory behavior of the vocal folds. In: *Dynamic Aspects of Speech Production*, edited by M. Sawashima, & F. S. Cooper., pp. 13-27. University of Tokyo Press, Tokyo.

Ishizaka, K. (1981). Equivalent lumped-mass models of vocal fold vibration. In: *Vocal Fold Physiology*, edited by K.N. Stevens and M. Hirano, pp. 231-241. University of Tokyo Press, Tokyo.

Ishizaka, K. (1985). Air resistance and intraglottal pressure in a model of the larynx. In: *Vocal Fold Physiology: Biomechanics, Acoustics and Phonatory Control*, edited by I.R. Titze and R.C. Scherer, pp. 414-424. The Denver Center for the Performing Arts, Denver.

Ishizaka, K. and Flanagan, J.L. (1972). Synthesis of voiced sounds from a two mass model of the vocal cords. *Bell Sys. Tech. J.* 51:1233-1268.

Ishizaka, K. and Matsudaira, M. (1972). Fluid Mechanical Considerations of Vocal Cord Vibration. *SCRL Monograph* No. 8. (Speech Communications Research Laboratory, Inc., Santa Barbara).

Kline, S.J. (1959). On the nature of stall. *J. Basic Eng.*, Trans. Am. Soc. Mec. Eng.. 81:305-320.

Koizumi, T., Taniguchi, S., and Hiromitsu, S. (1987). Two-mass model of the vocal cords for natural sounding voice synthesis. *J. Acoust. Soc. Am.* 82:1179-1192.

Scherer, R.C. (1981). *Laryngeal Fluid Mechanics: Steady Flow Considerations Using Static Models.* Ph.D. Thesis. The University of Iowa, Iowa City.

Scherer, R.C. (1983). Pressure-flow relationships in a laryngeal airway model having a diverging glottal duct. *J. Acoust. Soc. Am.* 73(S1):S46(A).

Scherer, R.C. and Titze, I.R. (1982). A new look at van den Berg's glottal aerodynamics. In: *Transcripts of the Tenth Symposium: Care of the Professional Voice*, edited by V. Lawrence, pp. 74-81. The Voice Foundation, New York.

Scherer, R.C. and Titze, I.R. (1983). Pressure-flow relationships in a model of the laryngeal airway with a diverging glottis. In: *Vocal Fold Physiology: Contemporary Research and Clinical Issues*, edited by D.M. Bless and J.H. Abbs, pp. 179-193. College-Hill Press, San Diego.

Scherer, R.C., Titze, I.R. and Curtis, J.F. (1983a). Pressure-flow relationships in two models of the larynx having rectangular glottal shapes. *J. Acoust. Soc. Am.* 73:668-676.

Scherer, R.C., Titze, I.R., Linville, R., Hueffner, D., and Shaw, K. (1983b). The effects of vocal fold growths on pressure-flow relationships in the larynx. In: *Transcripts of the Eleventh Symposium: Care of the Professional Voice*, edited by V. Lawrence, pp. 25-36. The Voice Foundation, New York.

Taylor, J.R. (1982). *An Introduction to Error Analysis.* University Science Books, Mill Valley, California.

Titze, I.R. (1973). The human vocal cords: A mathematical model. Part 1. *Phonetica* 28:129-170.

Titze, I.R. (1974). The human vocal cords: A mathematical model.Part II. *Phonetica* 29:1-21.

Titze, I.R. (1986). Mean intraglottal pressure in vocal fold oscillation. *J. Phonetics* 14:359-364.

Titze, I.R. (1988). The physics of small-amplitude oscillation of the vocal folds. *J. Acoust. Soc. Am.* 83:1536-1552.

Titze, I.R. and Talkin, D.T. (1979). A theoretical study of the effects of various laryngeal configurations on the acoustics of phonation. *J. Acoust. Soc. Am.* 66:60-74.

Wegel, R.L. (1930). Theory of vibration of the larynx. *Bell Sys. Tech. J.* 9:207-227.

12

Effects of Downstream Occlusions on Pressures Near the Glottis in Singing

Donald G. Miller and *Harm K. Schutte

*School of Music, Syracuse University, Syracuse New York, USA and *Voice Research Lab., University of Groningen, University Hospital Groningen, The Netherlands.*

In this paper we shall attempt to take a close look at some details of vocal fold oscillatory movements on the basis of measurements of vocal fold contact area and air pressures immediately above and below the glottis. These details occur within the larger cyclical movement of the vocal folds, which can be roughly represented by a triangular waveform. In Figure 1 we have given a few examples of such a waveform representing the movement of a single vocal fold (the other vocal fold describes a symmetrical movement) with respect to the midline of the glottis. In very breathy voice (Figure 1a) our vocal fold can oscillate without reaching the midline, while in tight voice (Figure 1b) the open phase, in which the vocal fold moves away from and towards the midline, may only be a fraction of the whole cycle. Intermediate adjustments are, of course, also possible. In the case of tight voice we give a revised waveform (Figure 1c), reflecting the greater movement of the vocal fold during the "free" open phase and its more restricted movement in the closed phase, which is represented here as a negative displacement. This movement in the closed phase, which probably includes a vertical component, results from the momentum acquired by the vocal fold in the closing phase, and it is opposed by elastic forces, which then reverse the movement, restoring the mass of the vocal fold to a position where the next open phase can begin.

Adjustments in this vocal fold cycle will play a large role in the search for improved or optimal phonation, and it is well to consider what adjustments are at the speaker's or singer's disposal. Although adjustments *within* the glottal cycle are not possible, the speaker/singer can make voluntary, if not always conscious, adjustments in four basic factors: subglottal pressure (P_{sub}), vocal fold adduction/stiffness, fundamental frequency (F0), and, by means of vocal tract articulations, the acoustic impedance of the vocal tract. The first two of these factors have a high degree of interdependence (in order to create high P_{sub}, one must restrict flow at the glottis), but a skilled singer can learn to vary them with a certain limited degree of independence (Rubin et al., 1967). The acoustic impedance of the vocal tract, which we shall consider below in detail, has a less direct, but still important, effect on vocal fold motion. Note, however, that these "voluntary" adjustments are far from being entirely free. The desired phonation intensity, generally regulated by a combined adjustment of P_{sub} and vocal fold adduction/stiffness, is often imposed by external circumstances. F0 is limited by the physical nature of the given voice, social/aes-

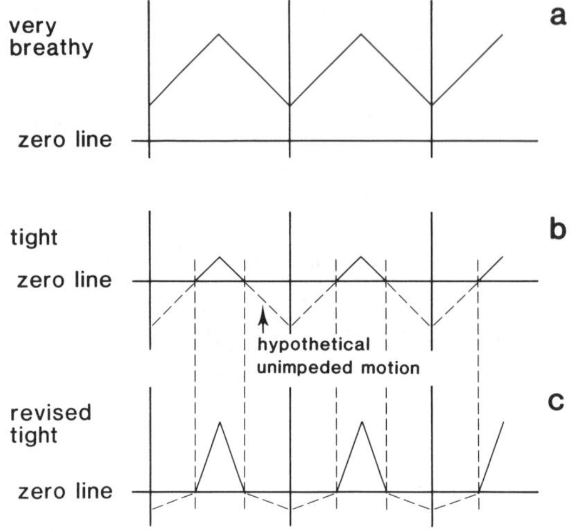

Fig. 1. Representation of oscillatory motion of a vocal fold. In very breathy voice (**a**) the adducted vocal fold does not reach the midline. In tight voice (**b**) the greater part of the cycle occurs in the closed phase. In (**c**) the tight-voice pattern is adjusted to reflect freer movement of the vocal fold in the open phase.

thetic considerations, and, in singing, precisely by prescription of the composer. The conventions of language determine, to a large extent, the articulation, and thus the acoustic impedance of the vocal tract.

The movement of the vocal folds in the closed phase is only a damped continuation of that generated in the open phase; the open phase, however, has a number of indeterminate features, including the speed and excursion of the vocal folds as well as the abruptness and precise timing of closing and opening, all of which can have important effects on the sound produced. These features are determined in part by the aerodynamic driving pressure in the open glottis, which is also the source of energy for vocal fold oscillation. This pressure (P_g) is given, according to Titze (1988), by the equation:

$$P_g = P_{supra} + (P_{sub} - P_{supra})(1 - \frac{a_2}{a_1}) \qquad (1)$$

where P_{supra} is the input pressure to the vocal tract, P_{sub} is the subglottal pressure, a_1 is the glottal entry area and a_2 is the glottal exit area (see Figure 2). Thus the term P_{sub} - P_{supra} is the transglottal pressure (P_{trans}) and a_2/a_1 is the glottal convergence ratio. As Titze (1985) explains, this ratio has a value of zero at the moment of opening and rises to >1 at closing, which explains why P_{trans} is effective in driving the vocal folds apart in the opening phase, but not in the closing phase, in spite of its typically high value at the moment of closing.

We can imagine, theoretically, a favorable configuration of pressures to drive the vocal folds, which would entail not only a continuing oscillation of adequate amplitude, but also, in the case of singing, the timing of the moments of opening and closing to drive the desired acoustic standing wave in the vocal tract. The complexity of this task becomes evident when we consider that the time-varying P_g is a function of covariation of (prescribed) F0, as well as (modifiable) P_{sub} and P_{supra}, pressures whose variations in time are functions of sub- and supraglottal formants, respectively. Since the subglottal formants are fixed, modification of supraglottal formants, particularly F1, offers the best means of controlling P_g.

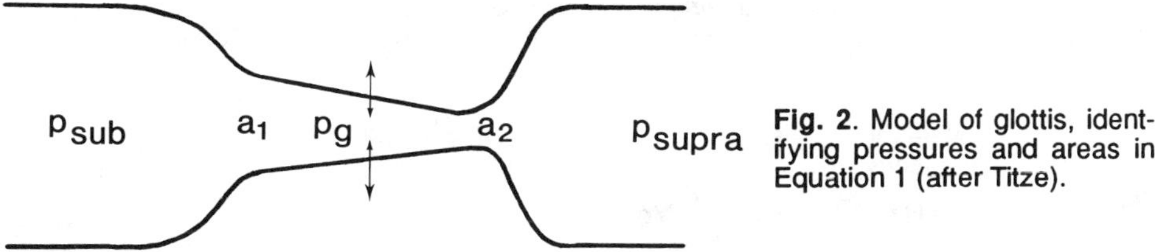

Fig. 2. Model of glottis, identifying pressures and areas in Equation 1 (after Titze).

METHOD

Our intention is to measure at certain points in the glottal cycle the changing pressures in Equation 1, and to consider what effects these may have on the oscillatory movement of the vocal folds. Pressures are measured by wide-band miniature pressure transducers on a catheter introduced through the nose and inserted through the glottis (Miller and Schutte, 1984), allowing direct measurement of the relevant pressures in our equation. Since we have no means of measuring the glottal entry and exit areas, a_1 and a_2, there can be no question of calculating a continuous numerical value for P_g, but from what is understood about vocal fold movement, we can presume that the glottal convergence factor, a_2/a_1, will be zero just before the upper edges of the vocal folds start to separate, after which it will rise to 1.0 at some point in the open phase, thus eliminating, at the closing of the glottis, P_{trans} as a positive component of the glottal driving pressure P_g. Because of this the moments of opening and closing provide the best opportunity of calculating P_g, following Equation 1.

Monitoring the changes in vocal fold oscillation as aerodynamic driving pressure varies is done by the electroglottograph (EGG), type Laryngograph. The shape and relative amplitude of the EGG-signal, and especially the details of the slopes around the points of closing and opening, allow us to make inferences about vocal fold vibratory behaviour. Rothenberg (1988) has given an example of such inferences in his study of detuning the soprano (falsetto) voice, while the present study deals with chest register only. Because they clearly and thoroughly reorganize the composite factors that govern the supraglottal pressure, we have chosen to examine voiced stops in vowel context. In order to facilitate comparison, all the examples we present here, which we consider representative of the phenomenon under discussion, are produced, in singing, by a single bass-baritone male singer in his normal, fairly "tight" (closed quotient ca. 2/3) chest register. The vowel is always /i/, and F0 ranges between medium and medium-high (given precisely in our examples). The occlusions are the bilabial /b/ and a "finger trill" produced by placing the index finger along the opening between the lips and moving it vertically, yielding a stop, designated in this paper by /b'/, alternating with a vowel at the rate of about 10 Hz, which is rapid enough to preclude voluntary adjustments of the vocal folds or vocal tract. The phonations considered consist of two ascending scales, one (/bibi/) with each successive note articulated by a single stop, and the other, also on the vowel /i/, with a continuous "finger trill", thus designated as /b'ib'i/.

Table 1. *Fundamental frequencies and pressures measured from the signals in Figures 3 to 6. Pressures at opening point are marked O and at closing point C, in Figures 3 to 6.*

	Fundamental frequency F0 Hz			Pressure at opening point H_2O						Pressure at closing point	
				Vowel			Occlusion			Vowel	Occlusion
	Before b/b'	During b/b'	After b/b'	P_{supra}	P_{trans}	P_g $=P_{sub}$	P_{supra}	P_{trans}	P_g $=P_{sub}$	$P_g = P_{supra}$	
/ibi/ mid	225	185	215	6	20	26	-3	32	29	-1	11
/ib'i/ mid	202	181	202	7	21	28	1	29	30	-2	10
/ibi/ high	300	272	307	5	38	43	1	41	42	-2	6
/ib'i/ high	307	270	307	12	41	53	-1	55	54	-9	9

RESULTS

From these two scales come the moments shown in Figures 3 to 6, each displaying a voiced occlusion and its vowel context. In all of them, the change from vowel to occlusion, which is accomplished within a few cycles, is characterized by a phase shift in P_{supra}: during the vowel, P_{supra} is very near a minimum at the closing point; during the occlusion it is close to a maximum. This phase shift results in a marked reduction in peak P_{trans} as well as an increase in P_{trans} at the point of opening. Further general effects of the occlusion are a small increase in average P_{supra} and a reduction in the peak-to-peak amplitude of the EGG signal.

In Table 1 we have assembled, along with F0 data, measurements of pressures at representative points of opening and closing in the four examples (marked O and C, respectively, in Figures 3 to 6). We have also calculated the driving pressure on the vocal folds, P_g, by applying Equation 1 in a simplified form by letting the glottal convergence factor, a_2/a_1, equal zero at opening and 1.0 at closing.

The evidence of change in vocal fold movement during occlusion will be found in the EGG curves, where each of the occlusion types has its characteristic pattern. The /b/ is the longer occlusion, having a superimposed low-frequency fall (not shown) and rise in the EGG curve, reflecting the movement of the larynx in executing the maneuver. Within the occlusion the closing slope is shorter and less steep, and the peak-to-peak amplitude is noticeably diminished, since the vocal fold contact area begins to fall just after the closing point. In the shorter /b'/ of the finger trill, the effects are similar, but less pronounced.

In both occlusions there may also be a marginally higher open quotient, but the evidence for it is not conclusive.

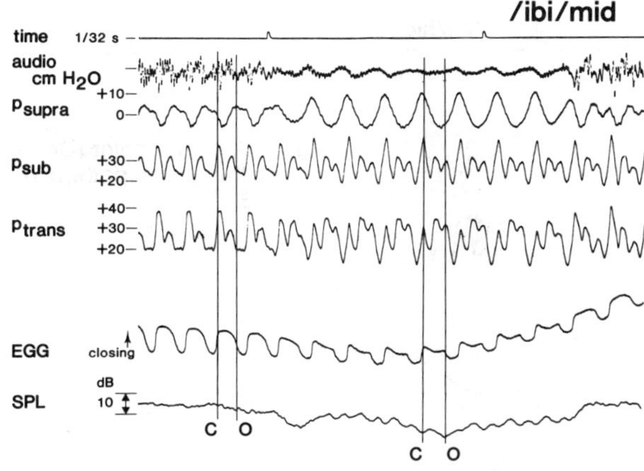

Fig. 3. The transient /b/ in the context of the stable vowel /i/ in ascending scale (here at the transition A3 to B3-flat). The signals, in descending order, are from a microphone 30 cm in front of the subject, supraglottal and subglottal pressures from transducers on a transglottal catheter, transglottal pressure (Psub - Psupra), vocal fold contact area (EGG), with greater contact showing a positive value, and sound pressure level, derived from the microphone signal. Characteristic points of closing, C, and opening, O, are identified and connected by drawn vertical lines.

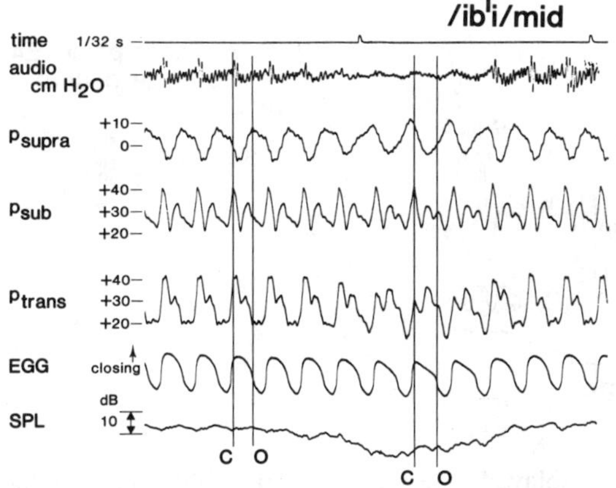

Fig. 4. The transient occlusion (/b'/) in the context of the stable vowel /i/ in an ascending scale with "finger trill" (here at the point A3-flat); signals as in Figure 3.

DISCUSSION

Vowel versus occlusion

Both the weakened closing slope and the diminished vocal fold contact area in the closed phase of the /b/, as compared to the /i/, are consistent with the high positive P_{supra} at closing in the occlusion. In the vowel the (normally) negative and falling P_{supra} help to propel the vocal folds together, and their "overshoot" results in increased contact after the closing point. The braking effect of the positive P_{supra} at or near closing (consistently ca. 10 cm H_2O in these four cases in spite of considerable differences in average P_{sub}) hinders this overshoot.

The relative prominence in the EGG curve of the opening moment during occlusion is probably not the result of altered P_g (this does not differ much from the opening in the vowel, although its P_{trans} component is greater), but is due to the fact that the opening occurs in the context of diminished, and apparently rising, vocal fold contact area in the closed phase.

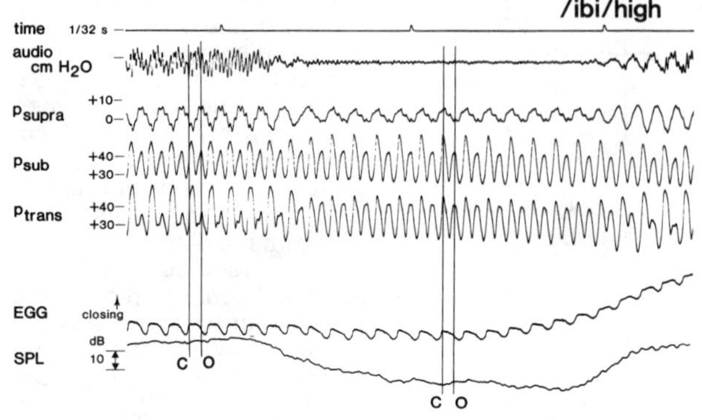

Fig. 5. A higher point (D4 to E4) in the scale pattern of Figure 3.

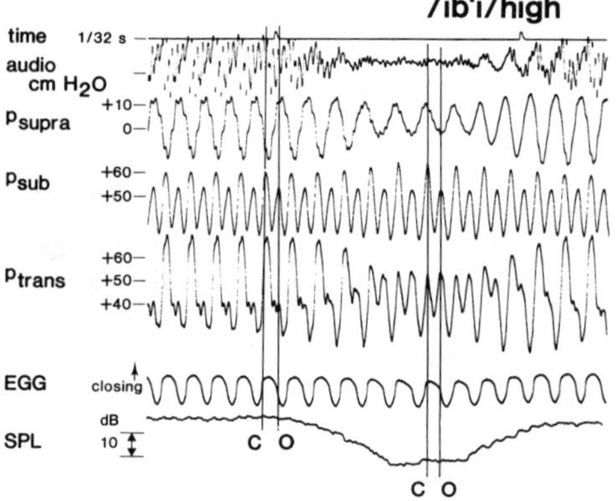

Fig. 6. A higher point (E4-flat) in the scale pattern of Figure 4.

High versus mid

The frequencies of the phonations displayed here were chosen to illustrate how the first formants of both supra- and subglottal vocal tracts (F1 and F'1, respectively) interact with F0. In the examples of lower F0, F1 of the vowel is substantially higher than F0, and the lowering of F1 in the occlusion brings improved tuning of the vocal tract with respect to F0, as evidenced in the increased amplitude of the P_{supra} wave. In the examples of higher F0, on the other hand, F1 is tuned to F0 during the vowel and detuned in the occlusion.

The interaction of F0 with the fixed *subglottal* first formant shows an interesting feature: during the occlusion the opening point occurs close to a peak in the P_{sub} waveform, either the second or third peak in the examples shown. This means that F0 during the occlusion, which is musically not prescribed, falls in the case of the lower /b/, from 225 Hz during the vowel to 185 Hz in the /b/, so that the opening can occur on the third P_{sub} peak. Two tones higher up the scale (not shown here) it rises from 249 Hz during the vowel to 277 Hz during the /b/, so that the opening can fall on the second peak. The point of this appears to be to produce an adequate P_{trans} component in the vocal fold driving force on opening. This condition does not apply to the opening moment in the vowel, which can happen at or near minimal P_{trans}, as in both of our lower examples here.

/bibi/ versus finger trill

As F0 increases, the peak-to-peak amplitude of the EGG waveform decreases during the occlusion for the /bibi/, but not the /b'ib'i/ (finger trill) phonation.

The high arch of the EGG waveform of the latter in the closed phase indicates, as we interpret it, larger, and/or freer, movement of the vocal folds. The larger "overshoot" in the EGG could result from higher momentum of the vocal folds in the closing phase and/or smaller vocal fold adduction, leaving more room for movement in the closed phase. This appears to confirm Titze's prediction, that a favorable pattern of P_g would make reduced vocal fold adduction both possible and desirable (Titze, 1985).

Voices with relatively high closed quotients are not infrequent among singers, especially males. They face a problem, particularly in the upper part of the range, in the basic adjustments of P_{sub} and vocal fold adduction/stiffness: if vocal fold adduction is increased to restrain flow when P_{sub} is high, then P_{sub} must in turn be increased to move the vocal folds, making still greater adduction necessary, etc. This can result in reduced vocal fold movement, such as we find here in the upper range of the /bibi/ scale. The rapidly recurring downstream occlusions of the finger trill, while only producing a minimal rise in mean P_{supra}, give a reactive backpressure that apparently relieves the adductive burden of the vocal folds in restraining high P_{sub}. The effect of this backpressure bears comparison with that of F1=F0 tuning in falsetto, where the flow in the open phase is restrained by considerably higher P_{supra} than is evident here in chest register (Schutte and Miller, 1986). In the present case the result of this backpressure is a vowel with a higher F1 peak-to-peak amplitude (25 cm H_2O for P_{supra} in Figure 6 versus 18 cm H_2O in Figure 5), produced by an apparently larger vocal fold oscillation in spite of a higher (by ca. 20%) P_{sub}, and having a more favorable vocal fold driving pressure at the closing (-9 cm H_2O versus -2).

CONCLUSIONS

The evident changes in the vocal fold vibratory pattern, induced by vocal tract loading from a downstream occlusion, point to the importance of using an interactive model of the voice, as both Titze and Rothenberg have done, when considering singing. The covariation of sub- and supraglottal formants, as well as fundamental frequency, however, is quite complex, and we should not be surprised to find considerable variation in the way these coalesce in actual voices, as opposed to models. In particular it should be noted that our examples are specific to chest register, where the pattern of interaction between vocal fold motion and vocal tract pressures differs substantially from that of falsetto.

A second conclusion is that favorable vocal tract loading appears to produce a larger vibratory movement, allowing reduced adduction of the vocal folds, as predicted by Titze. The experiment also indicates that this factor may be of importance in relieving the excessive adduction of a "tight" chest voice in singing, and perhaps in speaking as well.

ACKNOWLEDGEMENTS

This work was (partially) supported by the Foundation for Linguistic Research, which is funded by the Netherlands Organization for Scientific Research (NWO); by the National Institutes of Health research grant NS 08919 to Syracuse University, and the assistance of the College of Visual and Performing Arts, Syracuse University, Syracuse New York USA. The authors appreciate the assistance of Frouke Wildeboer, Franka Steenhuis, and, last but not least, Meindert Goslinga in preparation of the manuscript and figures.

REFERENCES

Miller, D.G. and Schutte, H.K. (1984). Characteristic patterns of sub- and supraglottal pressure variations within the glottal cycle. In: *Transcr XIIIth Symp Care Prof Voice*, edited by Van L. Lawrence, pp. 70-75. The Voice Foundation, New York.

Rothenberg, M. (1988). Acoustic reinforcement of vocal fold vibratory behavior in singing. In: *Vocal Physiology: Voice Production, Mechanisms and Functions*, edited by O. Fujimura, pp. 379-389. Raven Press Ltd, New York.

Rubin, H.J., LeCover, C.M., and Vennard, W. (1967). Vocal Intensity, Subglottic Pressure and Air Flow Relationships in Singers. *Folia Phoniatr*. 19:393-413.

Schutte, H.K. and Miller, D.G. (1986). The effect of F0/F1 coincidence in soprano high notes on pressure at the glottis. *J. Phonetics*. 14:385-392.

Titze, I. (1985). The importance of vocal tract loading in maintaining vocal fold oscillation. In: *Proc. Stockholm Music Acoustics Conf.*, edited by A. Askenfelt, S. Felicetti, E. Jansson, and J. Sundberg, pp 61-72. Royal Swedish Acad. Music, No 46, Vol I, Stockholm.

Titze, I. (1988). A framework for the study of vocal registers. *J. Voice* 2:183-194.

13

Numerical Simulations of Glottal Flow

Johan Liljencrants

Dept. of Speech Communication and Music Acoustics, Royal Institute of Technology, S-100 44 Stockholm, Sweden

Classical work such as van den Berg et al. (1957) describes the glottal pressure drop using empirical terms like entry and exit recovery coefficients. These are difficult to predict since they vary with the channel shape. The details of glottal airflow are also hard to access experimentally due to the small dimensions.

This study illustrates features of the glottal flow by numerical simulation of the fluid motion, an alternate experimental method. Viscosity is accounted for and is of primary importance to the flow phenomena. For practical reasons the scope of the present study is otherwise limited but still covers many important effects: The channel is given a static shape; in reality the walls of the channel move, but with a velocity a few orders of magnitude lower than the air velocity, so dynamic behaviour can largely be inferred from static data sequences. The flow is taken as two-dimensional, with the two dimensions lying in the coronal plane, thus assuming the flow to be invariant along the slit, that is, in the posterior-anterior direction. The medium is taken to be incompressible since the differential pressures are two orders of magnitude below the static atmospheric pressure.

SIMULATION METHOD

The simulations have been carried out as outlined by Roache (1972) using the Navier-Stokes equations (N-S) cast as a transport equation for vorticity ω:

$$\frac{\partial\omega}{\partial t} = -u\,\frac{\partial\omega}{\partial x} - v\,\frac{\partial\omega}{\partial y} + \frac{\mu}{\rho}\left(\frac{\partial^2\omega}{\partial x^2} + \frac{\partial^2\omega}{\partial y^2}\right) \tag{1}$$

This is the central vehicle of the simulation as it shows the development in time of the vorticity ω (which is a scalar property measuring the local shear rate) under influence of the particle velocity components u, v [m/s] in the x, y directions; u, v are in turn found from space differentiation of the stream function Ψ which describes the velocity field. μ [Ns/m^2] is the dynamic viscosity and ρ [kg/m^3] is the density. The first two terms on the right-hand side of the equation are called the convection terms and show how the vorticity pattern is carried along by the flow. The last term is the diffusion term and shows how inhomogeneities in vorticity will spread out into their vicinity. The relative importance of the terms depends on the Reynolds number.

A geometrical mesh for the bounding walls and the enclosed simulation area is laid out on a 65 by 49 point matrix in the axial and cross directions. The mesh is elastically distorted so that the upper and lower rows of nodes are located on the boundaries. This curved mesh enhances resolution at critical locations and is computationally economic, but causes technical difficulty in evaluating differences. Each node entry in the matrix specifies the x and y coordinates and some reasonable vorticity ω and stream function Ψ. In the present program, coded in C language for the Domain Apollo DN10000 computer, all simulation procedures can be geared to use a resolution reduced by the factors 2, 4, or 8. This is useful for debugging and test runs since each doubling in resolution will increase computation time 16-fold. Gearing is also used to quickly arrive at an approximate solution which is subsequently interpolated and refined at higher resolution.

Once the mesh has been established the actual simulation is done following these three basic steps:

1. Establish boundary values of Ψ and ω. Along the walls the stream function Ψ has a constant value determined by the total flow. Poiseuille flow (the classical flow in a straight channel with a parabolic velocity profile over the cross section) is assumed at the inflow boundary, while Ψ at the outflow boundary is determined by extrapolation from the interior. Vorticity ω is generated due to viscous shear at the walls and is evaluated from the stream function and the condition of zero velocity at the wall. This vorticity generation actually drives the simulation problem.

2. Transport the vorticity. At all interior nodes the velocities u and v are evaluated from Ψ and the transport equation is applied to find ω at a later time $t + \Delta t$. Initially vorticity will spread to the interior nodes by diffusion from the walls. Interior vorticity will diffuse further and is also convected downstream with the flow.

3. Modify the stream function. With the new vorticity distribution ω the stream function has to be modified at all internal nodes so that the Poisson equation $\partial^2\Psi = \omega$ (from the definition of vorticity) is satisfied. This is done with successive over-relaxation, a rapidly converging iteration algorithm. Despite its efficiency it consumes a major part of the total computing time.

These steps are reiterated until a sufficient time span has been covered. Sometimes the process converges into a stable solution, while in others the solution may vary with time; the flow problem itself is often unstable.

The pressure contour along the walls is finally integrated from $\frac{\partial P}{\partial s} = \mu \frac{\partial \omega}{\partial n}$, where s and n are the directions along and normal to the wall; the interior pressure field is found from surface integration of the fundamental N-S equations from the now known Ψ and ω.

The output obtained consists of sequences of graphs of field variables; examples are shown in Figure 1.

RESULTS

It is illuminating to note how flow variable images can show the effective distribution in space of resistance and inductance, conventionally modelled as discrete circuit elements.

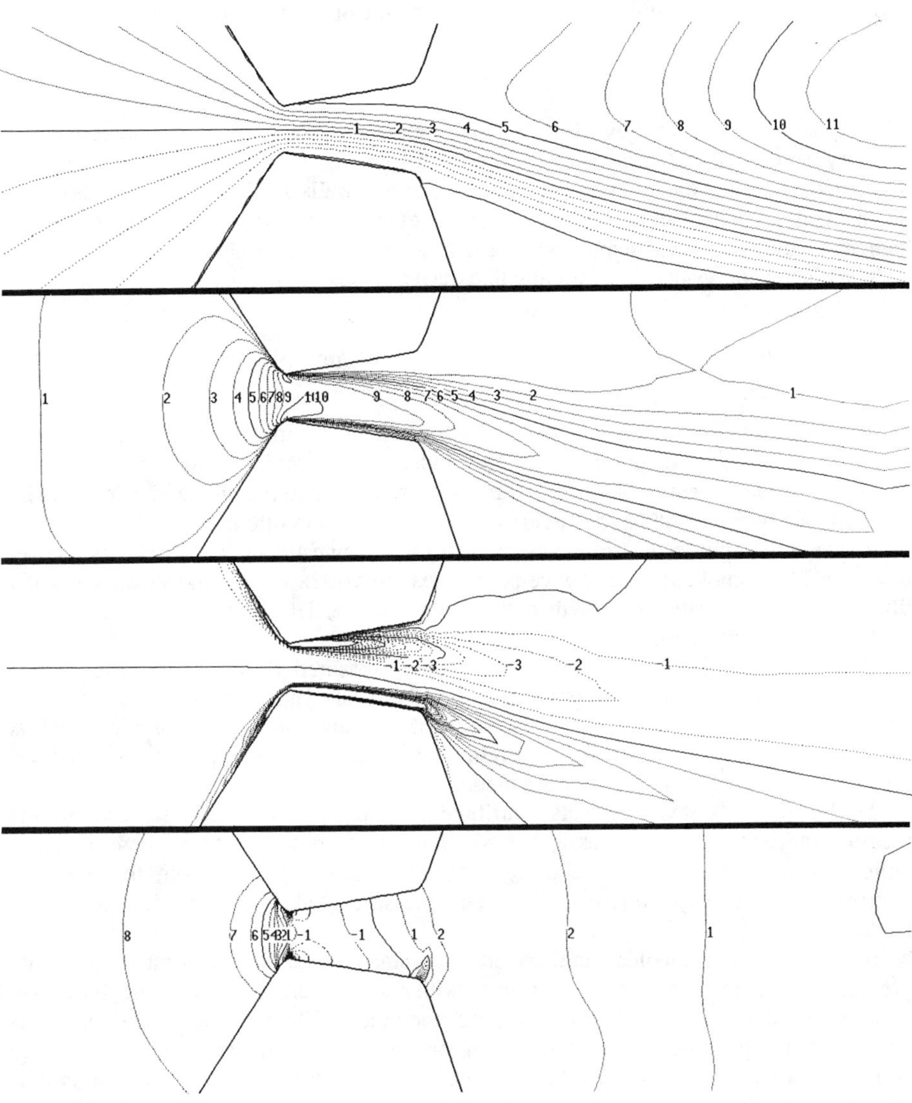

Fig. 1. Iso contours of field variables 25 ms after onset of the unstable flow through a diverging slit. The average velocity is 20 m/s in the constriction, corresponding to a Reynolds number of 1300, based on the cross width of 1 mm at the narrowest point. From top to bottom: stream function (streamlines), velocity in steps of 2 m/s, vorticity, and pressure in steps of 20 Pa (2 mm H_2O).

Within a small volume with essentially unidirectional sheared flow we can develop an expression for the dissipation in Watts per unit volume of the medium, namely

$$W_d = \mu\left(\frac{\partial u}{\partial n}\right)^2 \qquad [\mathrm{Nm/sm^3 = W/m^3}] \tag{2}$$

where n is normal to the flow. But for this laminar flow $\partial u/\partial n$ by definition equals the vorticity, so the *vorticity squared* will directly display the regions where flow energy is dissipated, mostly in the boundary layer at the passage walls and in the outer edges of the downstream jet. This can be seen in Figure 1c, even though the vorticity is not squared here, and would in a sense display where the flow resistance is located.

The kinetic energy density, formally like the dynamic pressure, is

$$P_k = \frac{1}{2}\rho u^2 \qquad [\mathrm{Ws/m^3 = Nm/m^3 = Pa}] \tag{3}$$

and the *velocity squared* shows this to be located in the middle of the passage and downstream in the jet, compare Figure 1b. Modelling with an inductance is problematic because of the nonlinearity. A linear inductance would require pressure and velocity to be proportional; here we will have to assume an inductance proportional to u.

In the initial phase a strong vortex is formed downstream of the slit as the jet develops, like a smoke ring. In low velocity cases this vortex widens and slows down and the flow becomes stationary. With higher velocities the jet often oscillates and sheds vortices to alternate sides.

Gauffin and Liljencrants (1988) show some measured data for similarly shaped channels, where the drop is not proportional to the ideal dynamic pressure. Drop versus velocity characteristics also differ in slope depending on whether the channel is convergent, straight, or divergent. Preliminary results of the present simulations essentially conform with these measurements.

To illustrate how several effects contribute to the pressure drop, Figure 2c shows the pressure profile in a straight passage. A sharp drop occurs at the entry where the air is violently accelerated. Inside the entry corner the flow separates from the wall but reattaches after a very short distance. Then pressure gradually drops due to viscous friction.

In case of low Reynolds numbers and consequently no flow separation the axial pressure profile can be basically constructed with a one-dimensional reasoning. It has two components, one from the friction losses and one kinetic. The loss component manifests with an axial pressure gradient that is proportional to velocity, while the kinetic component is the Bernoulli effect and reflects the velocity squared. The friction is thus relatively more important with low Reynolds numbers due to the different proportionality. At higher Reynolds numbers this simple reasoning breaks down as the lateral velocities become important, see for instance the local pressure minima created by the centrifugal force on the air close to the passage entry corners.

Also, when a jet is formed after flow separation the pressure becomes constant to a first approximation, for instance pressure does not reflect the wide variation in velocity within and outside the jet. The pressure variations in the wide outlet area are generally small, even in presence of fairly strong irregular vortices. Eventually some pressure is however recovered downstream as the jet diffuses and slows down.

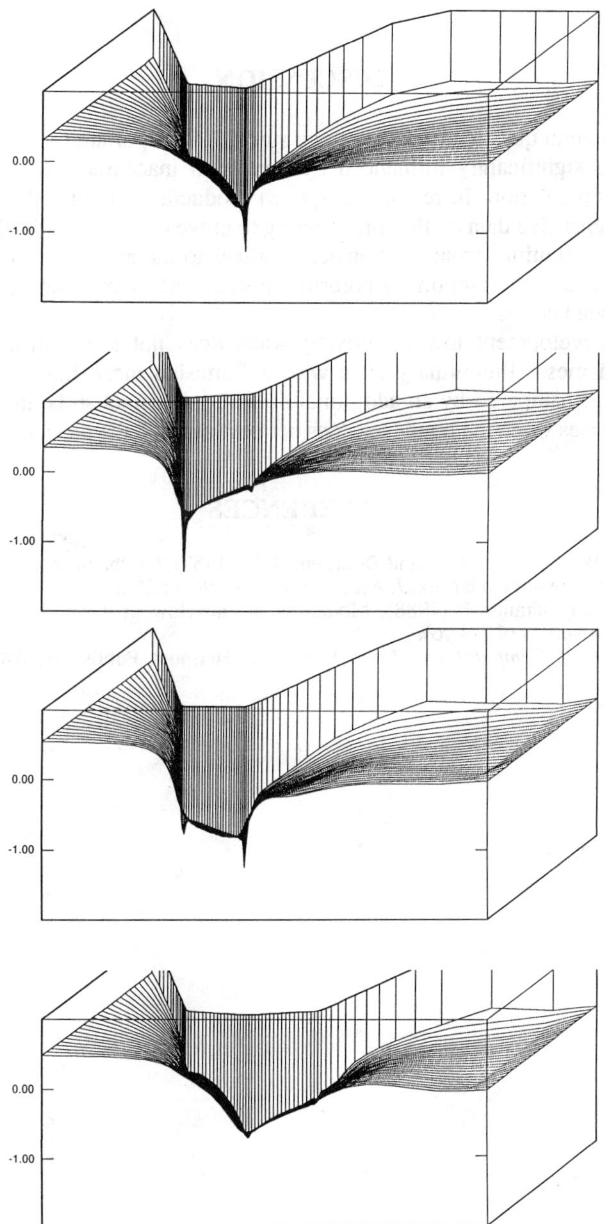

Fig. 2. Pressure distributions in four differently shaped slits: convergent, divergent, straight, and combined convergent-divergent. The average velocity vo is 6 m/s in the constriction, corresponding to a Reynolds number of 400, based on the minimum cross width which is 1 mm for all the shapes. The vertical scale is in units of nominal dynamic pressure 0.5 ρv_o^2 and the geometric area is displayed in perspective, from the center line to the wall.

DISCUSSION

There are several questions left for future study. It is important to determine if the jet oscillations are significantly influenced by numerical inaccuracy, for instance, in the Poisson equation solution. In relation to speech production, continued simulations may provide comprehensive data on the forces acting to move the vocal folds, they may reveal the possible contributions from the transient vortices to the excitation of the vocal tract, and they may shed some light on the notorious problem of source amplitude and location for flow-generated noise.

A further development toward moving walls does not seem attractive using the present curved mesh. Preliminary tests with a Cartesian mesh have given promising results, but were hampered by an additional difficulty to establish boundary conditions. The problem arises when the boundary does not pass through the mesh nodes.

REFERENCES

van den Berg, J.W., Zantema, J T., and Doornenbal, P. (1957). On the air resistance and the Bernoulli effect of the human larynx. *J. Acoust. Soc. Am.* 29(5):626-631.

Gauffin, J. and Liljencrants, J. (1988). Modelling the air flow in the glottis. *Ann. Bull. RILP* 22:39-50. (University of Tokyo).

Roache, P.J. (1972). *Computational Fluid Dynamics.* Hermosa Publishers, Albuquerque, New Mexico.

14

Damping-Biomechanics of Vocal Fold Oscillation

Philippe H. Dejonckere

Department of Phoniatrics, University Hospital, NL-3508 GA Utrecht, The Netherlands.

It is well known that vocal fold vibration in modal register involves, in addition to the gross opening and closing movements, a wave-like motion of the looser mucosa relative to the stiffer underlying tissues. This has led to theoretical approximation of vocal fold motion by mathematical two-mass (or two rows of masses) models (e.g. Titze, 1973; 1974), where the superficial row of masses represent the "cover", and the deeper row the "body" (see Figure 1).

Histological sections indicate that the membranous portion of the vocal fold should be considered as a layered structure (Hirano, 1974; 1977; 1988), which consists of :

1. The stratified squamous epithelium, about 50µm in thickness (7 to 8 layers of squamous epithelium).
2. The superficial layer of the lamina propria (Reinke's space), loose in fibrous components and very pliable. Its average thickness is 0.3 mm.
3. The intermediate layer of the lamina propria, consisting chiefly of elastic fibers, resembling rubber bands.
4. The deep layer of the lamina propria, with twisted collagenous fibers that can be likened to cotton thread. The intermediate and deep layers together are called the vocal ligament, which has a thickness of 0.8 mm.
5. The vocalis muscle, located underneath the lamina propria. It is the main body of the vocal fold; its stiffness depends on the degree of contraction.

The fibers of the vocal ligament insert into the vocalis muscle at many places and merge in the connective tissue between bundles of the muscle fibers. So, the vocal ligament is rather tightly connected to the vocalis muscle.

From a mechanical point of view, the five histological layers can be reclassified into three sections: The cover consisting of the epithelium and the superficial layer of the lamina propria, the transition consisting of the intermediate and deep layers of the lamina propria, and the body consisting of the muscle.

Furthermore, in an excised human larynx, Hirano (1977) showed that the load-strain curves are different for each layer (strain = elongation per unit of length). The strain for the cover is much greater than that for the body. The strain for the transition is closer to

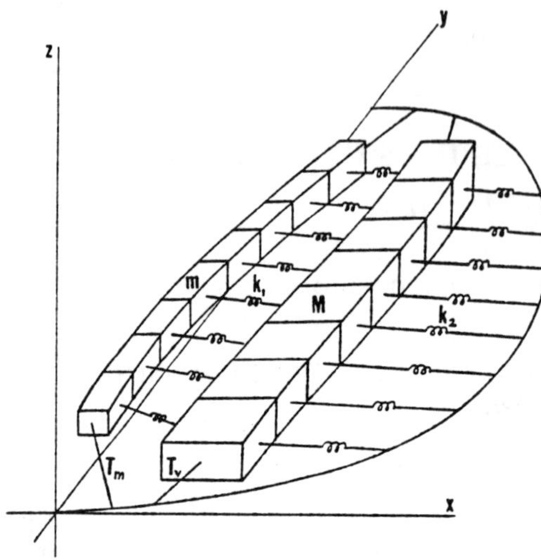

Fig. 1. Schematic model of the vocal fold, with two rows of masses, one superficial (m) and one deep (M), and viscoelastic connections. The orientation of the y-axis is antero-posterior (from Titze, 1973).

that of the cover. The ratio of strain for the body to that for the transition to that for the cover is approximately 1 to 8 to 10. This ratio changes as activation of the laryngeal muscles varies the mechanical properties of the larynx.

The present work deals with quantitative measurements *in vivo* about damping of the vocal oscillator, due to internal and external frictional forces, when the energy supply is ceasing. It may be expected that this damping does not occur as in a classical mass-spring system with friction. Differential components may be identified, with variations that are a function of well-defined conditions of voice production.

While stiffness and muscular tension play an essential role in regulating pitch, damping constants are fundamental for mechanical efficiency of vocal fold oscillation.

MATERIAL AND METHODS

Technique

The amount of light transmitted vertically through the glottis was measured by a photodiode (Centronic OSD 15 - ST), with an active area of 15 mm^2, applied onto the skin of the neck at the inter crico-thyroid level, while the larynx was illuminated and observed from above with a rigid 90° Hopkins endoscope. The light source was a tungsten lamp powered by a stabilized DC power supply. The amount of light transmitted through the glottis was thus proportional to the glottic surface area.

The photodiode signal was amplified by a current amplifier, so that the output voltage was also proportional to the glottic area. Then the signal was sampled at a rate of 10 kHz (12 bits), after an anti-aliasing filtering (F0 = 5 kHz), and displayed with a resolution of 200 x 640 pixels. An Olivetti XT personal computer was used.

Subjects

Five normal male subjects, aged from 25 to 40 years, were investigated. They were all trained vocalists but not professional singers. Further, similar data were collected, for comparison, from eight subjects with voice pathology, either organic or functional.

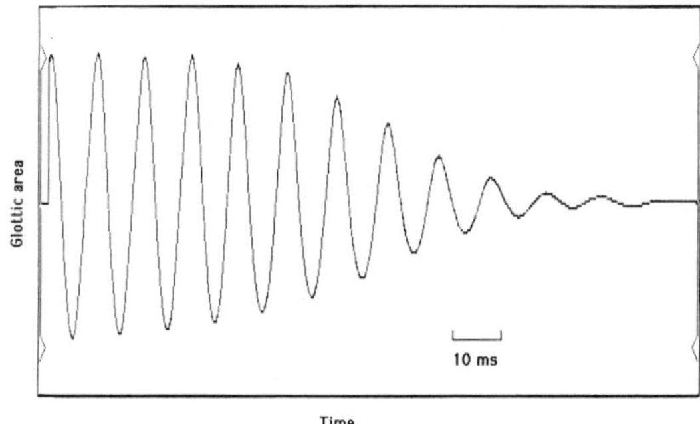

Fig. 2. Glottic area as a function of time (photoglottogram), at the end of the emission of an /a/ by a normal male subject (modal register, loudness 64 dBA at 30 cm, pitch 105 Hz), showing how the vocal folds still oscillate freely during several cycles after their last contact, i.e., after the last closure plateau. The slow component, corresponding to vocal fold abduction, is filtered out.

Protocol

In each subject, large series of photoglottographic recordings were made from terminal parts of sustained vocalic emissions on /a/, in modal and falsetto registers, at different sound pressure levels. Further, soft and breathy attacks were also analyzed.

RESULTS

The general patterns were found to be similar in all five normal subjects. An actual tracing (AC) is shown in Figure 2. Characteristic graphs are presented in Figures 3a to 3e. In each of them, the horizontal axis represents the number of periods and the vertical axis the logarithm of the maximal amplitude of glottic area (arbitrary linear units). Figures 3a to 3e correspond to end phases with damping; Figure 4 is a breathy attack. Figure 5 is an actual tracing of an end phase in a hoarse female patient with functional insufficient glottic closure.

In modal register, the essential characteristic of all recordings of good technical quality is that roughly two distinct phases appear in the glottal amplitude, at both the end of vocal fold oscillation (Figures 3a and 3b) and the beginning (Figure 4). Various curve fitting procedures were tried in each case: usually, the logarithmic decrement or increment in amplitude optimally fits with two linear phases, the second one showing a clearly steeper slope than the first. The breakpoint is most obvious when the voice is loud, as depicted in Figure 3b, and also in some breathy onsets (Figure 4).

The hypothesis is suggested that these phases are related to distinct mechanical components in the oscillator, that is, the vocal fold. The body of the vibrating fold is fixed in depth and becomes thinner near the free edge. So it may be supposed that, in the very last as well as in the very first oscillations, only the most superficial layers (cover) are involved. When voice intensity increases, the free edge of the fold becomes thicker, and a larger vibrating mass of body seems to be associated with reduced damping and a prolonged first phase (Figure 3b). At very low intensity, the first phase cannot be distinctly recognized, and no break is found (Figure 3c).

Also by contrast, in falsetto, no clear-cut break is observed between the components. The transition appears very progressive, suggesting that here body and cover are rather tightly connected (Figure 3d). The influence of intensity is similar to that in modal

a Modal register ; normal loudness ; normal male

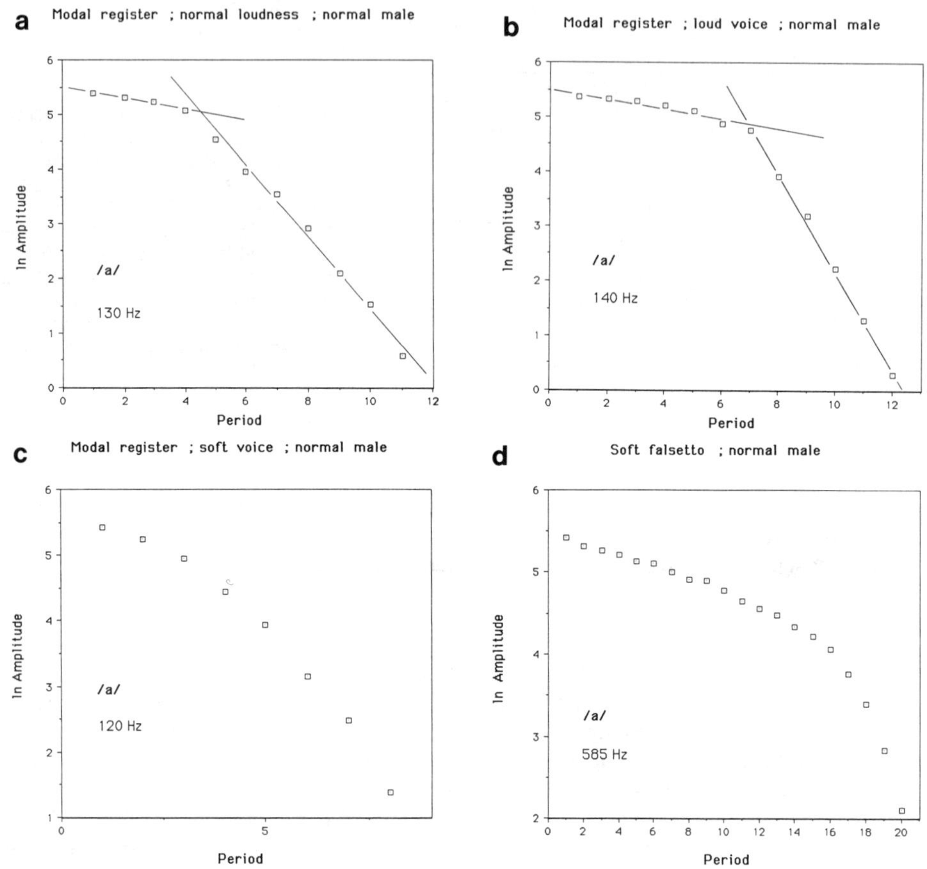

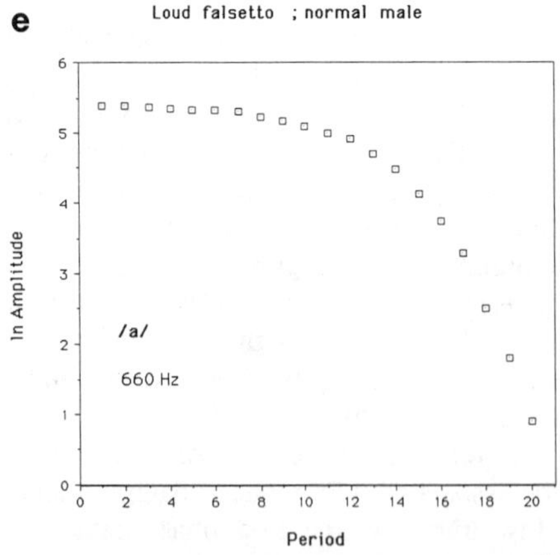

ln Amplitude — Period — /a/ — 130 Hz

b Modal register ; loud voice ; normal male

ln Amplitude — Period — /a/ — 140 Hz

c Modal register ; soft voice ; normal male

ln Amplitude — Period — /a/ — 120 Hz

d Soft falsetto ; normal male

ln Amplitude — Period — /a/ — 585 Hz

e Loud falsetto ; normal male

ln Amplitude — Period — /a/ — 660 Hz

Fig. 3. End phase of a spontaneous vocal emission on /a/. Natural logarithm of the max. amplitude of the glottic area (arbitrary linear units) period by period.
(**a**). Normal voice (66 dBA at 30 cm) . Evidence of two phases in the damping of the oscillation.
(**b**). Loud voice (96 dBA). The duration of the first phase is longer, and the damping is very slight during this first phase.
(**c**). Soft voice (56 dBA). The first phase of damping cannot be clearly recognized.
(**d**). Soft falsetto voice (60 dBA). There is no clear-cut separation in two phases: The damping constant gradually increases at the end.
(**e**). Loud falsetto voice (90 dBA). The beginning of damping is slighter than in soft falsetto.

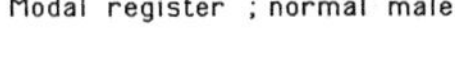

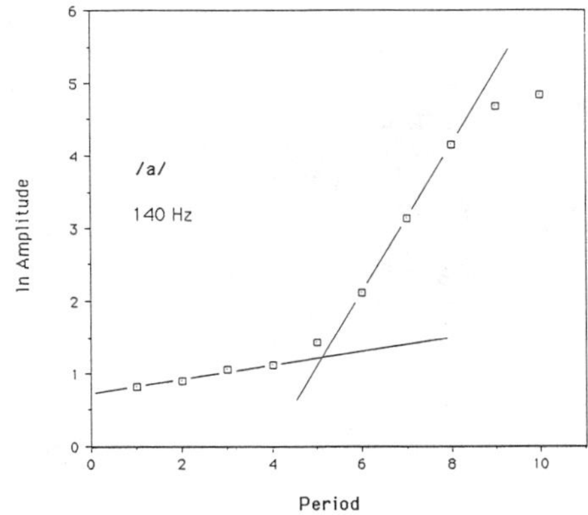

Fig. 4. Beginning of vocal fold oscillation during a soft/breathy attack. Normal spontaneous voice (65 dBA at 30 cm). Natural logarithm of the max. amplitude of the glottic area (arbitrary linear units), period by period.

register (Figure 3e). As soon as vocal function is disturbed (due to either a lesion or dysfunction) shimmer makes calculations of damping constants impossible (Figure 5).

DISCUSSION

It is obvious that the damping of the vocal oscillator differs from that of a single oscillating mass with a spring and a damping force. In the latter case, the formula for the envelope should be:

$$x = Ae^{-bt/2m} \quad \textbf{or} \quad x = Ae^{-\beta t} \quad \textbf{or} \quad \ln\frac{A}{x} = \beta t$$

$$\beta = \frac{b}{2m}\,(s^{-1})$$

where

x represents the displacement (m)
A represents the initial amplitude of the oscillation
e is the base of natural logarithms (2.718)
b represents a coefficient of friction (kg s^{-1})
t represents the time (s)
m represents the oscillating mass (kg)
β represents the damping constant.

β depends on friction forces but also on mass. This formula is graphed in Figure 6. A reasonable criterion for small damping is that the energy loss in one period be a small fraction of the total energy. For larger values of b, the system is critically damped or overdamped, and no oscillation occurs.

The total mechanical energy of the system is,

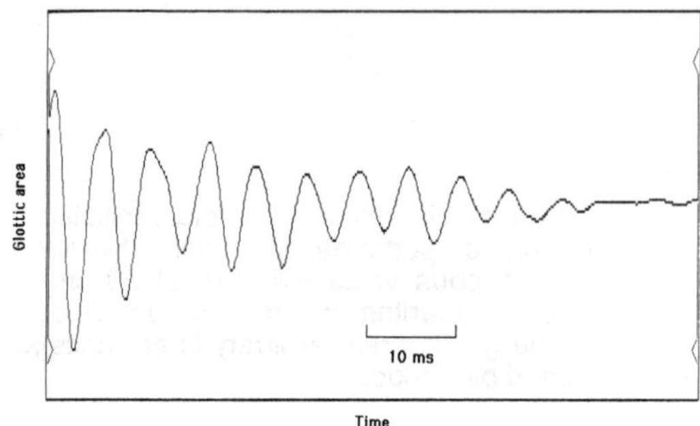

Fig. 5. Glottic area as a function of time, at the end of the emission of a spontaneous /a/ (loudness 63 dBA at 30 cm, pitch 172 Hz) in a female patient, with a low, hoarse voice, and a diagnosis of functional hypokinetic dysphonia, characterized by an incomplete posterior glottic closure. The damping phase is affected by a significant "shimmer" .

$$E = \frac{1}{2} mv^2 + \frac{1}{2} kx^2$$

where
v represents velocity
k represents the spring constant

The rate of change of mechanical energy is

$$\frac{dE}{dt} = \frac{1}{2} m\,(2v\,\frac{dv}{dt}) + \frac{1}{2} k\,(2x\frac{dx}{dt}) = v\,(m\,\frac{dv}{dt} + kx)$$

But we know that

$$m\,\frac{dv}{dt} + kx = -\,bv^2$$

Thus,

$$\frac{dE}{dt} = -\,bv^2$$

The rate of change of mechanical energy is just the power input, which is negative at the end of voicing (due to the damping force), but positive at the onset of vibration, during a soft or breathy vocalic attack. This has an importance in relation to the mechanical efficiency of the vibratory movement.

Now, for our trained vocalists, when we consider the decay from cycle to cycle, we obtain values for β from about $3s^{-1}$ to about $200\ s^{-1}$. In modal register, we may approximate a mean value from 7 to $10\ s^{-1}$ for the first component, with the rather gentle slope, and a mean value from 60 to $100\ s^{-1}$ for the second one, with the steeper slope (see Figures 3a and 3b). It may be assumed that the first component is related globally to body and cover, while the second is related to the superficial cover alone. The fact that β depends not only on friction forces but also on mass probably plays an important role in explaining these differences.

It is well known that the different layers undergo different physical adjustments from the laryngeal muscles (Hirano, 1982; 1988). The mechanical properties of the cover and

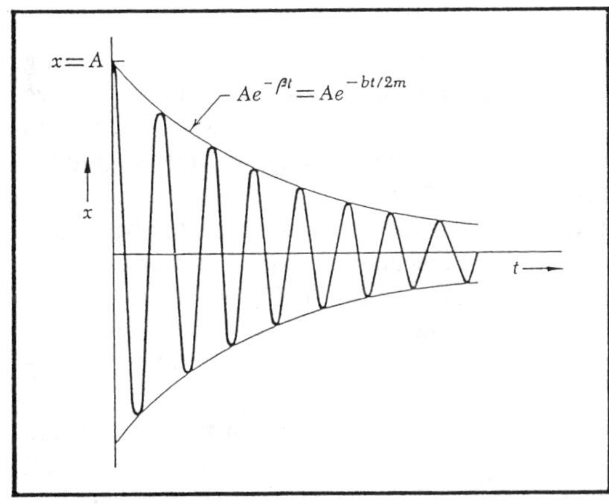

Fig. 6. Amplitude vs. time for a hypothetical harmonic oscillator with light damping.

transition as a vibrator are passively controlled by all the laryngeal muscles, whereas those of the body are controlled actively by its own contraction as well as by passive regulation of the activities of the other muscles.

Observation of histological specimens obtained from vocal folds fixed during electric stimulation (canine larynges) has led Hirano to the following schematic conclusions about the effect of the different intrinsic muscles on the morphology of the fold (1988) :

Effect on Vocal Fold	Muscle Activity
Elongation :	cricothyroid and posterior cricoarytenoid
Shortening:	vocalis
Thinning:	cricothyroid
Thickening:	vocalis
Sharpening of the edge:	cricothyroid
Rounding of the edge:	vocalis

The body of the oscillator is passively stiffened by the cricothyroid and actively stiffened by the vocalis, that is, the body itself. The cover of the oscillator is stiffened by the cricothyroid, whereas it is slackened by the vocalis.

Thus, it also seems likely that the coupling stiffness between the body and the cover is influenced by these muscular regulations. This determines to what extent it will be possible to individualize, for the very last or very first oscillations, mechanical characteristics of the cover alone.

In modal register at high intensity, both phases of the damping are better differentiated than at normal intensity (compare Figures 3a and 3b). The musculus vocalis is the intrinsic muscle exhibiting the greatest variation in activity with changes in intensity. Its activity changes markedly in proportion to the vocal intensity, while cricothyroid activity is often inversely related to the vocal intensity; this seems in agreement with a greater mechanical dissociation between cover and body, the latter becoming much stiffer. The oscillating mass (essentially the body) is also larger when the voice is louder.

With respect to register regulation, the cricothyroid activity is dominant over the vocalis activity in falsetto, whereas the vocalis activity is dominant over the cricothyroid activity in chest voice. In falsetto, the entire vocal fold is strongly stretched.

In falsetto register, as a general rule, no clear "break" is observed in the damping phase. This suggests that cover and body move rather as one single unit. The progressive increase in damping at the end of vibration may be related to a progressive decrease in vibrating mass. In falsetto register, the cross-sectional area of the vocal fold is thinned and the sharpened edge shows a roughly triangular surface.

When a comparison is made between the end of the oscillation and the beginning (breathy attack), it must be pointed out that the electrical activity in the intrinsic laryngeal muscles may be different. There is always a prephonatory "tuning", with significant electrical activity often occurring at the moment of vocal onset. During voice emission, and especially at the end of sound production, the electrical activity often slightly decreases.

Furthermore, in most cases of voice pathology, the damping constant, considered globally, was found to be increased (i. e. increased friction forces and/or decreased vibrating mass) (Dejonckere and Lebacq, 1984). The irregularity of the damping, comparable with the irregularity from cycle to cycle during sustained phonation, makes it impossible to differentiate a body-pathology from a cover-pathology.

CONCLUSIONS

1. The observation of vocal fold oscillation during a soft / breathy voice onset, and during the damping phase at the end of a sustained /a/ in modal register, suggests that at least two distinct mechanical components are present in the oscillating vocal fold, with different damping constants. The damping constant is directly related to the friction forces of the oscillator, and inversely related to the vibrating mass.
2. Muscular regulations and adjustments, in relation to various voice conditions (register changes, intensity changes), influence the relative importance as well as the degree of differentiation (coupling stiffness) of these two mechanical components.
3. In several pathological conditions, differential degrees of damping are masked by shimmer.

REFERENCES

Dejonckere, P.H. and Lebacq, J. (1984). Damping coefficient of oscillating vocal folds in relation with pitch perturbations. *Speech Communic.* 3:89-92.

Hirano, M. (1974). Morphological structure of the vocal fold as a vibrator and its variations. *Folia Phoniatr.* 26:89-94.

Hirano, M. (1977). Structure and vibratory behavior of the vocal folds. In: *Dynamic Aspects of Speech Production*, edited by M. Sawashima and F. S. Cooper, pp. 13-27. University of Tokyo Press, Tokyo.

Hirano, M. (1982). The role of the layer structure of the vocal fold in register control. *Papers in Speech Research* 5:49-62. (Institute of Finnish Language and Communication, University of Jyväskylä)

Hirano, M. (1988). Vocal mechanisms in singing : Laryngological and phoniatric aspects. *J. Voice* 2:51-69.

Titze, I. R. (1973). The human vocal cords. A mathematical model. Part I. *Phonetica* 28:129-170.

Titze, I. R. (1974). The human vocal cords. A mathematical model. Part II. *Phonetica* 29:1-21.

15

Voice Source Variations in Running Speech

Anders Löfqvist and *Richard S. McGowan

*Department of Logopedics and Phoniatrics, University Hospital, S-221 85 Lund, Sweden, *Haskins Laboratories, 270 Crown Street, New Haven, CT 06511-6695, USA*

Studies of the voice source during speech have mostly been concerned with variations in fundamental frequency and amplitude. Thus, there exists a large body of work on fundamental frequency changes related to intonation at the word and sentence levels. However, the source variations in normal speech also include the spectral characteristics of the source signal and the relationship between harmonic and non-harmonic components of the source. These aspects of source variations have mostly been investigated in relation to their linguistic function in different languages (e. g., Ladefoged, 1983; Ladefoged et al., 1988). In addition, they have been the focus of clinical investigations of aberrant voice function (e. g., Yuomoto, et al., 1982; Hammarberg, et al., 1984; Hirakoa, et al., 1984; Kasuya, et al., 1986; Muta, et al., 1988). However, variations in the spectral composition and the harmonics-to-noise ratio also occur in normal speech without necessarily having any phonological status or being related to abnormal voice function. In particular, such variations can be expected to occur at onsets and offsets of voicing at the transitions between voiced and unvoiced sounds. Incidentally, one aspect of source changes occurring at these very points has received considerable attention over the years, i. e., fundamental frequency changes induced by consonants (e. g., Hombert, et al., 1979; Ohde, 1984; Löfqvist, et al., 1989). Only recently have other types of source variations than fundamental frequency and amplitude been studied in connected speech (e. g., Gobl, 1988; Gobl and Ní Chasaide, 1988; Löfqvist and McGowan, 1988). The present experiment was designed to continue this line of investigation by providing measurements of peak and minimum flow during individual glottal cycles at transitions from vowels to consonants, and from consonants to vowels.

METHOD

In order to obtain information on the aerodynamic properties of the source signal, air flow was recorded using a face mask and a sensitive differential pressure transducer (Glottal Enterprises) according to the method described by Rothenberg (1973). Part of the mask was covered with a wire mesh providing a linear flow resistance. The system has a flat frequency response from DC to above 1 kHz. The flow was calibrated using a rotameter. A conventional acoustic recording was also made. The signals were recorded on a multichannel FM tape recorder.

Table 1. *The linguistic material. Underlining marks the syllable carrying the sentence stress of the utterance.*

Ma pa ma ma <u>a</u> ma
Ma pa ma ma <u>ba</u> ma
Ma pa ma ma <u>ma</u> ma
Ma pa ma ma <u>ha</u> ma
Ma pa ma ma <u>va</u> ma
Ma pa ma ma <u>sa</u> ma
Ma pa ma ma <u>pa</u> ma
Ma pa ma ma <u>spa</u> ma

The flow signal was inverse-filtered to recover the glottal pulse. This procedure requires that the inverse filter be adjusted to cancel the acoustic effects of the transfer function of the vocal tract. Since we are interested in studying source variations when the transfer function is changing rapidly, the filtering can be done interactively on a period-by-period basis (cf., Gobl, 1988). In the present case, this would have been prohibitively time consuming, however, so we adopted another strategy. We used reiterant speech modeled after the sentence *Its raining in Oslo*, cf., Table 1. An open vowel was used to ensure that the first formant was considerably higher than the fundamental. A hardware inverse filter was set at a constant setting during the recording session to cancel the first and second formants during the steady state portion of the vowel. This necessarily left traces of the formants in the filtered signal. In order to remove the remaining effects of the formants, the signal was digitally low-pass filtered with a linear phase low-pass filter using the LFI and FLT routines of the ILS signal processing package. Before filtering, the flow signal was sampled at 10 kHz with 12 bits resolution (no preemphasis); the sampling rate was chosen to provide good temporal resolution.

A female native speaker of American English (RSS) and a male native speaker of Swedish (AL) served as subjects. Twelve repetitions of the material listed in Table 1 were obtained. The cut-off frequency of the low pass filter was chosen individually for each subject so as to be below the first formant. The linear-phase filter was designed using the Remez exchange algorithm, which provides a least-squares fit to the ideal low-pass filter. These filters also have equal ripple characteristics. Transition bands were 1 kHz to 1.2 kHz for RSS, and 560 Hz to 640 Hz for AL. The stop bands for the resulting filters were 30 dB down from maximum for RSS, and 25 dB down from maximum for AL. While one might argue about the validity of inverse filtering a rapidly changing speech signal in the manner described here, the low pass filtering effectively removed all but the first four or five harmonics in the signal. Furthermore, the measurements we made are related to gross properties of the source pulse, such as peak and minimum values, that would not be very much affected by the filtering.

Measurements were made interactively on a computer and consisted of marking relevant points in the signal. As illustrated in Figure 1, these points were peak flow, and the onset and offset of the closed phase during each period, respectively. The closed phase was defined as the portion of the signal parallel to the x-axis. We should note that this definition of the closed phase allows flow to be non-zero during the closed phase. Minimum

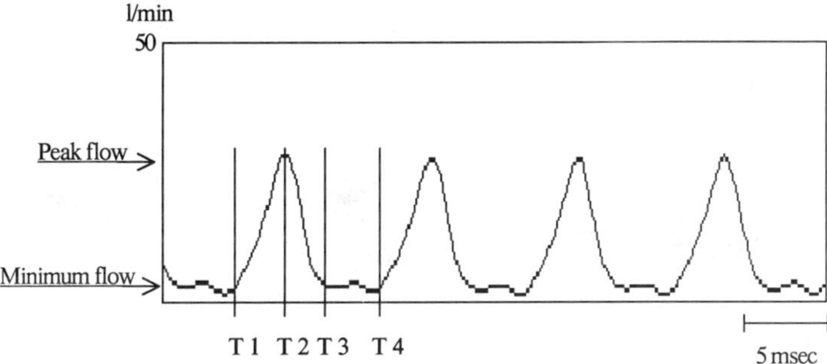

Fig 1. The inverse-filtered and low-pass filtered signal with markers during a single pulse.

flow during each cycle was taken as the average of the flow at points T1 and T3. The measures shown in Figure 1, of peak flow, and minimum flow were then calculated automatically, and the discussion will be restricted to these two measures; other measures are presented in Löfqvist and McGowan (in press). The measurements were made at the offset and onset of the vowels preceding and following the consonant in the syllable carrying sentence stress, respectively. The identification of offsets and onsets were unproblematic in most cases. For the laryngeal fricative /h/, glottal vibrations generally continued uninterruptedly during the consonant. Here, the offset was taken as the last period during the increase in air flow, and the onset as the first period during the decrease in air flow. For the voiced consonants /b, v, m/, the vibrations also continued during the consonant. In these cases, we used changes in the amplitude of the flow signal at onset and offset of closure/constriction to decide on the last and first glottal period, respectively. In order to keep the measurement task manageable, 8 periods before the offset of voicing, and 19 periods after the onset of voicing were measured.

RESULTS

In the following plots, the leftmost part of the x-axis shows the periods before voice offset and the rightmost part the periods after voice onset. Since the fundamental frequency differs for the two subjects, 210 Hz for RSS and 120 Hz for AL, the same number of pitch periods does not correspond to the same temporal interval. Each data point represents the mean of 12 measurements. For the different measurements, we shall first discuss the transition from a vowel into a consonant and then the events at the onset of the vowel following a consonant. Generally, as will be shown, the source changes associated with transitions to and from voiceless consonants tend to be more marked than those associated with transitions to and from voiced consonants. The glottal stop /ʔ/ and the laryngeal fricative /h/ also have large influences on the source properties; in the present context, they can be regarded as a hard and a breathy onset of phonation, respectively. Figures 2a and b show variations in peak flow before vowel offset and after vowel onset. Peak flow increases before the consonants /s, sp, h/ while it decreases before the glottal stop /ʔ/. It shows a small decrease before /p, b, v/ and almost no change before /m/. At periods -9 and -8 in Figure 2a, we see that peak flow at these points tends to be higher be-

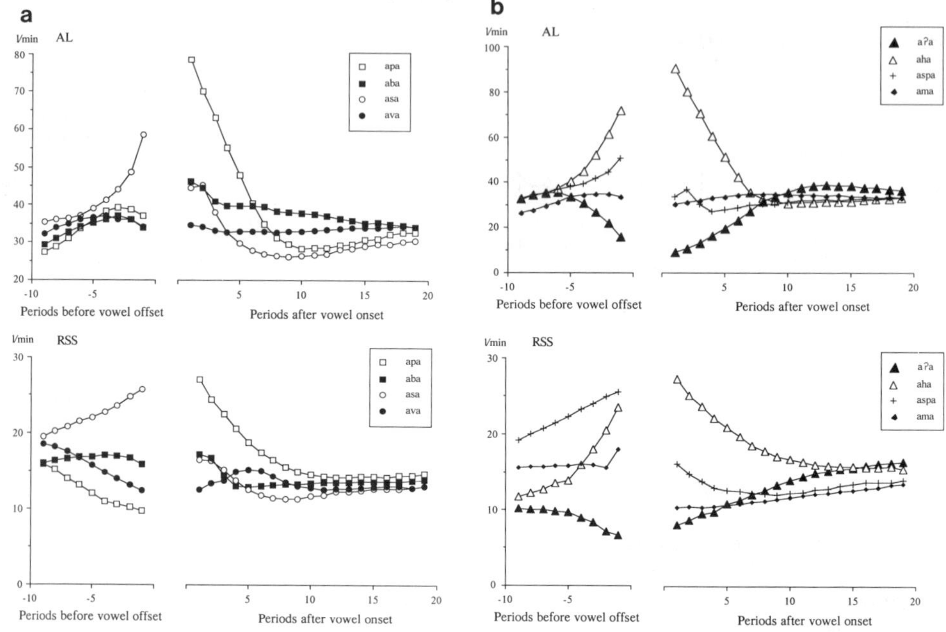

Fig 2. (a) Peak flow before vowel offset and after vowel onset for /apa/, /aba/, /asa/, and /ava/ for male subject AL and female subject RSS.

(b) Peak flow before vowel offset and after vowel onset for /a?a/, /aha/, /aspa/, and /ama/.

fore fricatives than before stops. For both subjects, peak flow in anticipation of the fricative /s/ is already higher at the 8th period before voicing offset; the same is true before /sp/ for RSS in Figure 2b, while for AL the curves for /ʔ, h, sp/ begin to diverge at the 5th period before voicing offset. The source variations during the transition from a consonant into a vowel generally persist for at least 15 periods after voicing onset; then, the curves associated with different consonantal contexts converge. This is the case for subject AL, whereas for RSS the curves usually have not converged at period 19. Recall that the fundamental frequency differs for the two subjects.

Peak flow is very high at voicing onset after /p, h/ and then decreases during the following periods. Some variations in peak flow also occur following /b, s, v/; here, there is a small decrease after voicing onset. At voicing onset for the hard attack /ʔ/, peak flow is low and increases. Following the nasal consonant /m/, the variations are very small. If we look at peak flow well into the vowel, at periods 15-19 (Figure 2a), we see a manner effect for RSS but not for AL. For RSS, peak flow is lower following fricatives, whereas for AL it is lower following voiceless consonants irrespective of manner of production.

Another feature is also evident in Figure 2. Following the voiceless consonants /p, s, h/ and to some extent /sp/, peak flow is high at voicing onset and then decreases. Concentrating on the curve for the syllable /pa/ of AL in Figure 2a, we see that it reaches a minimum at period 10 and then shows a small increase. The same is true for the curve /sa/ for the same subject, where the minimum occurs at period 9. The same pattern also occurs

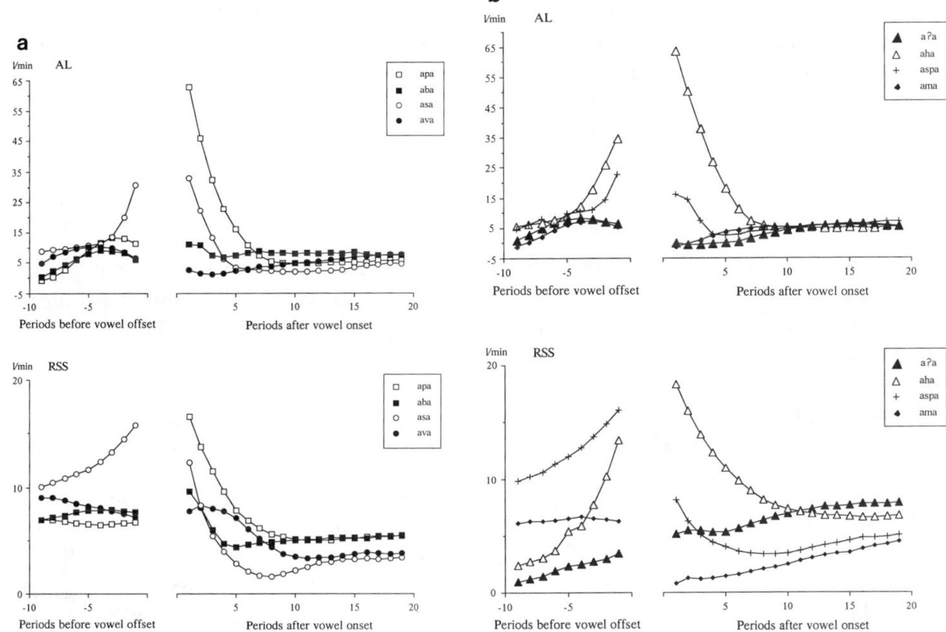

Fig 3. (a) Minimum flow before vowel offset and after vowel onset for /apa/, /aba/, /asa/, and /ava/.

(b) Minimum flow before vowel offset and after vowel onset for /aʔa/, /aha/, /aspa/, and /ama/.

for subject RSS. In her case, a minimum occurs at period 9 following the voiceless fricative /s/, whereas it is less clear following the voiceless stop /p/. When we look at the variations during the hard attack /ʔ/ for AL in Figure 2b, we find that peak flow is initially low and increases to reach a maximum at period 13; during the following periods, peak flow shows a small decrease.

Minimum flow is shown in Figure 3a, b. The variations in minimum flow are very similar to those in peak flow. Thus, minimum flow increases before /s, sp, h/ but it does not vary much before the other consonants. Also for minimum flow, the leftmost data points in Figure 3a show it to be higher when the following consonant is a fricative than when it is a stop. At voicing onset, minimum flow is high following /p, s, h/ and then decreases. For subject RSS, minimum flow shows a decrease during the first 5 to 10 periods in all consonantal contexts in Figure 3a. Again, at period 15 the pattern of minimum flow differs depending on consonantal context for the two subjects. For AL, minimum flow is lower following voiceless consonants, whereas for RSS it is lower following fricatives. There is also a tendency for minimum flow to show a decreasing-increasing pattern following the voiceless consonants in Figure 3a. Thus, for AL there is a minimum at period 10 and 11 following the fricative and the stop, respectively. For RSS, a minimum occurs at period 8 following the fricative /s/.

When we compare the results for the two speakers, we see that the male subject, AL, has larger values of peak flow due, presumably, to the larger dimensions of the male larynx (cf., Holmberg, et al., 1988). The results for the female subject RSS show that minimum flow never goes to zero, cf., Figure 3. This might indicate an incomplete closure. There is some evidence that female voices may have higher minimum flow than male voices (cf., Karlsson, 1988), although Holmberg et al. (1988) did not find any such difference in their study of male and female voices.

DISCUSSION

The present results complement and extend other studies of source variations at vowel-consonant and consonant-vowel transitions. In particular, they show that source changes occur well in advance of an upcoming consonant and persist for 10 to 15 periods following voicing onset.

The factors governing these source variations are the degree of glottal adduction, the transglottal flow, the properties of the vocal fold tissue, and the temporal phasing of oral and laryngeal articulatory gestures at the transitions from vowel to consonant, and from consonant to vowel.

For the voiceless consonants, the vocal folds are abducted to suppress glottal vibrations and contribute to the increase in oral pressure by decreasing laryngeal resistance to air flow. This laryngeal gesture is appropriately phased with the making and breaking of the oral closure and constriction for stops and fricatives, respectively (cf., Löfqvist and Yoshioka, 1984). In addition, recent electromyographic studies suggest that voiceless consonants are produced with higher activity of the cricothyroid muscle than their voiced cognates. This difference most likely reflects an increased longitudinal tension of the vocal folds that is made to arrest the glottal vibrations in combination with aerodynamic factors (Löfqvist et al., 1989).

For the voiceless stop /p/, the vocal folds are abducted at the same time as the oral closure is made. The vibrations cease as the transglottal pressure drop decreases; peak flow and minimum flow decrease at the consonant-vowel boundary. At the release of the oral closure, the glottis is still wide open, since the stops in English and Swedish are postaspirated in word-initial position. There is thus a high rate of air flow through the glottis as the folds are being adducted. Hence, at voicing onset a breathy type of phonation is found as evidenced by high values of peak and minimum flow. The breathy phonation gradually changes into a modal type during the first 10 to 15 periods after voicing onset. At the acoustic level, a comparison between a modal and a breathy type of voicing generally shows the latter to have a higher level of the fundamental and an increased tilt of the source spectrum. Noise components may also appear in the breathy phonation due to turbulence in the open glottis, and additional resonances due to tracheal coupling may also be present (cf., Klatt and Klatt, 1990). In the cluster /sp/, the voiceless stop is unaspirated. Here, the glottis begins to close at the transition from the fricative to the stop and is in a position suitable for voicing at the release of the stop closure (e. g., Löfqvist and Yoshioka, 1980; Yoshioka, et al., 1981). The pressure drop across the glottis is rapidly established after the release of the /p/ closure, and the variations in the source are confined to the first 3 to 5 periods after voicing onset.

For the voiced stop /b/, the glottal vibrations may continue uninterruptedly. No specific gross laryngeal adjustments appear to be made except for a reduction in the activity of the cricothyroid muscle to sustain voicing during oral closure (cf., Löfqvist, et al., 1989). At release, transglottal pressure is rapidly established. The effects on the source following oral release are transient in nature and confined to the first 3 to 5 periods.

The voiceless fricative /s/ is also produced with a glottal abduction/adduction gesture. The phasing of the oral and laryngeal gestures is such, however, that there is an increase in air flow at the transition from the vowel to the consonant and from the consonant to the vowel. As air flow continues during the abduction of the folds, both the offset and onset of phonation are breathy, cf., the measures of peak flow, and minimum flow. In the sequence /aspa/ the offset of phonation before the consonant shows the same pattern as for the single /s/.

The laryngeal consonants /ʔ/ and /h/ show opposite patterns of glottal activity. For /ʔ/, the glottis is tightly adducted and the transglottal flow stops. In contrast, the /h/ is produced with an open glottis and high air flow rate. The uninterruped air flow during the /h/ allows glottal vibrations to continue. The source is characterized by breathy phonation before, during, and after the laryngeal fricative. For the glottal stop, the effects of the tight glottal adduction are seen in the low values of peak and minimum flow.

The voiced fricative /v/ and the nasal consonant /m/ do not affect the source very much. The airflow continues during these consonants. There is a small build-up of oral pressure for the voiced fricative due to the increased resistance to airflow at the point of constriction. The source variations following /v, m/ are small and only occur during the first glottal periods. They are most likely related to aerodynamic changes at the release of the oral constriction/closure.

Another feature of the source variations following some voiceless consonants and the glottal stop is also worth mentioning. The measures of peak and minimum flow show a decreasing-increasing pattern after voiceless fricatives and aspirated stops. That is, after an initial decrease in these measures during the first periods, they show a small increase. This pattern most likely reflects small changes in the degree of glottal adduction following the voiceless consonants. In particular, the glottis is open during the consonant and then adducted for the upcoming vowel. The adduction gesture makes the folds come forcefully together and the resulting tight glottal closure is seen in the present set of measurements. The degree of glottal adduction then returns to a value appropriate for phonation during the vowel. Following the unaspirated stop in the cluster /sp/, this pattern is less clear, however, since the adduction gesture is almost completed before the release of the stop closure. Another factor possibly contributing to this pattern is the reduction in subglottal pressure that is commonly observed at the onset of a vowel following voiceless fricatives and aspirated stops (cf., Löfqvist, 1975).

An inverse pattern is seen following the glottal stop. Here peak and minimum flow show an initial increase followed by a small decrease. Most likely, this pattern reflects the loosening of the tight glottal closure during the period of voicelessness and its return to a setting appropriate for the vowel.

In summary, the measures that we have used make it possible to follow and document subtle variations in glottal behaviour. The source changes we have been concerned with have perceptual effects (cf., Ringo, 1988), and may also be incorporated in speech synthesis to improve on quality and naturalness.

ACKNOWLEDGMENTS

This work was supported by NINCDS Grant NS-13617, and BRS Grant RR-05596 to Haskins Laboratories.

REFERENCES

Gobl, C. (1988). Voice source dynamics in connected speech. *STL-QPSR* 1: 123-159. (Dept. of Speech Transmission and Music Acoustics, Royal Institute of Technology, Stockholm).

Gobl, C., and Ní Chasaide, A. (1988). The effects of adjacent voiced/voiceless consonants on the vowel voice source: A cross language study. *STL-QPSR* 2-3: 23-59.(Dept. of Speech Transmission and Music Acoustics, Royal Institute of Technology, Stockholm).

Hammarberg, B., Fritzell, B., and Schiratzki, H. (1984). Teflon injection in 16 patients with paralytic dysphonia: Perceptual and acoustical evaluations. *J. Speech Hear. Dis.* 49: 72-82.

Hirakoa, N., Kitazoe, Y., Ueta, H., Tanaka, S., and Tanabe, M. (1984). Harmonic-intensity analysis of normal and hoarse voices. *J. Acoust. Soc. Am.* 76: 1648-1651.

Holmberg, E., Hillman, R., and Perkell, J. (1988). Glottal airflow and transglottal air-pressure measurements for male and female speakers in soft, normal, and loud voice. *J. Acoust. Soc. Am.* 84: 511-529.

Hombert, J-M., Ohala, J., and Ewan, W. (1979). Phonetic explanations for the development of tones. *Language* 55: 37-58.

Karlsson, I. (1988). Glottal waveform parameters for different speaker types. *STL-QPSR* 2/3: 61-67. (Dept. of Speech Transmission and Music Acoustics, Royal Institute of Technology, Stockholm).

Kasuya, H., Ogawa, S., Mashima, K., and Ebihara, S. (1986). Normalized noise energy as an acoustic measure to evaluate pathologic voice. *J. Acoust. Soc. Am.* 80: 1329-1334.

Klatt, D., and Klatt, L. (1990). Analysis, synthesis and perception of voice quality variations among female and male talkers. *J. Acoust. Soc. Am.* 87:820-857.

Ladefoged, P. (1983). The linguistic use of different phonation types. In: *Vocal Fold Physiology: Contemporary Research and Clinical Issues.*, edited by D. Bless and J. Abbs, pp. 351-360. College-Hill Press, San Diego, CA.

Ladefoged, P., Maddieson, I., and Jackson, M. (1988). Investigating phonation types in different languages. In: *Vocal Physiology: Voice Production, Mechanisms and Functions.*, edited by O. Fujimura, pp. 297-317. Raven Press, New York.

Löfqvist, A. (1975). A study of subglottal pressure during the production of Swedish stops. *J. Phonetics* 3: 175-189.

Löfqvist, A., Baer, T., McGarr, N., and Seider Story, R. (1989). The cricothyroid muscle in voicing control. *J. Acoust. Soc. Am.* 85: 1314-1321.

Löfqvist, A., and McGowan, R. S. (1988). Voice source variations during consonant-vowel transitions. *J. Acoust. Soc. Am.* 84: S85 (A).

Löfqvist, A., and McGowan, R. S. Influence of consonantal environment on voice source aerodynamics. *J. Phonetics*, (in press).

Löfqvist, A., and Yoshioka, H. (1980). Laryngeal activity in Swedish obstruent clusters. *J. Acoust. Soc. Am.* 68: 792-801.

Löfqvist, A., and Yoshioka, H. (1984). Intrasegmental timing: Laryngeal-oral coordination in voiceless consonant production. *Speech Comm.* 3: 279-289.

Muta, H., Baer, T., Wagatsuma, K., Murakoa, T., and Fukuda, H. (1988). A pitch-synchronous analysis of hoarseness in running speech. *J. Acoust. Soc. Am.* 84: 1292-1301.

Ohde, R. (1984). Fundamental frequency as an acoustic correlate of stop consonant voicing. *J. Acoust. Soc. Am.* 75: 224-230.

Ringo, C. (1988). Enhanced amplitude of the first harmonic as a perceptual correlate of voicelessness in speech. *J. Acoust. Soc. Am.* 83: S70 (A).

Rothenberg, M. (1973). A new inverse filtering technique for deriving the glottal air flow waveform during speech. *J. Acoust. Soc. Am.* 53: 1632-1645.

Yoshioka, H., Löfqvist, A., and Hirose, H. (1981). Laryngeal adjustments in the production of consonant clusters and geminates in American English. *J. Acoust. Soc. Am.* 70: 1615-1623.

Yumoto, E., Gould, W., and Baer, T. (1982). Harmonics-to-nose ratio as an index of the degree of hoarseness. *J. Acoust. Soc. Am.* 71: 1544-1550.

16

Male and Female Voice Source Dynamics

Christer Gobl and Inger Karlsson

Dept of Speech Communication and Music Acoustics, Royal Institute of Technology, S-100 44 Stockholm, Sweden

Context-dependent temporal voice source variations and voice source differences due to different voice qualities are the center of interest in the present paper. Our approach here is to retain and optimize the voice source within the linear source-filter theory. In order to achieve this we analyzed recorded utterances (spoken by both adult male and female speakers) by means of inverse filtering and waveform parameterization. Temporal glottal pulse changes were measured by fitting a four parameter voice source model (the LF model) to the inverse filtered speech waveform. The results of the analysis provide a general idea of the range of pulse shape variation in normal speech. Significant changes in the glottal pulse shape are typically found at the onset and, particularly, at the termination of the voice source, and also at many boundaries between vowels and consonants. Different stress environments show major effects on the glottal excitation. Furthermore, differences in voice quality were correlated to parameter variations in the voice source.

The ultimate objective is a set of rules for the variation of the voice source model parameters according to the speaker's sex and voice quality, and to features like intonation, stress patterns, onset and termination of utterances, phonetic differences, etc. These rules could then be incorporated in text-to-speech synthesis.

METHODS

Speech materials

Seven adult female (F1-F7) and three adult male (M1-M3) speakers of Swedish with rather different voice qualities served as informants. For one female (F1) and the three male speakers the following voice source variations were studied: variation related to the stress pattern, variation between vowels and consonants, and variation for the transition between a vowel and a voiced or voiceless consonant. The seven female speakers have been classified as to perceived voice quality in terms of breathiness, sonority, etc. (see Karlsson, 1988). Relations between voice qualities and voice source parameters were established for these speakers.

Inverse filtering

The speech materials were recorded preserving a correct phase response even at the lowest frequencies, thereby minimizing the risk of distorting the glottal pulse shape. The speech waveform was then inverse filtered using an interactive computer program (cf., Gobl, 1988). After inverse filtering, the signal was band limited to 20-4000 Hz.

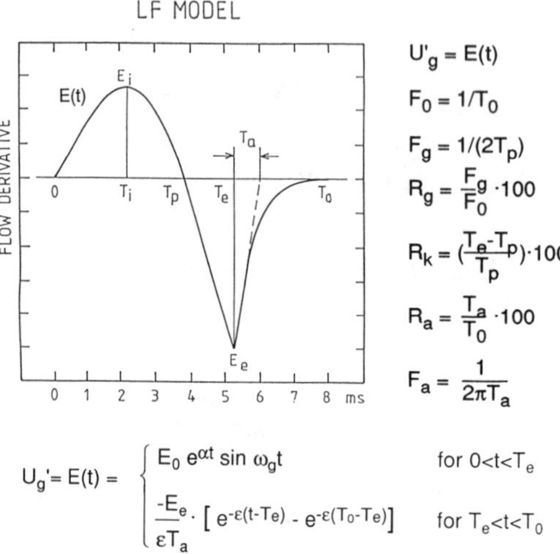

Fig. 1. The four parameter LF-model of differentiated glottal flow.

The voice source model

The model that we used for matching the inverse filtered waveform and measuring glottal parameters is a four parameter voice source model, named the LF-model. Its properties have been more fully described in Fant et al. (1985). The four parameters are used to model the differentiated flow rather than the real glottal flow. The model is presented in Figure 1. For the analysis, the parameters E_e, R_g, R_k and R_a were used, as these are more closely related to different properties of the voice source. The parameter E_e corresponds to the overall amplitude of the source while the three other parameters, R_g, R_k and R_a, influence the spectral content of the pulse. For these three parameters the differentiated flow and the flow spectrum for varying parameter values are shown in Figure 2. As can be seen in the figure, R_g has a small influence on the amplitude relationships of the lowest harmonics, increasing R_k boosts the lowest frequencies and increasing R_a attenuates the higher frequency region. A fuller description of the frequency correlates of the LF-model is given in Fant and Lin (1988). The LF-model glottal parameters were measured continuously through the analyzed utterances.

RESULTS

Two different sentences uttered by one female (F1) and three male speakers (M1-M3) were analyzed. In all these samples the end of a phrase is signaled by the voice source: E_e decreases, R_a and R_k are raised and R_g approaches 100 (see Figure 3; for further details and Gobl, 1988; Karlsson, 1989).

The Swedish word *behålla* was analyzed in three different stress contexts for one female (F1) and three male speakers (M1-M3). The three stress environments arose from repetitions of the utterance *Vi vill behålla honom*, read with emphatic stress on *vill* (*be-*

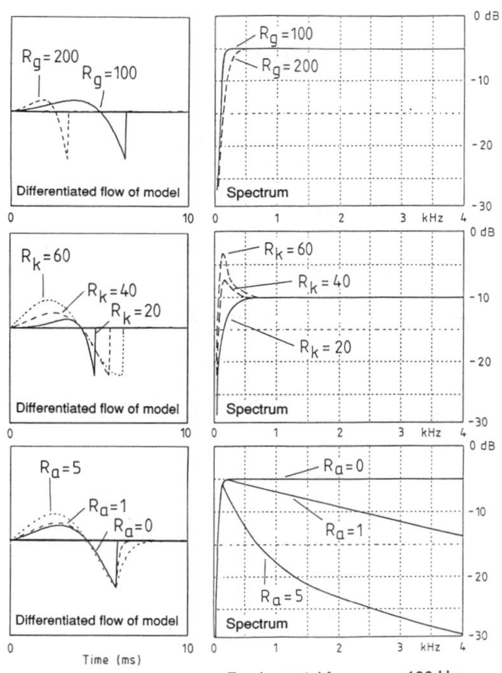

Fig. 2. LF-model pulse shape and corresponding spectrum for different values of R_g (top), R_k (middle), and R_a (bottom). The spectrum is lifted by +6 dB/octave.

hålla is in post-focal position), *behålla* (focal position) and *honom* (*behålla* is in pre-focal position). Some results are given in Figure 4. For all speakers, E_e exhibits a larger dynamic range in focal position: vowels are typically stronger and consonants are typically weaker. In Figure 4, this is most clearly seen for the male speaker, where most of the increase in dynamic range pertain to a lower E_e for the consonants /h/ and /l/. In some cases, as for the female speaker, R_a is also lower in focal position for the stressed vowel /o/. Furthermore, for all speakers, the highest E_e for the final vowel /a/ in *behålla* occurs when behålla is in pre-focal position. The E_e level seems to be affected by the emphatic stress of the following word (for further details, see Gobl, 1988; Karlsson, 1989).

Segment type variation

Two types of variations due to segment type can be detected: one is related to the segment itself, the other to coarticulation. Voiced consonants seem as a rule to have a lower E_e and also a slightly higher R_a than the vowels (see Figure 3). Voiced /h/ and voiced plosives tend to have both higher R_a and R_k than vowels (see Figures 4 and 5). This was also the case for voiced segments preceding a voiceless sound, such as an unvoiced plosive or fricative, which ends with a considerably raised R_a and R_k, and with a low E_e (see Figure 3, cf., Gobl, 1988; Gobl and Ní Chasaide, 1988).

Variations due to segment type were also studied in isolated vowels and vowels preceded by /h/ (voiceless). R_a was found to be higher for a more close/front vowel (see Figure 5). An initial /h/ will cause both R_a and R_k to begin at higher levels than in the isolated vowel (consistent with the higher values for voiced /h/ noted in the previous paragraph). The levels typical of isolated vowels are, however, obtained within the first

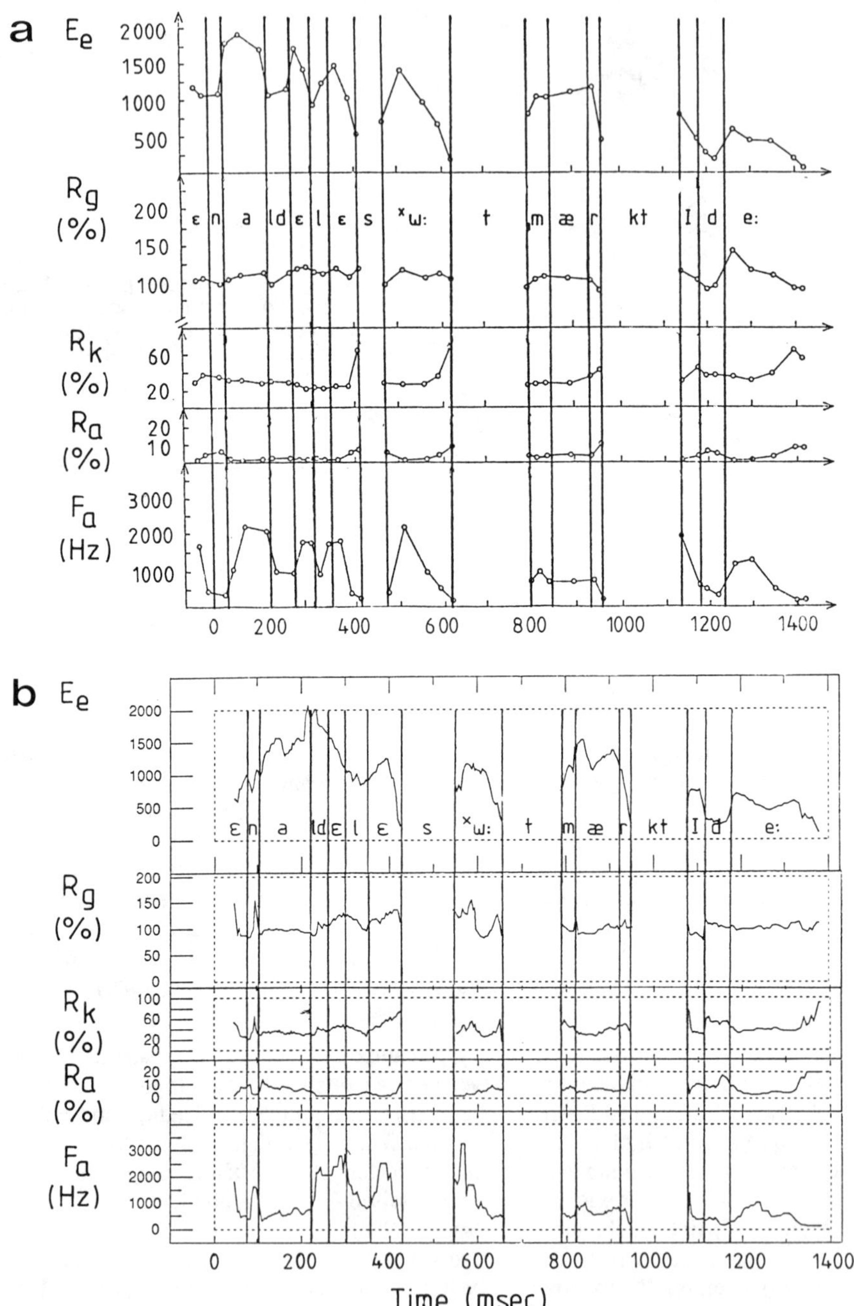

FIG. 3. Temporal variations of the analysis parameters of the Swedish sentence *En alldeles utmärkt idé* for (**a**) one male (M1) and (**b**) one female speaker (F1).

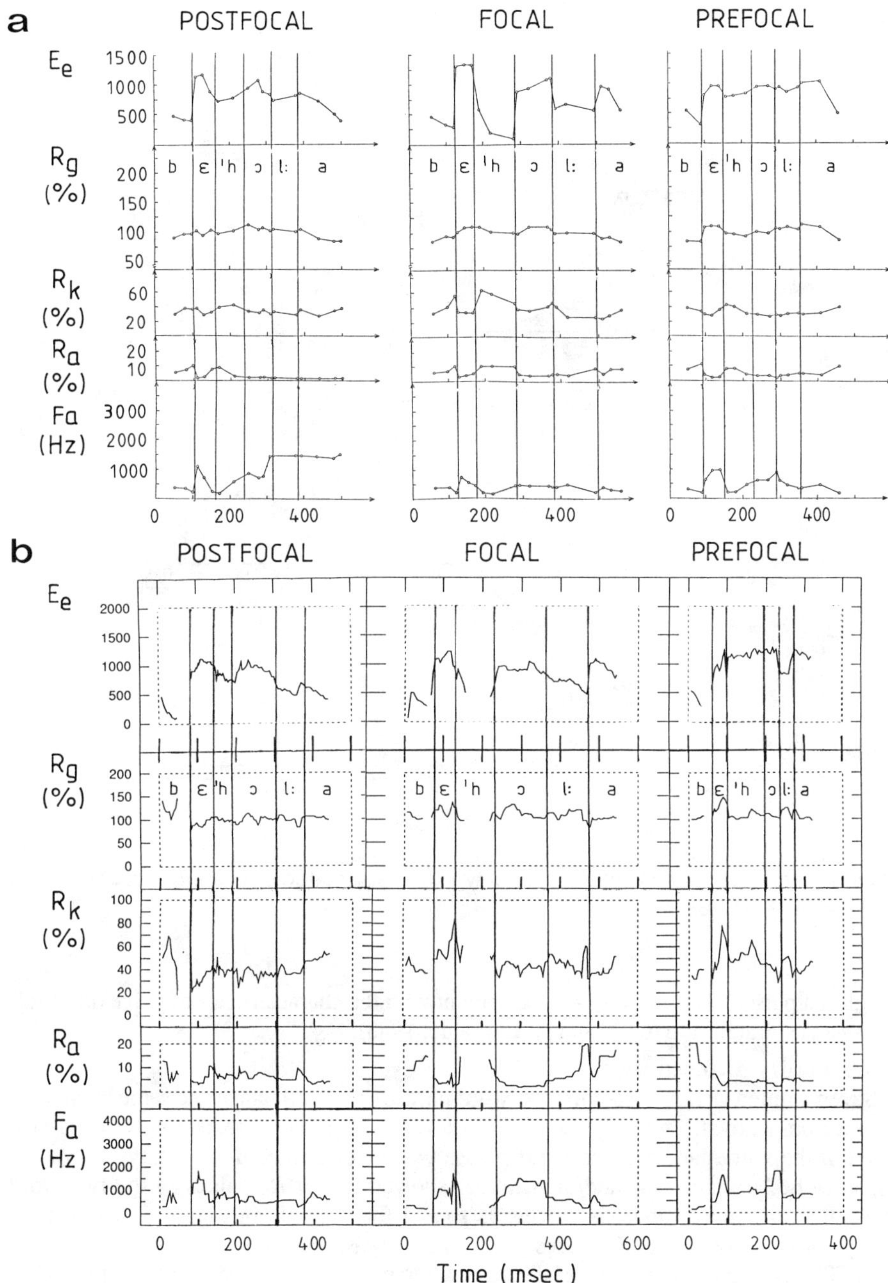

Fig. 4. The word *behålla* uttered with focal stress on the preceding word, postfocal position; on the word itself, focal position; and on the following word, prefocal position. Data are given for **(a)** one male (M1) and **(b)** one female (F1).

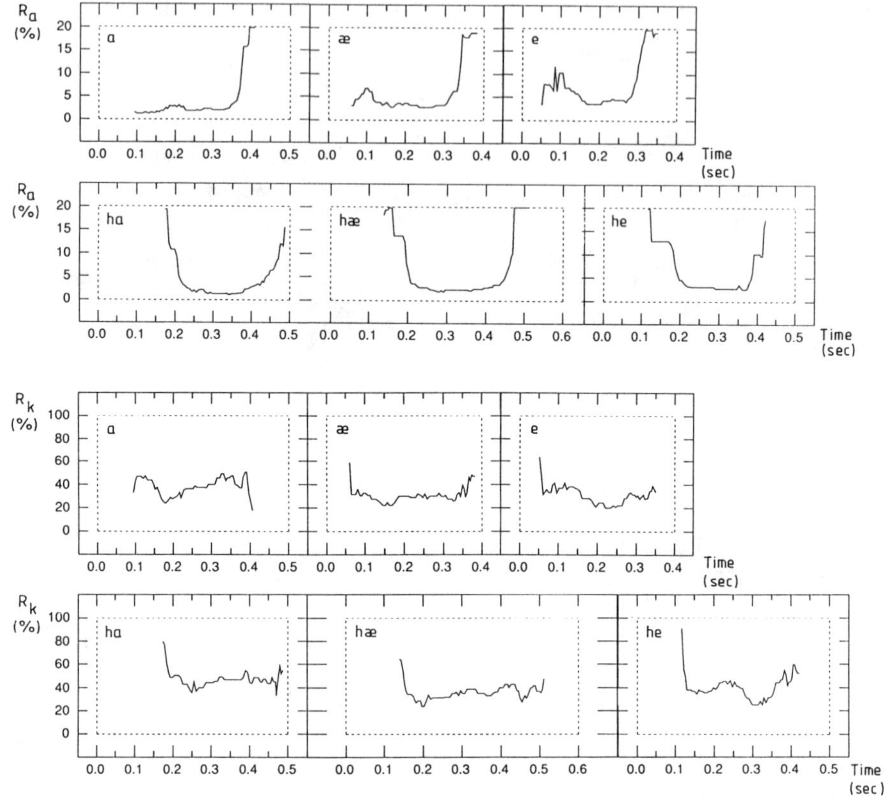

Fig. 5. R_a and R_k variations due to vowel type, either isolated or in an /hV/ context, for a female speaker (F1).

few glottal pulses. This finding is in agreement with the characteristics of voice onset following an aspirated stop (Gobl and Ní Chasaide, 1988).

Voice quality differences

Seven women (F1-F7) read the two-word phrase [ˈjɑ: aˈjø:] and at the same session an excerpt from a novel. The novel excerpt was used by a speech therapist to give a classification of the voices and the two-word phrase was inverse filtered and analyzed. Voices judged to be less sonorous and/or breathier showed higher R_a values in the two-word phrase than the more sonorous voices, as shown for example in Figure 6, and a more creaky voice showed lower R_k values (for further details, see Karlsson, 1988).

In Figures 3 and 5, examples of the same utterance by a male (M1) and a female (F1) speaker are shown. There seem to be no clear differences between the two sexes in these examples. However, the particular female speaker that is shown in these figures had a lower R_a (and higher F_a) than the six other female speakers in this study. (Speaker F1 was judged to have a "normal, somewhat tight and sonorous voice" in Karlsson (1988).)

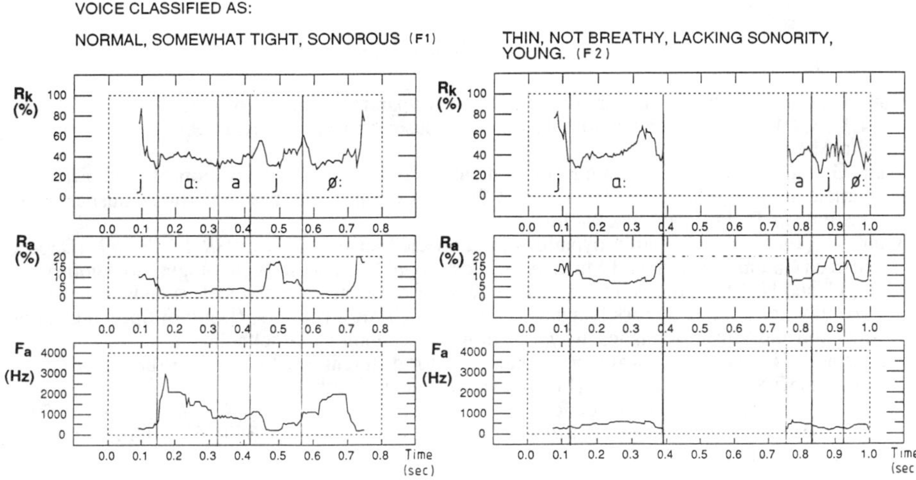

Fig. 6. Voice source parameters for two female speakers (F1, F2) with different voice quality.

Furthermore, in a study with 5 female and 7 male subjects (all different from the present study) the following differences were observed (Gobl and Ní Chasaide, 1988): R_a values for females were typically 2-4 times the male value; female R_g values tended to be 10 to 20% lower than for the males; R_k values were either about the same or slightly higher for the female speakers. Our conclusion is therefore that the average female speaker has higher R_a than the average male speaker.

CONCLUSIONS

Some relationships between the dynamic variations of the voice source and stress, segment, voice quality and sex have been demonstrated in this paper. The description given here is still at a very early stage and is far from complete. Further studies are needed in order to gain a more complete understanding of how the voice source is modulated, in terms of both linguistic and extra-linguistic factors.

ACKNOWLEDGMENTS

This study was in part supported by Swedish Telecom (Televerket) and the Swedish Board of Technical Development (STU).

REFERENCES

Fant, G., Liljencrants, J., and Lin, Q. (1985). A four-parameter model of glottal flow. *STL-QPSR* 4:1-13. (Dept. of Speech Communication and Music Acoustics, Royal Institute of Technology, Stockholm).

Fant, G. and Lin, Q. (1988). Frequency domain interpretation and derivation of glottal flow parameters. *STL-QPSR* 2-3:1-21. (Dept. of Speech Communication and Music Acoustics, Royal Institute of Technology, Stockholm).

Gobl, C. (1988). Voice source dynamics in connected speech. *STL-QPSR* 1:123-159. (Dept. of Speech Communication and Music Acoustics, Royal Institute of Technology, Stockholm).

Gobl, C. and Ní Chasaide, A. (1988). The effects of adjacent voiced/voiceless consonants on the vowel voice source: a cross language study. *STL-QPSR* 2-3:23-59. (Dept. of Speech Communication and Music Acoustics, Royal Institute of Technology, Stockholm).

Karlsson, I. (1988). Glottal waveform parameters for different speaker types. *Proc. SPEECH '88* (7th FASE Symp.), 1:225-231. (Institute of Acoustics, Edinburgh).

Karlsson, I. (1989). A female voice for a text-to-speech system. *Eurospeech, European Conference on Speech Communication and Technology,* Paris, Vol 1 pp. 349-352. CEP Consultans Ltd., Edinburgh.

17

Mechanisms Underlying the Control of Fundamental Frequency

Ingo R. Titze

Voice Acoustics and Biomechanics Laboratory, Department of Speech Pathology and Audiology, The University of Iowa Iowa City, Iowa 52242, and The Recording and Research Center, The Denver Center for the Performing Arts, Denver, Colorado 80204, USA

The purpose of this paper is to clarify and quantify three primary ways of regulating fundamental frequency: (1) by contracting the cricothyroid (CT) muscles, (2) by contracting the thyroarytenoid (TA) muscles, and (3) by changing lung pressure (P_L). All three of these mechanisms have been described phenomenologically for a number of decades, but only recently has the so-called body-cover hypothesis (Hirano, 1976; Fujimura, 1981) been stated in quantitative terms (Titze et al., 1987; Titze et al, 1989). On the basis of these first-round studies, the beginnings of a theory of F0 regulation is emerging. This discussion will focus on systematic integration of some of the individual F0 control mechanisms studied previously. Several parameters used in the body-cover model are still gross estimates. The reader is encouraged to view the results as trends, therefore, rather than as firm numerical predictions.

The mathematical development begins with an assumption that a continuous function for F0 can be written as

$$F0 = F0(a_{ct}, a_{ta}, P_L) \qquad (1)$$

where a_{ct} and a_{ta} are the normalized muscle activities of the CT and TA muscles, respectively, and P_L is the lung pressure. The normalized (non-dimensional) variables a_{ct} and a_{ta} range between 0 (no muscle activity) and 1 (maximum activity), and P_L can be expressed in any convenient unit. It is clear at the outset that this F0 model is restricted to intrinsic muscle activity of the laryngeal tensors and respiratory effort. Extrinsic muscle activity, such as that described by Honda and Fujimura (1991) is not explicitly included, but can be worked in later as an additional length-changing mechanism.

REGULATION OF VOCAL FOLD LENGTH

A relation between intrinsic muscle activity and vocal fold length was derived previously (Titze et al., 1987) on the basis of rotational equilibrium of torque produced around an axis through the cricothyroid joint:

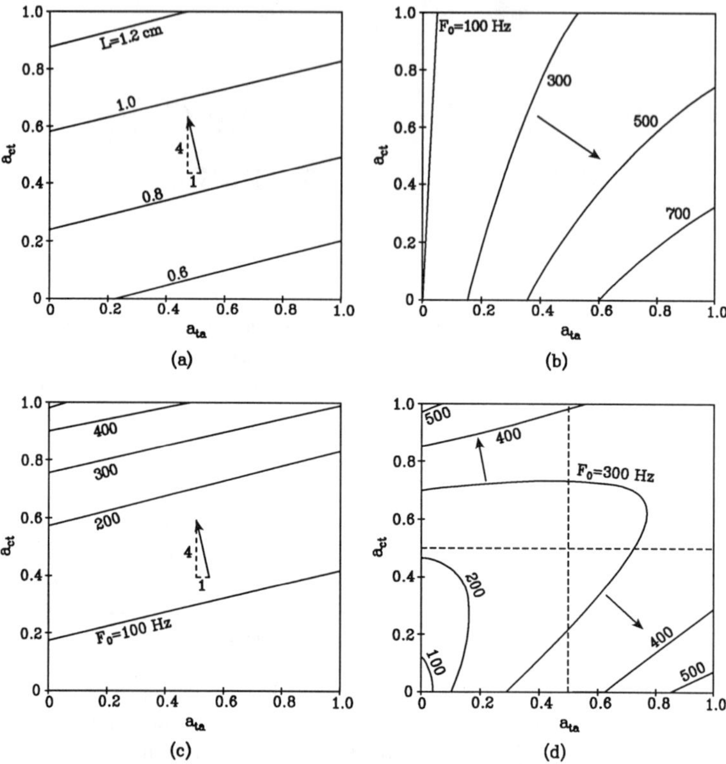

Fig. 1. Muscle Activation Plots (MAPS) for the laryngeal tensor muscles. On all plots, the ordinate is cricothyroid activity a_{ct} and the abscissa is thyroarytenoid activity a_{ta}. (**a**) Lines of constant vocal fold length are plotted using Equation 3. (**b**) Lines of constant F0 are plotted for the body model, Equation 7. (**c**) Lines of constant F0 are plotted for the cover model, Equation 10. (**d**) Lines of constant F0 are plotted for the body-cover model, Equation 13, with $\alpha = 0.3$.

$$L = L_0[\delta + G(Ra_{ct} - a_{ta})] \tag{2}$$

where L_o is the abducted membranous length of the vocal folds (1.6 cm on average for males and 1.0 cm for females), δ is the fraction of L_o to which the length is reduced by purely adductory means (with $a_{ct} = a_{ta} = 0$), G is a gain factor that determines how much length change can be achieved by extreme combinations of a_{ct} and a_{ta}, and R is a torque ratio that determines the mechanical advantage that CT has over TA in changing length. Values of R and G were obtained experimentally (on excised canine *in vivo* larynges) to be about 4 and 0.1, respectively, when δ was implicitly taken to be 1.0 (adducted and abducted lengths the same). There was no way to determine a δ in the previous canine experiment because lateral cricoarytenoid (LCA) muscle activity could not be produced separately from TA activity by recurrent nerve stimulation. In later attempts to match

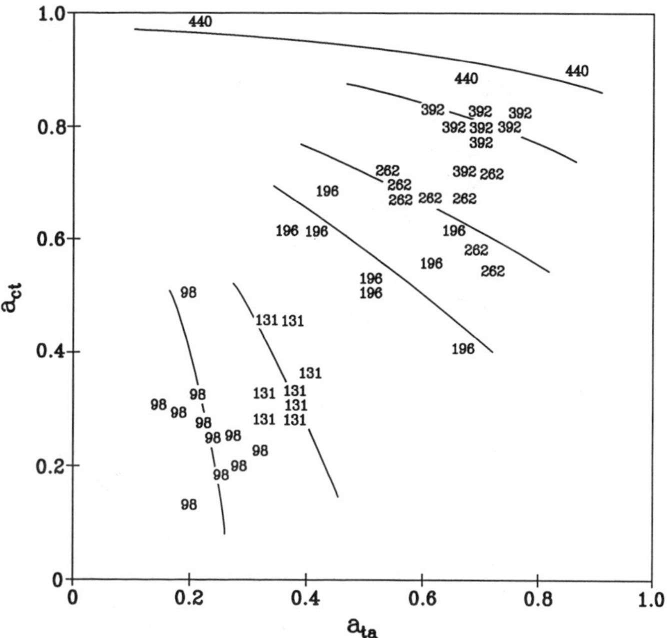

Fig. 2. Muscle Activation Plot (MAP) for a single human subject. Phonation frequencies are indicated in Hz and constant F0 lines are hand-drawn.

human data to an F0 model (Titze, 1989a; Titze et al., 1989), we introduced a δ of 0.377 (or $1 - \delta = 0.623$) in equations for elongation to keep approximately the same values of G and R. More anatomical and biomechanical measurements are presently being made to determine the values of δ, G, and R for both human and canine larynges.

With tentative one-significant figure values for δ, G and R, equation (2) assumes the form

$$L = 1.6\,[0.4 + 0.1(4a_{ct} - a_{ta})] \tag{3}$$

The total range of L, according to this model, is 0.5 to 1.3 cm. The lowest value is obtained by letting $a_{ct} = 0$ and $a_{ta} = 1$, whereas the highest value is obtained by letting $a_{ct} = 1$ and $a_{ta} = 0$. There is no guarantee, however, that these extreme lengths produce phonation; rather, they serve to bracket the length over laryngeal adjustments that include forced adduction (glottal stop) and hypertensing (devoicing). In phonation, Nishizawa et al. (1988) measured lengths that typically ranged from 0.7 cm to 1.2 cm, and there was considerable variation among subjects. Deductions from Hollien's (1960) data agree with this range of membranous vocal fold length (Titze, 1989b).

In previous work with laryngeal EMG (Titze et al., 1989), we found it convenient to plot a_{ct} against a_{ta} for various laryngeal adjustments. The resultant plot was called a Muscle Activation Plot (MAP). Such a plot is shown in Figure 1(a), with L being a parameter. Four isometric (constant length) lines are drawn, and an arrow indicates the direction of maximum length change (perpendicular to the isometric lines). Thus, Figure

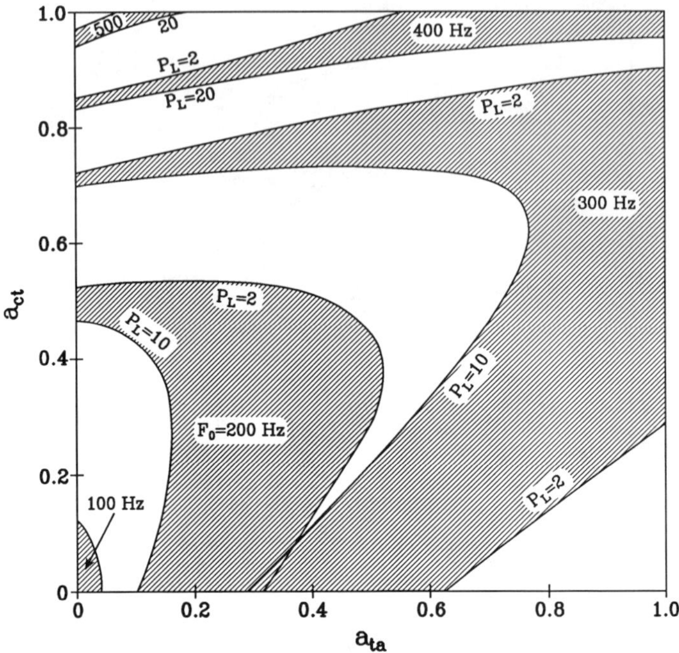

Fig. 3. Muscle Activation Plot (MAP) with constant F0 bands by the body-cover model. Lung pressure P_L is a new parameter that increases from one side of the band to the other as indicated. Values of P_L are in cm H_2O.

1(a) is a graphical representation of Equation (3), with the slope of the arrow being the torque ratio R=4, and the spacing between the isometric lines being proportional to the gain G. Note that an increase in a_{ta} always reduces the length (a lower isometric line is approached horizontally to the right), whereas an increase in a_{ct} always increases the length (a higher isometric line is approached vertically upward).

THE BODY MODEL

Consider now a vocal fold that is composed of muscle tissue only. (This may have some clinical relevance when the vocal fold has been surgically stripped of the cover; theoretically, it serves as an asymptotic condition for which a large portion of the TA muscle is in vibration.) Assume that muscle fibers course longitudinally from the arytenoid cartilage to the anterior portion of the thyroid cartilage. An ideal string model for F0 may then be used:*

* An ideal string model is not useful for elucidating the self-oscillating mechanism of vocal fold vibration, but a ribbon model is. To first order, F0 of a stretched ribbon is the same as that of a stretched string.

$$F0 = \frac{1}{2L}\left(\frac{\sigma}{\rho}\right)^{1/2} \tag{4}$$

where σ is the longitudinal stress (force per unit area) in the muscle, and ρ is the tissue density (a constant of about 1.03 g/cm^3). The longitudinal stress can further be written as

$$\sigma = \sigma_p + \sigma_{am}\, a_{ta} \tag{5}$$

where σ_p is the passive stress in the muscle's connective tissue and σ_{am} is the maximum active stress, developed in the muscle fibers when $a_{ta} = 1$. The passive stress is a strong nonlinear function of vocal fold length (Alipour-Haghighi et al., 1989). At typical lengths in phonation, σ_p is a small fraction of σ_{am}. The passive stress can then be neglected and the fundamental frequency becomes

$$F0 = \frac{\left(\dfrac{\sigma_{am}\, a_{ta}}{\rho}\right)^{1/2}}{2L_0\,[\delta + G\,(Ra_{ct} - a_{ta})]} \tag{6}$$

upon substitution of equations (2) and (5) into equation (4).

It is clear from equation (6), as well as from intuitive reasoning, that for typical values of δ, G, and R, the body model will produce an increase in F0 when a_{ta} is increased. A combined stiffening and shortening of the vibrating muscle fibers results in a profound F0 *increase* when the TA muscle is activated. Increased activity in the CT muscle, on the other hand, *decreases* F0 in the body model because the length increases while the longitudinal stress is negligibly affected. The fact that this somewhat surprising result is rarely (if ever) encountered in human phonation leads one to the conclusion that the body model is primarily of academic value. It shows extreme conditions that may be approached, but never quite achieved, in phonation.

With a numerical value of σ_{am} = 100 kPa = 10^6 dyn/cm^2 as reported by Alipour-Haghighi et al. (1989) for TA muscle tissue, and with other parameters as previously stated, equation (6) can be rearranged and numerically evaluated as

$$a_{ct} = \frac{770}{F0}\,(a_{ta})^{1/2} + 0.25a_{ta} - 1 \tag{7}$$

For any given F0, a tensor MAP can be drawn relating a_{ct} to a_{ta}. This is accomplished in Figure 1(b). Four constant F0 lines are shown, and the arrow depicts the direction of maximum F0 increase. Note that F0 will increase with either an increase in a_{ta} (horizontal component of arrow) or a decrease in a_{ct} (vertical component of arrow), or both.

THE COVER MODEL

If the body is not involved in vibration, but serves only to regulate the length, the F0 control mechanism is quite different. In equation (5), the passive stress becomes the stress in the cover, and the second term vanishes because there are no active fibers in vibration. The passive stress in the cover has been measured for canines (Perlman and Durham, 1987), but not for humans. We would expect σ_p to be greater, on the average, for humans becauseof the presence of the vocal ligament. Assuming an exponential stress-strain curve of the form

$$\sigma_p = 10^4 \, e^{13\varepsilon} \quad \text{dyn/cm}^2 \tag{8}$$

where the strain is

$$\varepsilon = G\,(Ra_{ct} - a_{ta}) \tag{9}$$

an F0 range of about 50-500 Hz is obtained. Explicitly, combining equations (2) and (8) with equation (4) yields

$$\text{F0} = \frac{98.5\, e^{6.5G(Ra_{ct} - a_{ta})}}{2L_0\,[\delta + G\,(Ra_{ct} - a_{ta})]} \tag{10}$$

The denominator is the same as in equation (6), but the numerator is very different. The change in length in the denominator with the term $G(Ra_{ct} - a_{ta})$ is more than offset by the same term in the exponent of the numerator. Thus, F0 *increases* with a_{ct} and *decreases* with a_{ta}. This is exactly opposite to the predictions for the body model.

A tensor MAP for the cover model is shown in Figure 1(c), with L, , G, and R as specified previously. Note the similarity between the constant F0 lines in this MAP and the isometric lines in Figure 1 a. The slopes are identical, but the spacing is different. The constant F0 lines are spaced nearly logarithmically because of the exponential term in equation (10). Thus, the change in F0 with an incremental length change is greater when the vocal folds are longer. Note also that the direction of maximum length change (shown by arrow) is almost 180° opposite that for the body model (Figure 1b).

THE BODY-COVER MODEL

When the body and cover are both involved in vibration, it is not easy to predict how the opposing F0-regulating mechanisms of the body and cover combine in a single diagram. A coupling parameter is needed that expresses the ratio of the relative cross-sections of tissues in vibration. This parameter was introduced previously (Titze et al., 1987) and will be given the symbol α here. It is hypothesized that α is proportional to the vibrational amplitude A. In other words, the depth to which the vibration extends into the body is reasoned to depend linearly on the displacement at the medial surface. A rough estimate of proportionality is

$$\alpha = \left(\frac{A}{0.5\ \text{cm}}\right) \tag{11}$$

suggesting that a typical 0.1 cm amplitude of vibration (for each vocal fold) would involve 20% of the muscle tissue in the vibrating cross-section. On the other hand, a more extreme 0.3 cm amplitude of vibration would involve 60% of the muscle tissue in the vibrating cross-section.

Equation (5) takes on the form

$$\sigma = \sigma_p + \alpha\sigma_{am}\, a_{ta} \tag{12}$$

with the introduction of the coupling parameter. The passive stress is for the cover, and the active stress is for the body. Substituting this into equation (4) yields

$$F0 = F0_p \left(1 + \alpha \frac{\sigma_{am}}{\sigma_p} a_{ta}\right)^{1/2} \tag{13}$$

for the body-cover model, where $F0_p$ is the "passive F0" for the cover as defined by equation (10). Thus, the second term in parentheses in equation (13) is the contribution of the body to F0. For $\alpha = 0$, the expression reduces to the cover model, and for $\alpha = 1$ and $\sigma_{am}/\sigma_p >> 1$, the expression reduces to the body model.

Figure 1(d) shows a tensor MAP for the body-cover model. The coupling parameter α is chosen to be 0.3. Note the highly curved nature of the constant F0 lines. Rather than rising linearly upward with a fixed slope, the constant F0 lines bend downward toward the horizontal axis, in some instances doubling back on themselves. This suggests that there may be two values of a_{ct} for a given value of a_{ta} for some fundamental frequencies.

If the body-cover MAP is divided into four quadrants as shown in the figure (Figure 1d), a better conceptualization of F0 regulation is obtained. In the upper left quadrant, the body-cover model asymptotes to the cover model. Here the vocal fold length is high and the passive stress in the cover overcomes the active stress in the muscle. The CT muscle dominates over the TA muscle. F0 increases toward the upper left corner (see arrow). In the lower right quadrant, on the other hand, the body model is approached asymptotically. Here the vocal fold is short and the cover is lax, allowing F0 to be controlled by the stress in the muscle fibers. F0 increases downward toward the lower right corner (see arrow). Thus, Figures 1(b) and 1(c) are special cases of Figure 1(d) for unbalanced muscle activity in the off-diagonal quadrants ($a_{ct} >> a_{ta}$ or $a_{ta} >> a_{ct}$).

For balanced muscle activity (near the diagonal, where $a_{ct} \approx a_{ta}$), F0 changes in different ways, depending on the curvature of the constant F0 lines. Some frequencies are difficult, if not impossible, to achieve along the diagonal (note the bulging of the lines). The explanation is that the two muscles are performing a nearly isometric exercise, with relatively little change in the stiffness of the vibrating tissue. Somehow, CT needs to be given an advantage over TA if F0 is to increase. Anatomically, the advantage comes with a greater torque ratio R. Physiologically, a gradual release of a_{ta} helps to approach the higher F0 curves above the diagonal in the upper right quadrant.

Figure 2 shows a tensor MAP obtained from measured EMG activities on a single male subject. Coordinates of a_{ct} and a_{ta} are entered as numbers that give the corresponding fundamental frequency of phonation. Experimental procedures for obtaining EMG and F0 are outlined in Titze et al. (1989). Maximum TA activity ($a_{ta} = 1$) was obtained from swallowing maneuvers and maximum CT activity ($a_{ct} = 1$) was obtained from the highest pitch the subject could produce. Fragments of constant F0 lines are hand-drawn through clusters of data points. Note that the lines are more vertical in the lower half of the MAP than in the upper half, in agreement with predictions (Figure 1d). Note also the tendency for this normal subject to stay slightly above the diagonal when F0 is raised, especially in the upper right quadrant. Little of the lower right quadrant is accessed by this subject. This is interesting in light of what Ludlow et al. (1989) found for spastic dysphonic patients, who often attempted to phonate in the lower right quadrant. The high upper left quadrant was accessed once by this subject in a falsetto tone at A4 (440 Hz). Results from other subjects have been reported elsewhere (Titze et al., 1989), and more are presently being analyzed.

F0 REGULATION BY LUNG PRESSURE

A critical parameter in the development of a quantitative F0 model is A/L, the vibrational-amplitude-to-length ratio of the vocal folds. This parameter is an indicator of the involvement of P_L in F0 control. As the vibrational amplitude increases with lung pressure and A/L approaches 0.1 or more, a dynamic vocal fold strain becomes important in relation to the static strain ε. The time-averaged value of this dynamic strain was previously derived to be

$$\bar{s} = \frac{1}{8}\left(\frac{\pi A}{L}\right)^2 \tag{14}$$

for a string model with variable tension (Titze, 1989a). A relation between lung pressure and vibrational amplitude was also obtained empirically (from excised canine larynx data):

$$A = (0.0862 - 0.0824\frac{L}{L_0})\sqrt{P_L} \tag{15}$$

By replacing ε in equation (8) with $\varepsilon + \bar{s}$, the combined static and dynamic strain, the stress σ_p in the cover and the fundamental frequency F0 can be made dependent on P_L through equations (14) and (15). This will then also make the coupling ratio α dependent on P_L through equation (11). The result is a splitting of the constant F0 lines into bands, as shown in Figure 3. In the upper half of the MAP, the bands are bounded by the lower pressure on top and the higher pressure on the bottom. This means that increased lung pressure raises F0, because less CT activity is needed for the same F0 if P_L increases. Hirano et al. (1970) observed such an inverse relationship between CT and P_L when a subject executed a crescendo at constant pitch.

In the lower half of the MAP, increased lung pressure shifts the constant F0 curves to the left, suggesting that less TA activity is needed to get the same F0. Thus, again, P_L raises Fo because the constant F0 lines shift toward the lower left corner and thus higher F0 values can be reached by the same range of a_{ct} and a_{ta}. Further predictions of the ways in which the constant F0 lines change with vocal intensity and P_L are difficult to make at this point because the parameters of the F0 model are still in need of further refinement.

CONCLUSIONS

A systematic development of a body-cover model for F0 regulation has been outlined. At this stage, the model is quantitative, but has arguable validity and accuracy. A number of key assumptions were made that need to be validated in future developments. The assumptions were (1) that the tension-carrying fibers in both body and cover course longitudinally so that a string model for F0 is applicable (i.e., lateral stiffness of the tissue was excluded); (2) effects of extrinsic laryngeal and pharyngeal muscle activity were omitted, but could be included later as a correction to length change; (3) acoustic loading effects of F0 by the vocal tract were omitted, but could be included later as a correction to amplitude of vibration; and (4) lateral depth of vibration into the tissue was assumed to be proportional to amplitude of vibration at the medial surface. In addition to these assumptions, the model may suffer from possible inaccuracy of certain anatomical and physiological parameters, such as the torque ratio and gain for rotation about the cricothyroid joint, the stress-strain curve for the human vocal fold cover, and the maximum active stress in the thyroarytenoid muscle. Further experiments are underway to refine these parameters.

With these stated limitations (and others that the author has perhaps overlooked), one might question the entire enterprise of attempting to relate F0 to muscle activity through a physical model. Perhaps a statistical model is the only viable one. The potential pay-off is too great, however, to consider an early bail-out. The establishment of causal relations between neural inputs to speech muscles and the resulting acoustic output is of great concern to virtually all speech and voice scientists today. At this stage, the model can explain (1) why the thyroarytenoid muscle is effective as an F0 raiser at low (speech) frequencies, but less effective at high frequencies, (2) why certain frequencies are difficult to achieve with nearly equal levels of activity in the cricothyroid and thyroarytenoid muscles, (3) why lung pressure raises F0 and allows higher frequencies to be achieved with the same laryngeal muscle activities, and (4) why certain frequencies may be attainable with multiple combinations of cricothyroid and thyroarytenoid activities. These results offer considerable encouragement to pursue this line of biomechanical modeling.

ACKNOWLEDGEMENTS

This work is supported by the National Institutes of Health, research grant No. DC 00159-09. The author expresses appreciation to Sharon Seymour and Linnie Southard for manuscript preparation and to David Druker for graphics work.

REFERENCES

Alipour-Haghighi, F., Titze, I., and Perlman, A. (1989). Tetanic contraction in vocal fold muscle. *J. Speech Hear. Res*, 32(2):226-231.

Fujimura, O. (1981). Body-cover theory of the vocal fold and its phonetic implications. In: *Vocal Fold Physiology*, edited by K. Stevens and M. Hirano, pp.271-281. University of Tokyo Press, Tokyo.

Hirano, M., Vennard, W., and Ohala, J. (1970). Regulation of register, pitch, and intensity of voice: An electromyographic investigation of intrinsic laryngeal muscles. *Folia Phoniatr.*, 22:1-20.

Hirano, M. (1976). Morphological structure of the vocal cord as a vibrator and its variations. *Folia Phoniatr.*, 26:89-94.

Hollien, H. (1960). Vocal pitch variation related to changes in vocal fold length. *J. Speech Hear. Res*, 3(2):150-156.

Honda, K., and Fujimura, O. (1991). Intrinsic vowel F0 and phrase-final F0 lowering: phonological vs. biological explanations. In: *Vocal Fold Physiology: Acoustic, Perceptual, and Physiological Aspects of Voice Mechanism*, edited by J. Gauffin and B. Hammarberg (this volume).

Ludlow, C., Sedory, S., Fujita, M. (1989). Correlations between intrinsic laryngeal muscles during different speech gestures. In: *Festschrift for Osamu Fujimura*, edited by S. Kiritani, H. Hirose, and H. Fujisaki, (in press). Ohmsha Publishers, Tokyo.

Nishizawa, N., Sawashima, M., and Yonemoto, K. (1988). Vocal length in vocal pitch change. In: *Vocal Physiology: Voice Production, Mechanisms, and Function,* edited by O. Fujimura, pp. 75-82. Raven Press, New York.

Perlman, A., and Durham, P. (1987). In vitro studies of vocal fold mucosa during isometric conditions. In: *Laryngeal Function in Phonation and Respiration*, edited by T. Baer, C. Sasaki, and K. Harris, pp. 291-303. Little and Brown, Boston.

Titze, I. (1989a). On the relation between subglottal pressure and fundamental frequency in phonation. *J. Acoust. Soc. Am.*, 85:901-906.

Titze, I. (1989b). Physiologic and acoustic differences between male and female voices. *J. Acoust. Soc. Am.*, 85(4):1699-1707.

Titze, I., Jiang, J., and Druker, D. (1987). Preliminaries to the body-cover model of pitch control. *J. Voice*, 1(4):314-319.

Titze, I., Luschei, E., and Hirano, M. (1989). Role of the thyroarytenoid muscle in regulation of fundamental frequency. *J. Voice*, 3(3):213-224.

18

Airflow-Based Analysis of Vocal Function

Martin Rothenberg and Karen Nezelek

Dept. of Electrical and Computer Eng., Syracuse University, Syracuse, New York 13244, USA

One of the few noninvasive methods available for obtaining a clinically useful estimate or description of the vibratory pattern of the vocal folds is the inverse filtering of either the airflow or pressure waveform at the mouth (Rothenberg, 1973, 1977), that is, the processing of the waveform at the mouth with a filtering system that has a transform approximately the inverse of that of the vocal tract between glottis and lips. For clinical purposes, inverse filtering of the airflow at the mouth rather than the pressure is preferable, since only the airflow method results in a known zero level and an easily calibrated airflow scale for the resulting glottal flow waveform. The circumferentially-vented wire-screen pneumotachograph mask has been shown to yield an oral volume velocity waveform adequate for inverse-filtering up to about 1 kHz to 2 kHz, depending on the mask configuration.

Though such a mask, combined with a manually-adjusted inverse filter, is now being used by many voice research laboratories and a small number of research-oriented clinical facilities, the necessity of properly adjusting the inverse filter parameters for each subject - to match the frequency and damping of the lowest one or two formants (vocal tract resonances) - makes this system impractical for general clinical use. To overcome this problem, a number of laboratories are attempting to develop computer-based, automated inverse filtering algorithms (for example, Javkin, et al., 1987 and Gauffin, et al., 1986). Though of possible value in the long term, presently proposed automated schemes can produce large errors if the program errs. This is likely to occur for grossly abnormal voices, such as highly breathy voices, or in the presence of significant nasality. Both of these conditions are counter to the assumptions upon which automated inverse-filtering schemes are normally predicated. Sophisticated schemes for automated inverse-filtering which are robust under a wide variety of voice conditions are yet to be developed.

This paper proposes a system for the airflow-based analysis of vocal function employing a processing scheme for airflow signals that appears to bypass the pitfalls inherent in standard inverse filtering and provide an easily used and robust method for obtaining from the oral airflow waveform those parameters of the glottal waveform having the most significance in clinical applications. The method uses the output of a wide-band circumferentially-vented wire-screen pneumotachograph mask during a spoken vowel having a high first formant, such as /æ/ or /a/ in English, to derive a set of parameters adequate for reconstructing a simplified or stylized version of the glottal waveform. These parameters are:

1. T_0, the fundamental period of each cycle of the quasiperiodic flow waveform.

2. P, the peak airflow attained during each period T_0.
3. L, the minimum (lowest) airflow during each period, sometimes referred to as the waveform offset from zero flow.
4. M, the mean or average airflow during each period.
5. Q_o, often referred to as the open quotient, which is the fraction of each period T_0 during which the vocal folds are essentially not in contact.

Each of these variables relates to physiologically significant variables of clinical interest: (1) The importance of T_0 as the primary determinant of voice pitch is unquestioned. (2) For a given subglottal pressure, the minimum flow L indicates the degree to which the vocal folds do not attain a complete closure during the vibratory cycle. (3) The peak flow P, or peak-to-peak flow P-L, would correlate well with the peak variation in glottal area and, therefore, with vocal fold mobility and oscillatory efficiency, assuming a given level of subglottal pressure and ab-adductory force. (4) The mean flow M determines the rate of deflation of the lungs. (5) The open quotient Q_o tends to reflect the degree of abduction or adduction of the vocal folds (as does P).

The proposed method is based on certain very general assumptions related to the nature of glottal waveforms, namely, that (1) the primary excitation of the vocal tract resonances for each glottal cycle occurs during the glottal closing phase, after the occurrence of the peak glottal flow, (2) the vocal tract resonances are more highly damped during the open phase of the glottal cycle, and (3) any strong waveform discontinuity in slope - most significantly the abrupt flattening of the waveform caused by the closing of the vocal folds over some portion of their length - will tend to occur near the smaller values of instantaneous airflow rather than the higher values. These assumptions are well supported in the literature and result from the basic physics of vocal fold vibration and vocal tract acoustics. Finally, we assume that for the clinical evaluation of vocal fold vibratory behaviour it is sufficient to record such behaviour during an open vowel, such as /æ/ or /a/.

Under these assumptions, reasonable estimates of the peak and minimum values of the glottal volume velocity waveform can be obtained by measuring the peak and minimum values of low-pass filtered versions of the flow waveform at the mouth. From the first two assumptions it can be inferred that there is little formant energy added to the glottal flow by the vocal tract at the instant of peak glottal flow; the formants would be stimulated just after the peak flow for the previous glottal cycle, and the resulting energy would have largely decayed by the time that the peak flow occurs, since the peak flow occurs near, usually just after, the instant of maximum glottal area. (See for example Rothenberg, 1973, Figure 16, or Rothenberg, 1977, Figure 8). Thus, a small amount of smoothing or low-pass filtering of the oral waveform, to further reduce formant energy during the glottal open phase, should be sufficient to yield a waveform with a peak value close to that of the glottal waveform. As we have previously shown, a low-pass filter with good phase response and little or no overshoot in its transient response, such as a Bessel-derived filter, can be used for this purpose, if the cutoff frequency of the filter is chosen to be above F0 but significantly below the frequency of the first formant F1 (Rothenberg, 1977, Figure 8).

The minimum value of the glottal waveform is especially well retained by such filtering, since, during the period of relatively constant glottal flow level during a closed phase, there is time for the low-pass filter output to approach this level. For waveforms with little or no closed phase, the low-pass filtering, as long as it is significantly above

F0, will still yield a reasonable minimum value, since the Fourier component at F0 will tend to dominate in both the oral and glottal waveforms.

We describe below two implementations of this procedure, as well as initial test results for speakers having a variety of voice qualities. In the implementations to be described, an approximate F1 inverse filter stage was added to the low-pass filtering to increase accuracy with very strong voices, that is, with voices having a relatively high amount of energy at the formant frequencies.

Method - first experiment

In our first experiment with the newly proposed method, we implemented an automatic parameter measurement system of the type outlined and compared the resulting parameter values with the values obtained by means of a standard inverse-filtering procedure in which the filter parameters are manually adjusted by a trained operator while observing the filtered waveform during a repetitive playback of the voice sample. The system was tested with 29 subjects having a variety of voice qualities.

The test system was implemented on a Data Precision DATA 6000 microprocessor-based waveform analyzer, with some of the signal filtering performed in analog form, before A-D conversion. The system is shown in Figure 1. The output of an airflow mask having a double layer of 500 mesh wire screen and a flow resistance of about 0.5 cm H_2O/liter per second (Glottal Enterprises model MA-2) and a Laryngograph electroglottograph were recorded on FM tape. The electroglottograph signal was included to allow independent measurements of T_0 and Q_o, though it was realized that measurements of Q_o derived from airflow and EGG signal could be quite different. The EGG signal was also used occasionally as an indication of the glottal closed period in setting the manual inverse filter parameters (Rothenberg, 1979).

During analysis, a 40 msec segment of each vowel to be tested was first captured on a two-channel, wide-bandwidth transient storage unit. This segment was then recorded in the DATA 6000 signal analyzer in four forms:

(1) On Channel 1, a manually inverse-filtered glottal waveform was recorded, using a standard analog filter (Glottal Enterprises model MSIF). Though four formants could be removed by this filter, only three zero pairs (antiresonances or antiformants) had any noticeable effect on the waveform for the voices tested.

(2) On Channel 2, an airflow signal was recorded that was passed through a single-formant approximate inverse filter set for the average first formant for the vowel /ae/ for adult males, adult females or children, depending on the subject, as taken from the classical study by Peterson and Barney (1952). The antiformant (complex zero) damping factor was set to zero, though it was later determined that a setting of about 0.5 in damping factor would have led to slightly more accurate values of L in some cases. An 8-pole Bessel low-pass filter with -3dB cutoff frequency set at 2/3 times the average formant frequency for that subject category (Male, Female or Child) was also used to further attenuate the formant energy, as required by the proposed system design for estimating the minimum glottal airflow parameter L. The Channel 2 signal was also used by the DATA 6000 for estimating the waveform period T_0 and the mean airflow M.

(3) On Channel 3, the airflow waveform was only slightly low-pass filtered, using an 8-pole Bessel filter set to -3dB at the relatively high value of 1.5 times the average F1 for the subject-age category. According to the system design, the maximum of this signal during T_0 would be used for estimating the peak glottal airflow P.

(4) The EGG waveform was recorded on Channel 4.

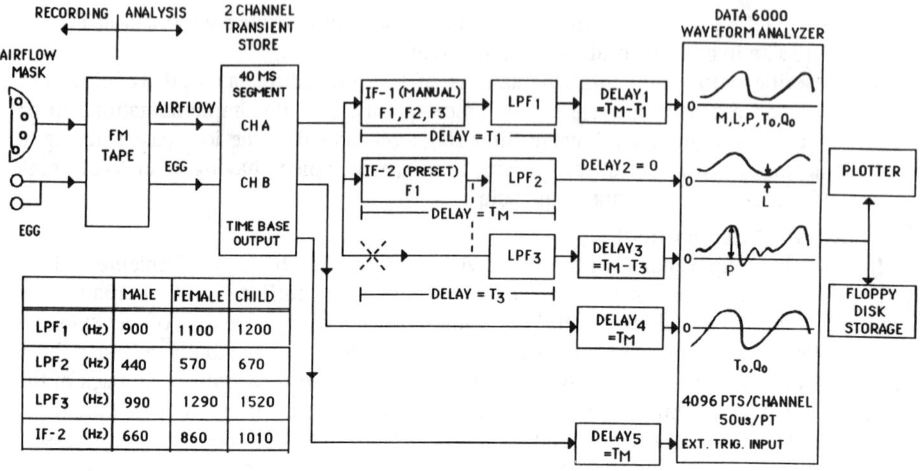

	MALE	FEMALE	CHILD
LPF1 (Hz)	900	1100	1200
LPF2 (Hz)	440	570	670
LPF3 (Hz)	990	1290	1520
IF-2 (Hz)	660	860	1010

Fig. 1. Analysis system used. The dashed lines show changes for the second experiment. Settings for LPF3 in the second experiment were changed to 660 Hz (Male), 850 Hz (Female), and 1010 Hz (Child). The time delay units were adjusted to put all waveforms in correct time alignment.

A program on the DATA 6000 automatically derived T_0, M, L, P and Q_o. T_0 was measured at a criterion level approximately half way between the maximum and minimum values of the captured sample in Channel 2, and M was computed as the mean of all data points in the Channel 2 waveform during the period T_0. L and P were measured according to the rules indicated in Figure 1.

The open quotient Q_o was estimated from the airflow parameters P, L and M by assuming a model for the glottal waveform of a sinusoid truncated at its lower extreme. According to this model, Q_o is uniquely related to P, L and M by the equation:

$$\frac{\sin(\pi Q_o) - \pi Q_o \cos(\pi Q_o)}{1 - \cos(\pi Q_o)} = \frac{\pi M}{P - L}$$

We found this equation to yield a reasonable first approximation for Q_o, given accurate estimates of P, L and M.

The system in Figure 1 was tested using 29 subjects as follows:

6 normal adult males
6 dysfunctional adult males
6 normal adult females
3 dysfunctional adult females
7 normal children (5 female and 2 male, 7 to 13 years old)
1 dysfunctional child (male, 11 years old).

The dysfunctional adults included cases of laryngitis, diplophonia secondary to laryngitis, Parkinson's disease, post-surgery-trauma-induced left vocal fold paralysis, trauma-induced breathiness, and simulated hyperfunctional-adducted phonation. The child's vocal dysfunction was caused by a vocal fold nodule. Each subject was asked to vocalize

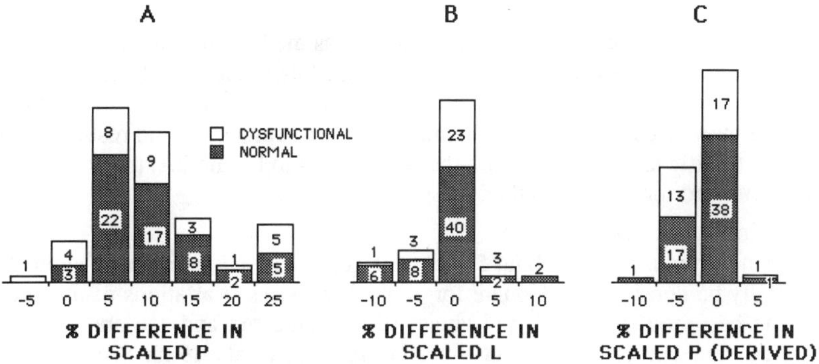

Fig. 2. Histograms showing the distribution of the percent difference between the automatic and manually filtered airflow waveforms. In all cases, the percent difference was scaled as a percentage of the manually filtered peak airflow value.

a short held /æ/ at a normal, conversational level, and at levels roughly 6dB above and below this level, as monitored by the subject on a digital (LED) level display. The subject's most comfortable pitch was used at each level. Twenty-eight subjects produced 3 loudness levels and 1 subject produced 4 loudness levels, resulting in a total of 88 data points. The manual inverse-filtering was performed by the second author or a graduate research assistant, with each previously trained in this task by the first author.

Results - first experiment

We now consider the accuracy of the test system, using the manual inverse filter result as a standard. We collapse our results across loudness, sex and age in the following discussions, since scatter plots for the measures discussed indicated that accuracy did not vary significantly with any of these variables, except for a slight tendency toward more variability in the case of loud phonation.

Measurements of T_0 in almost all cases showed differences of less than two percent from measurements made from the EGG waveform. This degree of accuracy would be expected from the results reported previously for airflow-derived T_0 measurements (Rothenberg, 1977). As would also be expected, measurements of mean airflow (M) made from the Channel 2 signal were essentially the same as those from the manually inverse filtered signal, since the filtering procedures have no effect on the mean airflow. Q_o measurements roughly agreed with the predictions from the EGG signal, but no quantitative estimate of the correlation was derived, since the accuracy of the flow-derived Q_o would depend greatly on the accuracy of the estimates of L and P.

Thus, the parameters of most interest in these tests were the peak and minimum values of airflow. In Figure 2A, the value of peak airflow P derived by the automatic procedure (Channel 3) is compared with the value obtained by manual inverse filtering. The percentage error was computed assuming the manual procedure to be the reference or accurate condition. It can be seen that the errors were generally positive, resulting in values about 10% too high. This error occurred for both normal and disordered voices.

As shown in Figure 2B, the error for the minimum value L was generally less than 5%, with the automated procedure tending to give values slightly less than the manual filtering. As in Figure 2A, the percentage calculation was made with reference to the peak value of the manually inverse-filtered waveform, since this reference reflects the scale of interest for a particular waveform. (Since minimum values can be very small, or even zero, using the more accurate minimum value for the denominator would result in "error" percentages with little meaning.) As with the peak values in Figure 2A, the accuracy was generally maintained for both normal and disordered voices.

Interpretation - first experiment

The error in minimum value, about 5% of peak flow, with a maximum of about 10%, would generally be considered adequate for clinical purposes. Variations of much more than 10% can be found among normal voices of the same sex and age and in a single voice within a sentence or at different times (Holmberg, et al., 1988; Karlsson, 1988; Schutte, 1980). The tendency for this error to be negative indicates that the errors may be largely due to remanent first formant energy not removed by the automated filtering. This might explain why there are proportionally more normal voices (with stronger F1 energy) that show the higher errors. Thus, some increase in the strength of the low-pass filtering, or a small reduction in the cutoff value, could conceivably reduce the error further and remove the negative bias.

The error in peak value *P* was of somewhat more concern, though the errors shown might still be acceptable for most applications. Because the error tended to be positive (from the approximately filtered waveform exceeding the assumed true glottal waveform), it was also deemed to be caused by some remanent F1 energy. This was verified by the data in Figure 2C, in which the peak of the more highly filtered Channel 2 waveform was used as the test value. It can be seen that the Channel 2 peak was generally within about 5 to 10% of the accurately filtered value, with a slight tendency toward a too negative value, as would be caused by the overfiltering of the waveform. Thus, an optimum filter for peak value would lie somewhere between those used for Channel 2 and Channel 3. This hypothesis was supported by the additional experiment to be described below.

Thus, Figure 2 indicates that if the average error could be removed, an accuracy of 10% when compared to actual peak airflow can be attained by the new automated system in almost all cases, with most measurements within 5%. However, the presence of a few outliers with possible errors of over 15% was disturbing, since a presumed advantage of the new system was its robust procedure, that is, the absence of any feature that could cause a large error in unusual cases. To probe this potential problem further, a few of the outlying measurements were examined by comparing the print-outs of the waveforms in each channel of the DATA 6000. In each case, the "error" was associated with a potentially incorrect manually inverse-filtered waveform; the vocalization did not have the long, clearly defined closed phase near zero flow that makes the inverse-filter settings unambiguous. For example, in some cases a detailed examination of the waveforms suggested that the Channel 2 low-pass filtered waveform better preserved the true minimum glottal flow than did the presumably accurate, manually filtered waveform.

It therefore appeared to us that some significant proportion of the variance in the "errors" reported in Figure 2 was, in actuality, caused by errors in the parameters of the reference waveform. To investigate this possibility, as well as to test a revised filtering procedure in Channel 3 for measuring *P*, as suggested above, the following additional experiment was performed.

Method - reevaluation experiment

In this second, reevaluation experiment, data from six of the original subjects, chosen to represent the widest variety of glottal waveform types, were reprocessed with the system revised as shown by the dashed lines in Figure 1. The same analysis procedure was used, except that the manual inverse filtering for each sample was performed independently by four members of the research staff, including the two persons performing the previous inverse filter adjustments. Each adjuster had extensive experience in this task.

In the revised system, the filtering for Channel 3 was altered to include the approximate F1 inverse filter, and had a reduced low-pass setting, according to our interpretation of the results in Figure 2, A and B, above. In addition, the damping factor of the approximate F1 inverse-filter was changed from zero to 0.5 to match the approximate average vocal tract damping with the mask in place. The multiple versions of the manual inverse filtering were meant to give some indication of the variability possible in the manually set antiformants and the resulting variability in the reference values of P and L.

Results - reevaluation experiment.

Results from the second experiment indicated that the biases in the estimation of both P and L are essentially removed in the revised system. An increased variability in the error values was found, since some of the more difficult-to-inverse-filter voices were included in the sample of six subjects; however, an appreciable part of this variability appeared to be due to inaccuracy in the manual inverse filtering of the reference waveforms, as discussed above. This conclusion is supported by the fact that the highest error values generally occurred with disordered voices that tended to be breathy. These waveforms usually had no clear, flat "closed" period near zero flow in the inverse-filtered waveform to act as a reference in the adjustment procedure. In addition, informal observations with other subjects confirmed that little variance between experimenters is present when there is a clear closed phase with little or no airflow, as was the case for our sample of a healthy male voice.

The variability in the formant settings for breathy voices is shown in Figure 3. The first-formant settings (the most significant formant in determining the waveshape) are shown for all four experimenters, for each of the six subjects. Also shown as a measure of relative breathiness is the ratio L/P, as averaged over all reference values. This ratio will be zero if a complete glottal closure is attained during the closed period and approaches unity for very breathy voices. It appears from the figure that the variability in the formant settings is to some extent correlated with this measure of breathiness.

To show the effect on the waveform of the range of formant settings obtained by the different adjusters, Figure 4 presents the manually inverse-filtered waveforms from a vocalization by an 11-year-old boy diagnosed as having a vocal nodule. Though the resulting waveforms are grossly the same, there would be a significant variance in the resulting values for the minimum value L and, to a lesser extent, for the peak value P. It should be emphasized that without further knowledge there is no way to choose with confidence the most accurate waveform among the four. Even a waveform that shows some residual F1 energy near its minimum value could be correct, since there could be (and probably is) some F1 energy passing through the open glottis during that time interval.

Reconstructing Idealized Waveforms

The airflow-based analysis system we envision would print out for each subject, in addition to the measured numerical parameter values, an idealized glottal airflow waveform

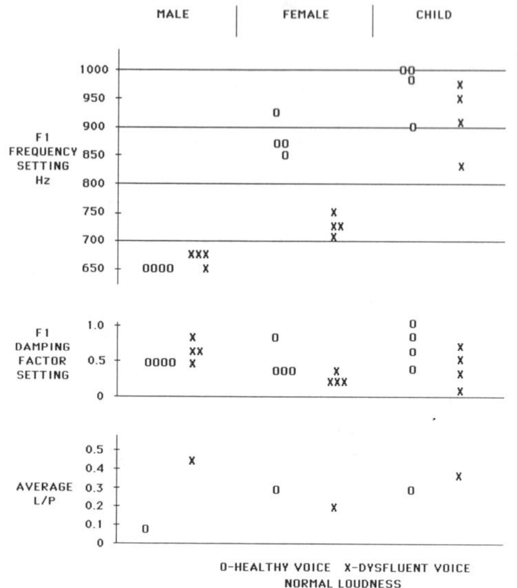

Fig. 3. Variation in the formant settings over four experimenters

Fig. 4. Variation between adjusters in the manually adjusted inverse-filter output for the 11-year-old boy with a vocal fold nodule.

that conforms to these values. This type of graphical printout would greatly simplify judgments of vocal function by making visually transparent the interrelationship of the various parameters and would also facilitate intra- and intersubject comparisons. In addition, when the analysis is performed separately for a number of consecutive glottal cycles, the resulting reconstructed waveform would exhibit more clearly the nature of any gross aperiodicities.

To test the viability of this type of graphical printout, the analysis results from three of the subjects were transferred manually from the DATA 6000 system to a microcomputer which generated the required idealized waveform, given the measured parameter values. To conform to the truncated sinusoidal approximation of the glottal pulse described above, the idealized glottal volume-velocity Ug is defined by

$$U_g = \frac{P-L}{1-\cos(\pi Q_o)}\cos\frac{2\pi t}{T_0} + P - \frac{P-L}{1-\cos(\pi Q_o)}$$

during the "open" periods, and remains at L during the "closed" periods. This equation results in a symmetrical waveform that has the required values of T_0, M, L, P, and Q_o. To show a diversity of waveform types, the subjects chosen for this exercise were an adult male known to have a strong, efficient voice, the adult male Parkinson's disease patient, and the 7-year-old healthy female child.

Parts A, B and C of Figure 5 compare the reconstructed glottal flow waveforms with the output of the manually-adjusted inverse-filter. The child's waveform is also shown with an enlarged flow scale, because of the much lower flow values. It can be seen from the figure that the reconstructed waveforms retain most of the significant properties of the manually obtained inverse-filtered waveforms, while eliminating many of the details -

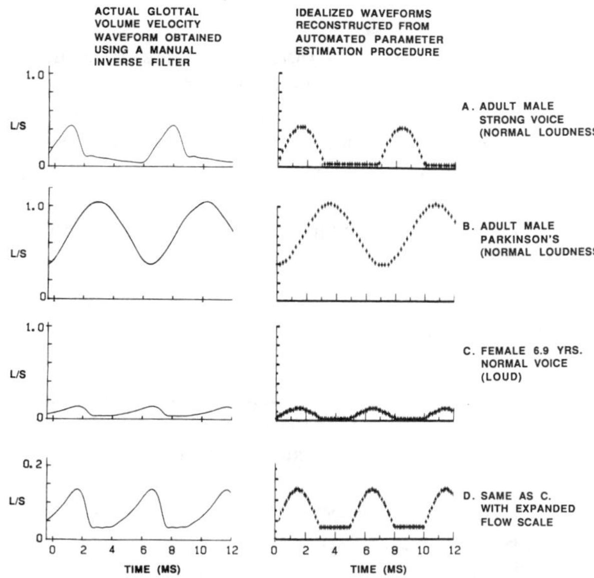

Fig. 5. Three representative reconstructed glottal flow waveforms as compared with the output of the manually adjusted inverse-filter.

such as a slight closed-period slope or remanent F1 energy - which would be of minimal interest to the clinician. The most notable exception is the asymmetry, or skewing to the right, of the glottal pulse that occurs in stronger voices; this is caused primarily by source-tract acoustic interaction and does not directly reflect vocal fold movements. However, if it is eventually found to be of interest clinically, this asymmetry could be inserted into the idealized waveform and the corresponding computation of Q_O, using a simple model of a source-tract interaction such as the one which was originally proposed by the author (Rothenberg, 1981) or a similar model proposed by Fant (1983). A measure of spectral balance or spectral slope for the mask waveform that reflected the relative strength of the higher frequency harmonics could also be used to help determine the degree of asymmetry, since a strengthening of the higher frequency harmonics is a primary correlate of this asymmetry.

CONCLUSIONS

The results described above indicate that an automated parameter extraction system similar to our revised system can be constructed that will have a standard deviation that is no more than 5% of the peak airflow value for measurements of both the minimum and peak flow values. This system will be robust in that it will rarely result in errors of more than about 10% of the peak flow value when used according to the designated protocol (mask seal adjusted for no leakage, vowel similar to /æ/ or /a/). More precise determinations of system error than those made in this project will be difficult to obtain without some independent verification of the actual glottal airflow waveform that is more accurate than manual inverse-filtering by a highly trained operator. There is no method now available for such a verification in the human vocal tract, though a model experiment (mechanical, animal or computer) might be possible.

However, as pointed out above, a variance of 5%, or even 10%, in the measured values is not unreasonable for a clinical system, given the larger variance found among normal voices or in the same voice at different times. The other side of this coin must be that there are clinically significant variations in these airflow parameters that exceed 5% to 10%. This is generally acknowledged for average airflow, which has long been easy to measure, and evidence that this is also true for the parameters of peak and minimum airflow is evolving in current studies of breathy, hyperfunctional and aging voice (Fritzell, et al., 1983; Hillman, et al., 1988; Higgins, 1989).

The extrapolation of Q_o from M, L and P also appears to be a reasonable alternative to other presently-proposed noninvasive procedures for estimating this variable.

ACKNOWLEDGEMENTS

The research reported here was supported by Research Grant NS-08919 to Syracuse University and by a Small Business Innovative Research (SBIR) Grant to Glottal Enterprises, both from the National Institutes of Health. The measurements reported were performed with the able assistance of Ashok Kalyanswamy, who was responsible for the implementation and monitoring of the DATA 6000-based analysis system and helped in the analysis procedure. Roy Thomas assisted in the design of the microcomputer-based system used for Figure 5. Richard Molitor was the fourth adjuster.

REFERENCES

Fant, G. (1983). Preliminaries to analysis of the human voice source. *Speech Communication Group Working Papers* 3, (Research Laboratory of Electronics, Massachusetts Institute of Technology).

Fritzell, B., Gauffin, J., Hammarberg, B., Karlsson, I., and Sundberg, J. (1983). Measuring insufficient vocal fold closure during phonation. *STL-QPSR* 4:50-59. (Dept. of Speech Communication and Music Acoustics, Royal Institute of Technology, Stockholm).

Gauffin, J., Hammarberg, B., and Imaizumi, S. (1986). A microcomputer based system for acoustic analsyis of voice characteristics. *Proc. ICASSP 86*, Tokyo, 1:681-684.

Higgins, M. (1989). *A Comparison of Selected Laryngeal Behaviors of Aged and Young Adult Healthy Speakers.* Unpublished doctoral dissertation. Syracuse University, Syracuse.

Hillman, R., Holmberg, E., Perkell, J., Walsh, M., and Vaughan, C. (1988). Objective assessment of vocal hyperfunction: an experimental framework and preliminary results. *Speech Commun. Group Working Papers,* 6:67-135. (Res. Lab. of Electronics, MIT)

Holmberg, E., Hillman, R., and Perkell, J. (1988). Glottal airflow and transglottal air pressure measurements for male and female speakers in soft, normal and loud voice. *J. Acoust. Soc. Amer.* 84:511-519.

Javkin, H.R., Antonanzas-Barroso, N. and Maddieson, I. (1987). Digital inverse filtering for linguistic research. *J. Speech Hear. Res.* 30:122-129.

Karlsson, I. (1988). Glottal waveform parameters for different speaker types. *STL-QPSR* 2-3:61-63. (Dept. of Speech Communication and Music Acoustics, Royal Institute of Technology, Stockholm).

Peterson, G. and Barney, H. (1952). Control methods used in a study of the vowels, *J. Acoust. Soc. Amer.* 24:175-184.

Rothenberg, M. (1973). A new inverse-filtering technique for deriving the glottal airflow waveform during voicing. *J. Acoust. Soc. Amer.* 53:1632-1645.

Rothenberg, M. (1977). Measurement of airflow in speech. *J. Speech Hear. Res.* 20:155-176.

Rothenberg, M. (1979). Some relations between glottal airflow and vocal fold contact area. Proceedings of the Conference on the Assessment of Vocal Pathology, *ASHA Reports* 11: 88-96.

Rothenberg, M. (1981). Acoustic interaction between the glottal source and vocal tract. In: *Vocal Fold Physiology*, edited by K.N. Stevens and H. Hirano, pp. 305-328, Tokyo Press, Tokyo.

Schutte, H. (1980). *The Efficiency of Voice Production.* Kemper, Groningen, Netherlands.

19

Intrinsic Vowel F0 and Phrase-Final F0 Lowering: Phonological vs. Biological Explanations

Kiyoshi Honda and *Osamu Fujimura

*Kanazawa Institute of Technology, Kanazawa Minami 921, Japan ,*Ohio State University, Speech and Hearing Science, Columbus, OH 43210, USA*

There have been observations in many languages that different vowels tend to exhibit slight but significant differences in F0 values, *ceteris paribus*, in speech utterances (Peterson and Barney, 1952; Lehiste and Peterson, 1961). Roughly speaking, high vowels tend to have a high F0, and low vowels have a low F0. An electromyographic study conducted by one of the authors at Haskins Laboratories (Honda, 1983) has provided some physiological explanation relating the tongue gestures inherent in vowel articulations to laryngeal positions, affecting F0 in the directions observed, resulting in inherent and largely universal F0 differences among vowels.

Figure 1 depicts such a mechanism of interaction between tongue gesture and laryngeal position, mediated by the hyoid bone. The tongue and the larynx are interconnected via the hyoid bone by means of a number of muscles and connective tissue. Because of these connections, the hyoid bone's position tends to change in accordance with tongue gesture. For example, in producing the high front vowel /i/, the hyoid bone moves forward and slightly downward due to the contraction of the posterior genioglossus. In contrast, for the low back vowel /ɑ/, the hyoid bone moves back and upward in conjunction with the pulled back position of the tongue. Since the whole larynx is suspended by the hyoid bone (among other structures), hyoid bone movements generally create some force to act on the larynx. The vertical component of the force causes a vertical movement of the larynx, and its horizontal component can rotate the thyroid cartilage around the cricothyroid joint. In particular, a forward movement of the hyoid bone rotates the thyroid cartilage forward, stretching the vocal folds (see below). This movement is equivalent to the action of the cricothyroid as far as raising F0 is concerned.

This interpretation is supported by electromyographic data (Alfonso et al., 1982; Baer et al., 1988). These studies used electromyographic data from four major extrinsic tongue muscles (anterior and posterior genioglossus, styloglossus and hyoglossus) that were collected simultaneously from one male speaker with those from the cricothyroid and the orbicularis oris. Among these extrinsic tongue muscles, the activity of the posterior genioglossus muscle showed a high correlation with the intrinsic vowel F0. Figure 2

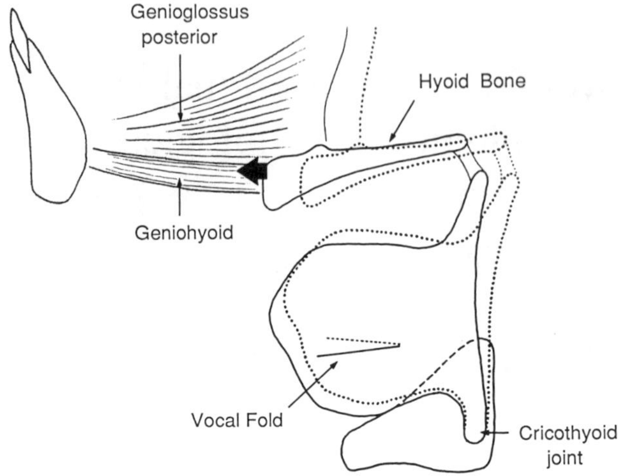

Fig 1. Supplementary tensor mechanism (Honda, 1986) which explains the biomechanical interaction between the tongue and the larynx. The geniohyoid muscle pulls the hyoid bone forward and causes the thyroid cartilage to rotate forward by pulling its superior horns, resulting in raising F0. Tongue gestures involve hyoid bone movement and thus activate this mechanism.

shows the relationship between the peak activity of the posterior genioglossus muscle for vowels and the intrinsic vowel F0 reported by Lehiste and Peterson (1961). This muscle is the largest among the extrinsic tongue muscles and the most important in determining the overall shape of the tongue. It is characteristically active for high vowels. Since the posterior genioglossus muscle ends in the posterior part of the tongue which has some tissue linkage to the hyoid bone, when it contracts it affects vowel F0 by pulling the hyoid bone forward.

Additional support for the relationship between hyoid bone position and vowel F0 is found in the electromyographic signals from the geniohyoid muscle. This muscle has a direct insertion into the hyoid bone and becomes active in phonations involving high F0. It is suggested that the geniohyoid contraction supplements the cricothyroid activity in raising F0 by pulling the hyoid bone forward. When the hyoid bone moves forward, the superior horns of the thyroid cartilage are pulled forward, tilting the cartilage forward. This function of the hyoid bone in F0 control is called "a supplementary tensor mechanism" (Honda, 1986). The posterior genioglossus muscle shows similar effects when it contracts. Thus, intrinsic vowel F0 can be explained by the biomechanical interaction between the tongue and the larynx, mediated by the hyoid bone.

However, by examining the same electromyographic data noted above in detail, we observed unexpected activity in the signals from the cricothyroid muscle, as shown in Figure 3. This activity varied across vowels and exhibited vowel-to-vowel variation similar to that of F0 measured from simultaneously recorded speech signals. Although vowel F0 in the data exhibited slight discrepancies with the intrinsic vowel F0 or the activity of the posterior genioglossus particularly in lax vowels /I/ and /U/ (which might be due to subject's experimental intention to produce acoustically homogeneous data), the activity of the cricothyroid muscle showed a higher activity in high vowels. Therefore, it might be assumed that the cricothyroid muscle alone determined vowel F0,

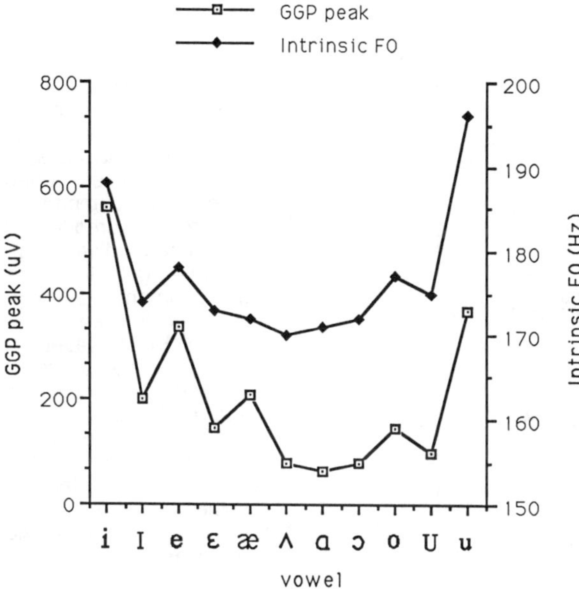

Fig. 2. The EMG activity of the posterior genioglossus muscle (GGP) during production of 11 English vowels in isolated /əpVp/ utterances (open squares) in comparison with the intrinsic vowel F0 (closed diamonds). "GGP peak" represents peak values of the ensemble average waveform of the EMG signals from GGP for ten repetitions, produced by one male speaker. "Intrinsic F0" is computed from the data by Lehiste and Peterson (1961), by averaging the F0 values of the vowels following /p/, /t/, and /k/.

whether the supraglottal influence existed or not. This argument does not explain, however, why the cricothyroid exhibits vowel-to-vowel variation in activity.

Our interpretation is that while the biological circumstances create a phonetic tendency for high vowels, for example, to be associated with high F0, such a tendency has to go through a process of phonologization to create a language-specific rule, in order to account for all aspects of observed characteristics associating intrinsic F0 with vowels in different languages. Once such phonologization takes place, not only can the same F0 effect be used perceptually as one of the cues for vowel features, but also, the same effect can be attained through other biological mechanisms that may be available. Thus the cricothyroid activity associated with high vowels "emulates" the biologically natural F0 rise due to hyoid bone movements.

PHRASE-FINAL F0 LOWERING

A similar argument may apply to an independent case of the so-called pitch declination: the universal tendency to observe a considerable descent in F0 toward the end of an utterance or of a major phrase (which may or may not be followed by a clear pause with an inhalation). Like vowel intrinsic F0, this phenomenon is only a tendency, and there are numerous cases where this does not take place. Even when it does take place, the physiological mechanism described below may not necessarily be the one responsible for the particular event or circumstance. Nevertheless, what follows seems to offer some plausible explanation (in addition to the commonly held notion that F0 generally tends to decline to some extent due to general relaxation) why there is a strong universal tendency for phonologies of different languages to follow this rule of intonation.

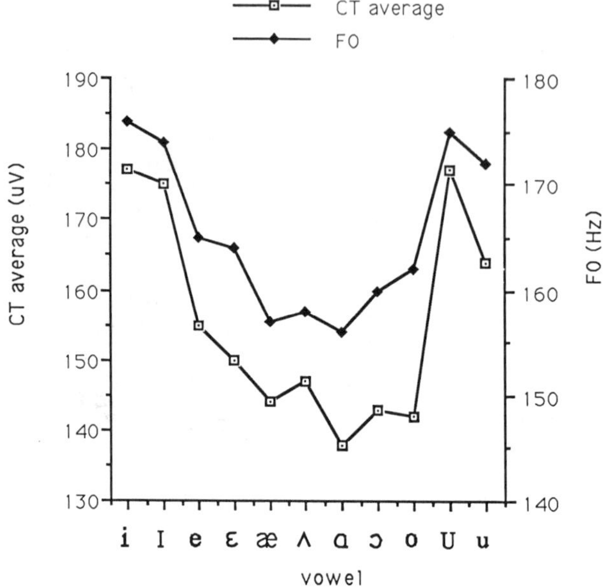

Fig. 3. The EMG activity of the cricothyroid muscle (CT) during productions of the vowels in isolated /əpVp/ utterances (open squares) in comparison with the measured vowel F0 (closed diamonds). "CT average" indicates the segment average values of the ensemble average EMG waveform from CT. The segment averages are computed using a 150-ms time window before the voice onset. "F0" represents the peak F0 values in the ensemble average waveform of vowel F0 in the utterances.

The biological basis for this phrasal declination has been studied by many researchers. Early studies (Ladefoged, 1961; Lieberman, 1967; Ohala and Ladefoged, 1970) proposed that F0 declination is based on relaxation of laryngeal muscles or decreasing pulmonary pressure and air flow. The speculation that there must be some biological basis for F0 descent in the phrasal domain is partly supported by acoustic characteristics of the infant's cry. The declining F0 pattern is always observed in vocalization of neonatal infants.

We can produce a sentence comprising two major phrases without taking a breath. In such a case, the second phrase can be initiated easily by reinforcing laryngeal muscular and/or expiratory activities. In many languages, if not universally, phonologies seem to specify a resetting of initial F0 values for a new major phrase, regardless of what happens to breathing. In contrast to these phrasal initiation effects, phrase final phenomena, in particular F0 lowering, cannot be explained from the same point of view, since the mechanisms for F0 lowering, such as cricothyroid relaxation, are not effective in very low F0 ranges beyond a certain degree of relaxation. On the other hand, F0 lowering can occur toward the end of a major phrase without being followed by inhalation or showing any sign of exhaustion of pulmonary pressure. Also, while the electromyographic signals from the cricothyroid muscle show activities directly related to accented (stressed) syllable nuclei, they do not exhibit high statistical correlations with F0 with respect to sentential declination (Collier and Gelfer, 1984; Gelfer et al., 1983). This is somewhat puzzling, given that most F0 descent throughout a sentence or a major phrase is ascribed to the accumulation of the F0-dropping effect of accents (*i.e.*, catathesis), in English and Japanese at least (see Poser, 1984; Pierrehumbert and Beckman, 1988). Presumably, the lack of any high correlation between laryngeal relaxation and F0 descent in the global domain of major phrases is largely due to phrase-final effects, which contribute poor

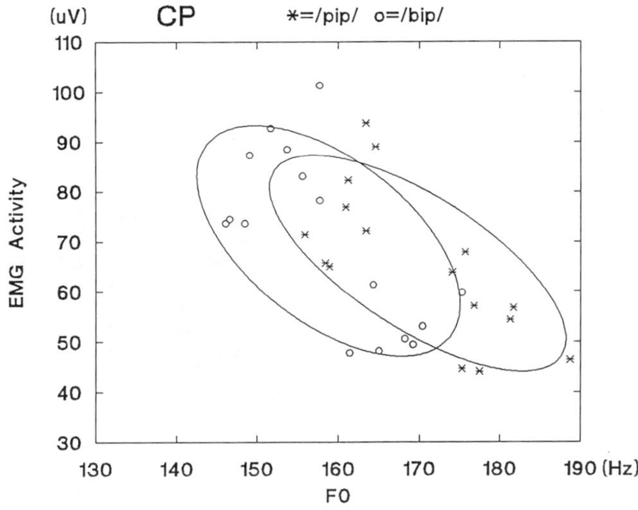

Fig. 4. The EMG activity of the cricopharyngeus (CP) during 16 repetitions of /pip/ and /bip/ utterances in a frame sentence, and the measured vowel F0. Segment averages which correspond to the vowel portion were also computed for both EMG and F0.

correlations to the overall statistics. Thus, the phrasal or configurational effect of F0 descent at the end of a phrase is yet to be accounted for from a physiological point of view. This effect must be set aside from a relatively small effect of true declination, which may remain after subtracting the accent-related catathesis effects.

One of the authors has proposed a new mechanism for F0 lowering (Honda, 1988). Among many laryngeal muscles studied electromyographically, the cricopharyngeus muscle demonstrated an activity which correlated inversely with F0. Figure 4 shows the relationship between the EMG activity of this muscle and vowel F0 in repetitions of word

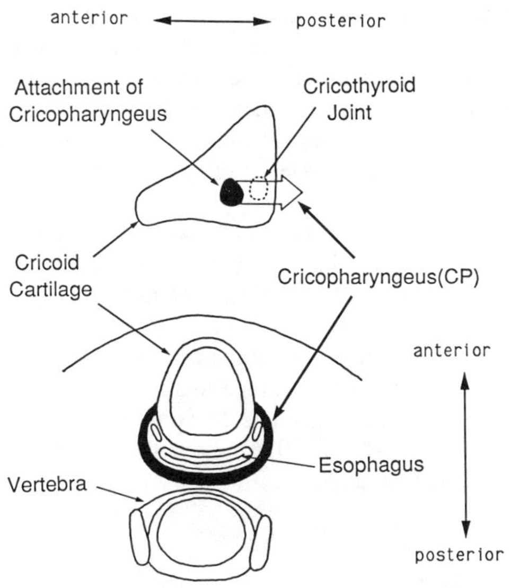

Fig. 5. Schematic drawings of the cricopharyngeus muscle (CP), showing the location of its attachment on the cricoid cartilage and the direction in which the main part of its muscle fibers runs.

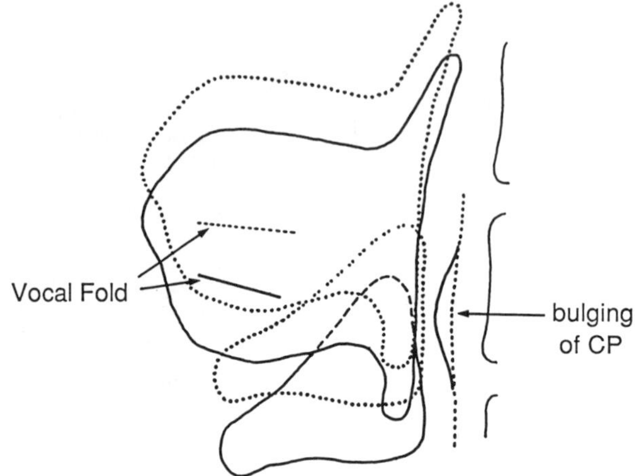

Fig. 6 The speculated mechanism of the crico-pharyngeus muscle for lowering F0. The contraction of CP causes the bulging of muscle belly at the postcricoid region. When larynx lowering takes place, the cricoid cartilage descends its posterior plate held against the slope formed by the bulging of CP, thus pushing the apex of the cricoid cartilage forward.

utterances produced by a male subject. The cricopharyngeus has attachments on the cricoid cartilage at both sides, running around the orifice of the esophagus, as shown in Figure 5. This muscle shows a continuous tonic contraction except for a moment of deglutition in order to function as the sphincter of the esophagus. Since the muscle fibers run semicircularly and the attachments on the cricoid cartilage are located very close to the cricothyroid joint, and since the linkage of this muscle to the posterior structures (including the vertebrae) is loose, a contraction of this muscle does not produce any significant force to pull the cartilage posteriorly. Even if it did, the posterior movement would be stopped by the stiffened muscle itself. Whatever the linkage is between the posterior surface of the muscle and the fixed wall (the vertebrae), the only effect of pulling the cricoid cartilage posteriorly by the semicircular muscle is to shorten the distance between the posterior edge of the cartilage and the center of the muscle, and there is no possibility of shortening the distance between the center of the muscle and the back wall. Unless there are deformable soft tissues that can be compressed significantly between the cricoid cartilage and the cricopharyngeus, there will be no posterior movement of the cartilage. Presumably, the structure lying between the cartilage and the muscle is mainly the esophageal tube, which is completely collapsed during speech, leaving little compliance for compression.

Instead of pulling the cricoid cartilage posteriorly, the bulging of the belly of this muscle by contraction results in a pressure exerted on the cartilage anteriorly. This effect may produce a forward movement of the cartilage. Furthermore, if the larynx is lowered by some other means simultaneously with the contraction of the cricopharyngeus, the result will be that the upper parts of the cricoid cartilage, accompanied by the arytenoids on top, move forward, as shown in Figure 6, tilting the cartilage in such a way that the vocal folds become shortened and slack. This mechanism is in conformity with the vertical movement theory for F0 lowering (see Ewan, 1976), even though the exact mechanism for laryngeal lowering is not yet well understood.

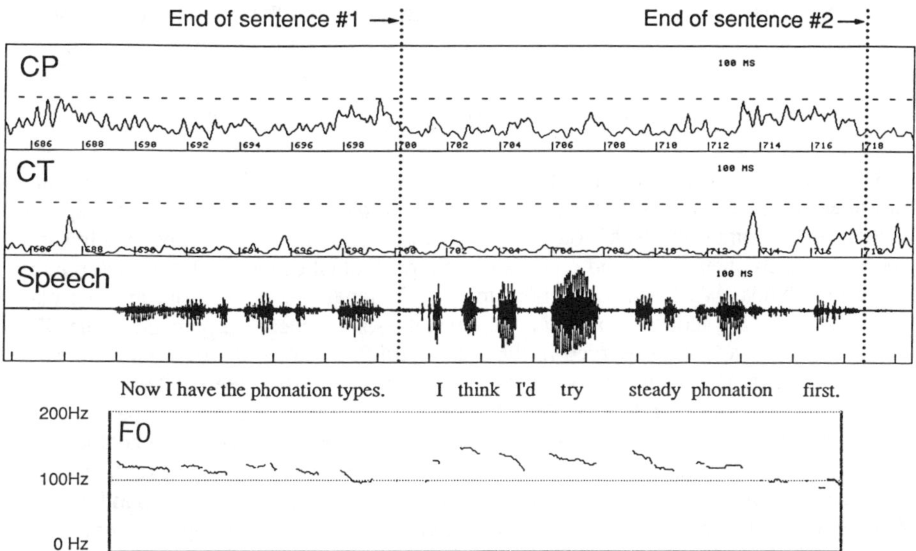

Fig. 7. Integrated EMG waveforms of the cricopharyngeus (CP, top panel) and the cricothyroid (CT, second panel) EMG signals, and the F0 contour (F0, bottom) during production of two declarative sentences. CP activity increases near the end of each sentence where F0 lowering takes place, while CT does not have clear activity change for F0 lowering, even showing paradoxical activities near the end of the second sentence.

The cricopharyngeus muscle shows increased activity during speech, particularly near the end of declarative sentences, as shown in Figure 7. Two sentences with different lengths are shown in the figure. At the end of both sentences, this muscle shows an increase in activity which is approximately twice as high as that for the preceding portions. The longer sentence shows a longer duration of the increased muscular activity. This informal observation suggests that the activity of the cricopharyngeus is relevant to phrase accent and/or final boundary tone (see Pierrehumbert and Beckman, 1988), but it is not clear whether or how its activity duration is related to utterance length. It also indicates the possibility that laryngeal adjustments for F0 are executed by different physiological mechanisms depending on the particular linguistic function, such as final lowering or accentual fall, even for the same physical effect, namely F0 lowering. Thus the use of the cricopharyngeus muscle near the end of a major phrase or an utterance may well be motivated by the fact that in the extremely low frequency range which is likely to be the case at the end of a phrase, this mechanism is the most effective and reliable to achieve F0 lowering required by the phonology of the language. On the other hand, it is also possible that such phonological rules specifying F0 descent at the end of a major phrase themselves may be motivated by a biological need associated with the anticipation of some nonspeech gestures, such as sphincteric closure of the glottis, involving the use of the cricopharyngeus muscle among others. If so, the use of entirely unrelated mechanisms for F0 lowering, such as cricothyroid relaxation (associated with a preceding contraction and resultant F0 ascent for accent manifestation), on the one hand, and cricopharyngeus contraction at the end of a major phrase, on the other hand, may seem only natural.

DISCUSSION

Some of the acoustic characteristics of speech, such as the intrinsic F0 of vowels and phrasal effects on F0, can be explained on the basis of biological characteristics of speech mechanisms. In other words, a biological mechanism generates a basic tendency in some aspect of speech phenomena and contributes to a perceptual cue as well as to naturalness of speech sounds. We learn such characteristics in language acquisition, and we may amplify the relevant acoustic characteristic when it is established as a perceptual cue. The vowel-to-vowel variation observed in the cricothyroid muscle is one of the examples of such phenomena. Once such a cue or its production counterpart constitutes part of the phonetic implementation rule of a phonological unit, the effect is robust. In pathological cases, when the mechanism originally responsible for the effect is not available, it is replaced by an alternative mechanism to produce the same effect. For example, good esophageal speakers can produce the intrinsic F0 of vowels properly (Gandour and Weinberg, 1980), even though there is nothing gained in terms of biological economy of vowel production by doing so. In normal speakers, there may well be different mechanisms employed for achieving the same acoustic characteristics or vocal tract configuration, depending on the particular speaker or particular phonological context, etc. This does not imply, of course, that all phonetic implementation must respect perceptual specifications. There is little doubt that production constraints and principles of economy play important roles in formulating the general strategy of pronunciation, most likely involving certain parameters of the individual speaker's choice. There is also no doubt that listeners are equipped with a powerful capability to cope with variation from speaker to speaker and from context to context under strong constraints in terms of production mechanisms and occasional deviations from the norm.

Considering the use of different biological mechanisms for different phonological elements in languages in typical or prototypical situations seems to help our understanding of the general tendencies observed in formulations of phonological systems, and may well dictate a particular representational framework for linguistic structures in general. However, attempting to rigidly associate particular physiological devices in speech production or, for that matter, particular perceptual patterns, to functional units in phonological specifications may not always be well motivated.

ACKNOWLEDGEMENT

This work is in part supported by NIH research grant NS-13617 to Haskins Laboratories (PI: K. S. Harris). All the data reported here were collected and processed at Haskins Laboratories. The authors are particularly grateful to Thomas Baer and Anders Löfqvist for serving as subjects for the experiments as well as for helpful discussions.

REFERENCES

Alfonso, P.J., Baer, T., Honda, K., and Harris, K.S. (1982). Multi-channel study of tongue EMG during vowel production. *J. Acoust. Soc. Am.* Suppl. 1, 71:S54.

Baer, T., Alfonso, P.J., and Honda, K. (1988). Electromyography of the tongue muscle during vowels in /əpVp/ environment. *Ann. Bull. of RILP*.22:7-20 (University of Tokyo).

Collier, R. and Gelfer, C.E. (1984). Physiological explanation of F0 declination. In: *Proceedings of the 10th International Congress of Phonetic Sciences, IIB*, edited by M.P.R. Van den Bröcke and A. Cohen), pp. 354-360. Foris Publications, Dortrecht.

Ewan, W. (1976). *Laryngeal Behavior in Speech.* Ph.D. dissertation, University of California, Berkeley.

Gandour, J. and Weinberg, B. (1980). On the relationship between vowel height and fundamental frequency: evidence from esophageal speech. *Phonetica* 37:344-354.

Gelfer, C.E., Harris, K.S., Collier, R. and Baer, T. (1983). Is declination actively controlled? In: *Vocal Fold Physiology: Biomechanics, Acoustics, and Phonatory Control*, edited by I. Titze and R. Scherer, pp. 113-126. Denver Center for the Performing Arts, Denver, CO.

Honda, K. (1983). Relationship between pitch control and vowel articulation. In: *Vocal Fold Physiology*, edited by D.M. Bless and J.H. Abbs, pp. 286-299. College-Hill Press, San Diego, CA.

Honda, K. (1986). *Biomechanical Interaction between Fundamental Frequency Control and Vowel Articulation.* Doctoral dissertation, University of Tokyo.

Honda, K. (1988). Various laryngeal mechanisms in controlling voice fundamental frequency. *J. Acoust. Soc. Am.* Suppl.1, 84:S82.

Ladefoged, P. (1961). Physiological studies of speech. *STL-QPSR* 3:16-21 (Dept. of Speech Communication and Music Acoustics, Royal Institute of Technology, Stockholm).

Lehiste, I. and Peterson, G.E. (1961). Some basic considerations in the analysis of intonation. *J. Acoust. Soc. Am.* 33:419-423.

Lieberman, P. (1967). Intonation, perception and language. *Research Monograph* No. 38, MIT Press, Cambridge, MA.

Ohala, J.J. and Ladefoged, P. (1970). Further investigation of pitch regulation in speech. *UCLA Working Papers in Phonetics* 14:12-24.

Pierrehumbert, J.B. and Beckman, M E. (1988). *Japanese Tone Structure* (Linguistic Inquiry Monograph 15). The MIT Press, Cambridge, MA.

Peterson, G.E. and Barney, H L. (1952). Control methods used in a study of the vowels. *J. Acoust. Soc. Am.* 24:184-195.

Poser, W.J. (1984). *The Phonetics and Phonology of Tone and Intonation in Japanese.* Ph.D. dissertation, Massachusetts Institute of Technology, Cambridge, MA.

20

Intrinsic Pitch of Vowels - a Complicated Problem with an Obvious Solution?

Erkki Vilkman, *Olli Aaltonen, **Unto Laine, and *Ilkka Raimo

*The Phoniatric Department of the ENT Clinic, Oulu University Central Hospital, Oulu, Finland, *Department of Phonetics, University of Turku, Turku, Finland, **Acoustics Laboratory, Helsinki University of Technology, Helsinki, Finland.*

It is well-known that vowels in comparable environments tend to have systematically different F0 values. This phenomenon is called the intrinsic pitch or F0 of vowels. Usually the highest F0 values have been reported for the vowels produced with high tongue positions (/i, u/) and the lowest for the vowels connected with low tongue positions (/a/) (e.g., Lehiste, 1970; Reinholt Petersen, 1978). In a recent study Ternström et al. (1988) found this phenomenon also in singing.

Many different explanations have been presented to explain the physiological background of vowel intrinsic F0 (c.f. Sapir, 1989). One line of discussion arises from acoustical explanations, i.e., F0 is supposed to be affected by vowel-specific changes in the vocal tract acoustics. This view was based on a one-mass model of the vocal fold vibrations in which the first formant (F1) "pulls" F0 up when it comes closer to F0 in high vowels (Flanagan and Landgraf, 1968). However, a simulation experiment based on a two-mass model (Ishizaka and Flanagan, 1972) showed a reversed relationship between vowel F0 and F1 (Guérin and Boë, 1980). Several studies on normal human subjects have failed to support the F0/F1 coupling hypothesis (Beil, 1962; Ewan, 1979).

On the other hand, it has been suggested that the articulatory movements connected with vowel production cause changes in the vibratory properties of the vocal folds. The classical tongue-pull hypothesis was based on the assumption that raising the tongue pulls the larynx upward and the tension of the vocal folds increases (Lehiste, 1970). This hypothesis is related to the finding that F0 correlates positively with larynx height in, for instance, untrained singers (Sonninen, 1968). However, X-ray studies have shown that the position of the hyoid-larynx column is lower during high vowel (/i,u/) than low vowel (/a/) production (Bothorel, 1978; Perkell, 1969). This discrepancy led to a modified version of the tongue-pull hypothesis which suggests that the tongue-pull causes a change in the vertical tension of the vocal folds (Ohala, 1977).

The present study comprises three separate experiments aimed at shedding light on different possible mechanisms underlying the vowel intrinsic F0 phenomenon. In the first experiment the acoustical vocal source-tract interaction was studied by connecting an artificial vocal tract to an excised human larynx with vibrating vocal folds. The changes in the phonation elicited by altered supraglottal acoustics were monitored. In the second experiment the tongue-pull hypothesis was simulated by recording the changes in the phonation of excised larynges while the vertical tension of the larynx was changed by lifting the hyoid bone. In the third experiment a patient with an inborn anomaly of the hyoid-larynx column was studied and compared to a normal subject in order to find out whether a tight mechanical coupling between the hyoid bone and the thyroid cartilage is necessary for intrinsic F0 production. In addition, the significance of the cricothyroid muscle activity in this respect was analysed.

EXPERIMENT I. ACOUSTICS VS. INTRINSIC F0

Material and methods

In this acoustical experiment excised human larynges were attached to an apparatus used in our earlier studies (see Laine and Vilkman, 1987; Vilkman, 1987; Vilkman and Laine, under publ., for detailed description). For the experiments the cricoid cartilage was attached firmly to a plate. The supraglottic tube (length 17.5 cm, inner diameter 2.9 cm) was supported by a holder, and an air-tight attachment to the thyroid cartilage was achieved by using rubber sealant. The glottal closure was obtained by moving the arytenoid cartilages towards midline with constant forces. The phonation was elicited by warmed and humidified air-flow.

Acoustical, EGG and pressure signals were recorded using an FM tape-recorder (Racal). The recorded signals were analyzed using a microprocessor-based F0 analysis program (ISA). The data base used in this part of the study is the same as that used in our forthcoming paper (Vilkman and Laine, under publ.).

In the experiment the supraglottal acoustic impedance was varied by moving two cylindrical blocks in the supraglottal tube. The diameter of the smaller block was 27 mm and of the bigger 28.8 mm (length 80 mm).

Summary of results

The results showed that the greatest rise in F0 in chest register phonation occurred when the block was inserted in the tube, and vice versa. For one larynx the maximum F0 change between the neutral tube and the medium block (diameter 27 mm; length 80 mm) inserted was an F0 rise of (X±SD) 3.8 ±0.9 Hz (n=16). An example of this can be seen in Figure 1. Generally the F0 changes associated with moving the block in the tube were small. The maximum F0 change measured was about 5 Hz for high (165 Hz) and somewhat pressed chest voice phonation. In this case the high front vowel (the block near the opening of the supraglottal tube) had a lower F0 than the low back vowel (the block deep in the supraglottal tube).

When the largest-diameter block was used a drop in F0 was noticed when the block was inserted. It was obviously acting as a DC resistance because it was difficult to insert and this configuration generated noise.

EXPERIMENT II. VERTICAL HYOID BONE DISPLACEMENT AND F0

Material and methods

The effects of vertical changes in the laryngeal tissues on F0 were studied by means of five excised human larynges. The apparatus described in our earlier studies (Vilkman, 1987) was used with some modification. The experimental arrangements as well as the

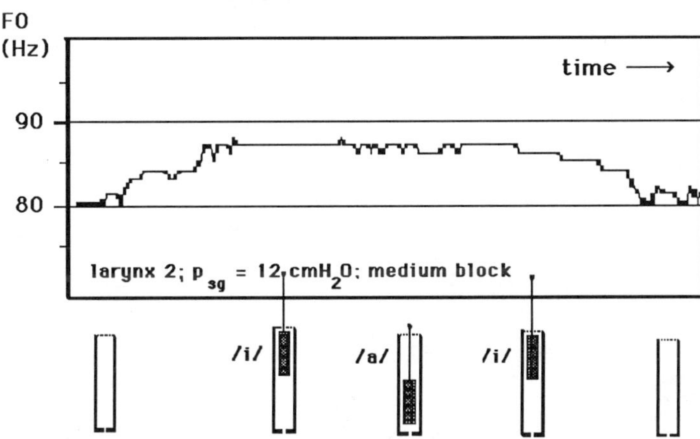

Fig. 1. Fundamental frequency changes due to moving a block in the supraglottal space. The schematic figures with corresponding "vowels" at the bottom illustrate the movement of the block. *N.B.* the initial F0 rise occurred when the block was inserted in the supraglottal tube, the final drop when the block was taken out. When the block was moved in the tube the F0 change was negligible.

main bulk of the results of Experiment II are described in detail in a recent article by Vilkman and Karma (1989).

At the dissection, the intralaryngeal structures as well as the hyoid bone with the hyothyroid ligaments and membrane were left intact. The suprahyoidal structures and the external laryngeal muscles were removed. The first tracheal ring was left in place. The connective tissues in both ends of the specimen were sutured to adjacent structures, i.e. to the cricoid cartilage and the hyoid bone. The technique of eliciting phonation as well as the recording and analysis procedures were the same as in Experiment I. The maximum F0 change was measured.

The cricoid cartilage was firmly attached to a plate, and the thyroid cartilage to the frame of the apparatus; the vertical tension of the laryngeal tissues was increased by lifting the hyoid bone with a calibrated spring. The vertical forces were increased gradually to 12 N. The experimental arrangements are shown in Figure 2.

Summary of results

When the hyoid bone was leaning upon the thyroid cartilage the ventricular and vocal folds were extremely folded. In many cases the ventricular folds tended to vibrate in this position. When the hyoid bone was lifted the epiglottis tilted ventrocranially, the vestibule of the larynx expanded, the ventricular folds abducted and the vocal folds also tended to abduct slightly.

The phonation of these specimens represent low chest register which was determined by both perceptual analysis as well as stroboscopic evaluation. The average F0 (X ±SD) was 83 ±48 Hz (range 40-192)(n=26). The increase in the vertical tension of the vocal folds always caused a rise in F0. The maximum average F0 rise, which was statistically significant, was (X ±SD) 8 ±8.4 Hz. This represents the difference between the minimum

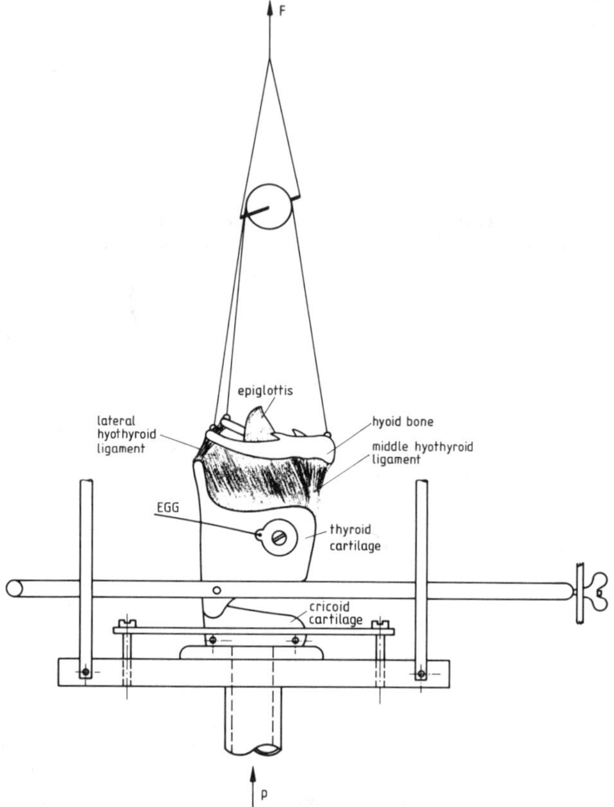

Fig. 2. The experimental arrangements for lifting the hyoid bone used to study the significance of changes in the vertical tension of the vocal folds. The anterior part of the thyroid cartilage was supported by the frame of the apparatus (not drawn) (from Vilkman and Karma, 1989, with permission).

and maximum vertical force. However, the greatest force (12 N) could not be used in all cases because of the opening of the glottis caused by hyoid bone elevation.

EXPERIMENT III. ABNORMAL AND NORMAL HYOID-LARYNGEAL COLUMN VS. INTRINSIC F0

Material and methods

This experiment used an abnormal female subject and a normal male subject. Both subjects read a list of nonsense VCCV (V=/i, u, æ, a/; C= /p, t, k, f, s, m, n, ng, l, r, ʔ/) words (e.g. /ippi/, /uttu/, /alla/ etc.) five times. The samples were recorded and the F0 analysis was carried out in the same way as in Experiments I and II. F0 peak values were measured.

The abnormal subject was examined clinically, with the findings discussed below, but only the acoustic recordings were made during the test utterances. The normal subject, in addition to being recorded, also was studied via simultaneous electromyography using hooked-wire electrodes of the cricothyroid (CT) muscle. The CT peak values were measured manually from rectified and integrated recordings. The CT examination could not be done to the patient because it could not be clinically motivated.

The results were analyzed by means of ANOVA.

Summary of results

In the first part, the vowel intrinsic F0 of a young female patient with an inborn anomaly of the larynx - hyoid bone column was studied. Initially she came to the Phoniatric Department because of voice problems. She reported no swallowing problems. Her profession demanded talking to clients 6-8 hours a day. In the clinical examination her voice was otherwise normal but the timbre was somewhat guttural. The palpation of the laryngeal structures and later the X-ray study revealed that the position of her larynx was exceptionally low. The distance between the corpus of the hyoid bone and the superomedial part of the thyroid cartilage was about 4 cm at rest. Under indirect laryngoscopy her larynx was functionally normal. In a videofluorographical examination made when the patient was producing Finnish vowels the hyoid bone was seen to move upward and forward during the vowel /u/ and backward and downward during /a/ production. On the horizontal plane the hyoid bone was most anterior for the vowel /i/. The movements of the larynx were small but the larynx was slightly lower for /u/ than for /æ/ and /a/. During swallowing her larynx was not moving vertically, instead, her hyoid bone moved caudally towards it which is opposite to normal.

The average F0 peak values (X±SD) for the vowels /i, u, æ, a/ were, respectively: 246.2 ±10.0 Hz; 248.7 ±10.8 Hz; 238.2 ±8.9 Hz and 237.4 ±8.0 Hz (n=55). The analysis of variance revealed among other things that the vowels /i/ and /u/ were statistically significantly higher than the vowels /æ/ and /a/ ($F(1)=65.6$; $p<0.01$).

For the normal subject the difference between the vowels /i, u/ and /æ, a/ (F0 in the same order: 118.0 ±7.9 Hz; 118.8 ±5.7 Hz; 113.8 ±6.4 Hz; 113.7 ±5.5 Hz) was also statistically significant ($F(1)=55.1$; $p<0.01$). The analysis of variance revealed that the CT peak values improved the fit of the linear model significantly ($F(1)=243.6$; $p<0.01$). The peak F0 and CT values are plotted separately for each vowel in Figure 3. See Vilkman et al. 1989 for further details.

DISCUSSION

The F0 changes associated with changes in supraglottal acoustics were greatest at the moment of the insertion of the block in the artificial supraglottal space connected to the excised larynx (Experiment I). From the point of view of the present study this finding has limited significance. The occasional measurable F0 changes connected with the simulation of front-back vowel distinction were in line with those measured by means of a two-mass model of the vocal folds (Guérin and Boë, 1980), i.e., F0 of the front vowel (block near the opening of the supraglottal tube) was lower than the back vowel (block deep in the tube).

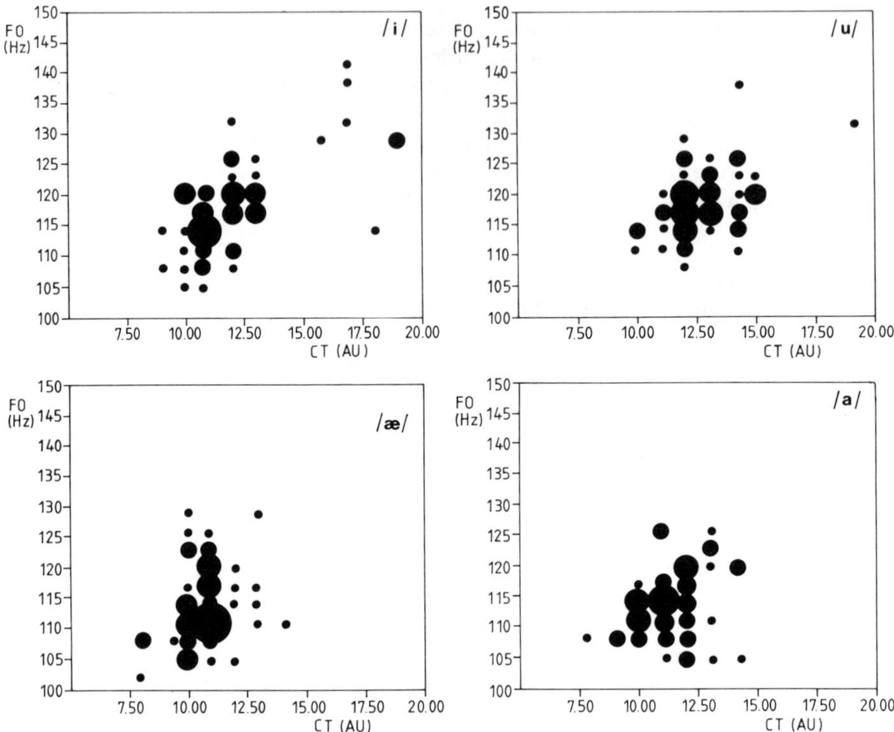

Fig. 3. A scattergram of peak F0 and CT values (AU = arbitrary units). The size of the dot corresponds to the number of occurrences.

The F0 rise as a result of increased vertical tension of the vocal folds (Experiment II) supports the modified tongue-pull hypothesis (c.f., Ohala, 1977). However, the soft tissue changes were somewhat exaggerated as compared to normal phonation in living subjects. The starting point in this experiment was a state of maximal folding, i.e. also the ventricular folds were adducted. In normal subjects this is more likely to be seen during swallowing than during phonation (e.g., Fink 1975). All in all, the F0 changes (range 1-17 Hz) measured in this experiment were too small to explain exclusively the extremes of the variation of the intrinsic F0. For instance, Reinholt Petersen (1978) reported that the F0 difference between /i/ and /a/ varied from 10 Hz to 35 Hz across subjects.

On the basis of the results of Experiment III it seems that a tight mechanical coupling between the hyoid bone and the thyroid cartilage is not a necessary condition for the production of a normal pattern of vowel intrinsic F0. This is, however, a precondition to Honda's (1983) explanations of the intrinsic F0 control mechanism. The CT muscle activity of the normal subject showed a significant relationship with the vowel intrinsic F0 variation. This relationship should be further studied in relation to the timing of articulatory events. CT muscle activity is probably also the mechanism by which the patient produced the normal intrinsic F0 pattern.

CONCLUSION

In conclusion, the acoustical vocal source-tract interaction seems to play no role in vowel intrinsic F0 production in the chest register. The activity of the CT muscle, on the other hand, is obviously an important contributing factor. However, the CT muscle activity did not completely explain the intrinsic F0 variation, so other mechanisms are likely to cause it also. One of these mechanisms emerges from the changes in the vertical tension or configuration of the vocal folds.

As to the question presented in the title of the present study, these results suggest once again a modified tongue-pull hypothesis according to which the vowel intrinsic F0 variation is to a great extent the result of compensatory CT muscle activity. It is well-known that the CT muscle is the main F0 controller in general. The reflex-like compensation by this muscle can be thought to occur when the tongue goes up for the high vowels: this movement causes a vertical stretch in the hyoid-laryngeal tissues which would, without extra support, tend to open the cricothyroid visor. This hypothesis naturally calls for further studies.

REFERENCES

Beil, R. (1962). Frequency analysis of vowels produced in a helium-rich atmosphere. *J. Acoust. Soc. Am.* 34:347-349.

Bothorel, A. (1978). Déplacement vertical de l'os hyoide et variation de la fréquence fondamentale. Travaux de l'institut de phonétique de Strasbourg 10:120-132.

Ewan, W.G. (1979). Can intrinsic vowel F0 be explained by source/tract coupling? *J. Acoust. Soc. Am.* 66:358-362.

Fink, B.R. (1975). *The human larynx. A functional study.* Raven Press, New York.

Flanagan, J., L. and Landgraf, L. (1968). Self-oscillating source for vocal-tract synthesizers. *IEEE Trans. Audio Electroacoust.*, 16:57-64.

Guérin, B. and Boë, L.J. (1980) Étude de l'influence du couplage acoustique source-conduit vocal sur F0 des voyelles orales. *Phonetica* 37:169-192.

Honda, K. (1983). Relationship between pitch control and vowel articulation. In: *Vocal Fold Physiology*, edited by D.M. Bless & J.H. Abbs, pp. 286-297. College-Hill Press, San Diego.

Ishizaka, K. and Flanagan, J.L. (1972). Synthesis of voiced sounds from a two-mass model of the vocal cords. *Bell Syst. Techn. J.* 51:1233-1268.

Laine, U. and Vilkman E. (1987). Acoustic-mechanical feedback in vocal source-tract interaction. In: *Proc. XIth ICPhS* vol. 5. pp. 19-22. Academy of Sciences of the Estonian S.S.R., Tallinn.

Lehiste, I. (1970). *Suprasegmentals.* The M.I.T. Press, Cambridge, Mass.

Ohala, J. (1977). Speculation on pitch regulation. *Phonetica* 34:310-312.

Perkell, J.S. (1969) *Physiology of speech production: results and implications of a quantitative cineradiographic study.* The M.I.T. Press. Cambridge, Mass.

Reinholt Petersen, N. (1978). Intrinsic fundamental frequency of Danish vowels. *J. Phonetics* 6:177-189.

Sapir, S. (1989). The intrinsic pitch of vowels: theoretical, physiological, and clinical considerations. *J. Voice* 3:44-51.

Sonninen, A. (1968). The external frame function in the control of pitch in the human voice. In: *Sound Production in Man*, edited by A Bouhuys, pp. 68-90. Annals of New York Academy of Sciences 155, New York Academy of Sciences; New York.

Ternström, S., Sundberg, J., and Colldén, A. (1988). Articulatory F0 perturbations and auditory feedback. *J. Speech Hear. Res.* 31:187-192.

Vilkman, E. (1987). An apparatus for studying the role of the cricothyroid articulation in the voice production of excised human larynges. *Folia Phoniatr.* 39:169-177.

Vilkman, E., Aaltonen, O., Raimo, I., Arajèrvi, P. and Oksanen, H. (1989). Articulatory hyoid-laryngeal changes vs. cricothyroid muscle activity in the control of intrinsic F0 of vowels. *J. Phonetics* 17:193-203.

Vilkman, E. and Karma, P. (1989). Vertical hyoid bone displacement and fundamental frequency of phonation. *Acta Otolaryngol.* 108:142-151.

Vilkman, E. and Laine, U. (under publ.). Supraglottal acoustics and F0 changes in excised larynges.

21

Comparison of Physiological Properties of PAG and Medullary Neurons Involved in Vocalization

Charles R. Larson, Elizabeth DeRosier, and Robert West

Depts. of Communication Sciences and Disorders and Neurobiology and Physiology, Northwestern University, Evanston, IL 60208

Brainstem mechanisms involved in vocalization have seen increased research emphasis over the past several years. Work in our laboratory has concentrated on the midbrain periaqueductal gray (PAG), an area demonstrated through several different methodologies to be important in vocalization (Adametz and O'Leary, 1959; Bandler and Carrive, 1988; Jürgens and Ploog, 1970; Jürgens and Pratt, 1979; Jürgens and Richter, 1986; Larson and Kistler, 1986; Magoun et al., 1937; Robinson, 1967). Although the results of our single unit recording studies in the PAG (Larson and Kistler, 1986) have provided important information regarding cell behavior in this region, the results have not led to major new insights of the PAG's function, in part due to the difficulties in establishing unequivocal relationships with output parameters. We have therefore begun recording cellular activity in and close to the nucleus ambiguus (NA). By analyzing single units related to vocalization in the medulla, we hope to determine the similarity between PAG and medullary units. This understanding should help to further define the function of the PAG cells as well as those in the medulla. In the present paper we compare results of recordings made in the PAG and medulla from different groups of monkeys and discuss possible functions of each group of cells.

METHODS

Five monkeys, one female *Macaca fascicularis* and four male *Macaca nemestrina*, were trained to vocalize for a food reward over a period of several months. Following training, the animals underwent three separate surgical operations, which have been described in detail elsewhere (Larson and Kistler, 1986). In the present study, electrodes were chronically implanted in the posterior cricoarytenoid (PCA; four monkeys), thyroarytenoid (TA), cricothyroid (CT), thyrohyoid (TH; four monkeys), diaphragm (D; four monkeys), intercostal, (IC; four monkeys), rectus abdominus (RA; four monkeys), and external abdominal oblique (EO; one monkey) muscles. For three monkeys, single neuron recording chambers were aimed at stereotaxic coordinates appropriate for the dorsolateral PAG. For the other two monkeys, the chambers were aimed at the reticular

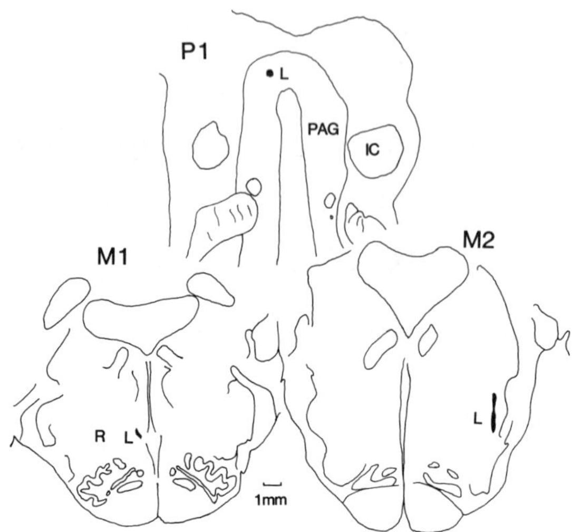

Fig 1. Drawings of three representative coronal sections from monkeys of this study. Monkey P1 shows a lesion (L) at the recording site from where most neurons were recorded in the PAG. Histological examination showed similar results for all three monkeys involved in PAG recording. In monkey M1, a lesion (L) was made 1 mm medial to the recording site (R) in the reticular formation 1-2 mm medial to the nucleus ambiguous. Monkey M2 shows a marking lesion directly in the NA region. Abbreviations: PAG-periaqueductal gray; IC-inferior colliculus.

formation region medial to the NA. For one of the latter two monkeys, after failing to find cells related to vocalization, the chamber was moved and directed towards the NA. Following the surgeries, animals were given pain killing drugs and antibiotics. Topical antibiotic ointment applied around the edges of the dental acrylic for the remainder of the experiments led to complete wound healing.

After recovery from the surgical procedures, the animals again entered the training apparatus, and while they vocalized, activity from single neurons was recorded with a tungsten microelectrode. For a complete description of recording, microstimulation and analysis techniques, see Larson and Kistler (1986, 1987). After several months of recording and exploration of the respective areas, a small marking lesion was made in the areas from which most neurons had been recorded, the animals were sacrificed, and their brains removed for histological verification of lesions sites.

RESULTS

From the five monkeys, 375 neurons, 214 from the PAG and 161 from the medulla, were recorded. Of this number, 305 were related to vocalization, i.e., they either increased or decreased their firing rate before or during vocalization. Sufficient data were recorded from 248 cells to create ensemble averages, 179 cells to do STA of muscle EMGs, and microstimulation was done at 192 electrode sites following recording.

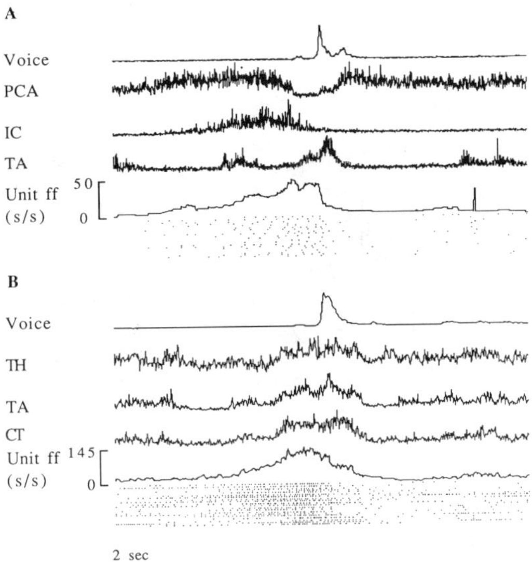

Fig. 2. Ensemble averages and dot-rasters for two representative cells. Cell in A was recorded in the PAG, while B was from the nucleus ambiguous. Voice and EMGs were full-wave rectified prior to averaging. Averages are from 20 vocalizations for each cell. Total time for each average is 2 s. Abbreviations: PCA-posterior cricoarytenoid muscle; IC-intercostal; TA-thyroarytenoid, TH-thyrohyoid; CT-cricothyroid. Line up point for averaging was at onset of vocalization.

From histological analyses, it was apparent that the recording sites in the PAG were very similar for all three monkeys (Figure 1). The dorsolateral region of the midbrain PAG has previously been demonstrated to contain neurons related to vocalization (Larson and Kistler, 1986). The recording site in the medulla differed for the other two monkeys. In one monkey, cells were recorded in the reticular formation between 1 and 2 mm medial to the NA. In the other monkey, cells were recorded directly in and immediately surrounding the NA.

The discharge properties relative to vocalization for most neurons from each region were quite similar. Figure 2 A and B illustrate ensemble averages from representative cells of the PAG and medulla. Each cell increased and then decreased its activity before vocalization. Other types of cells increased activity before vocalization and decreased their activity after vocalization, and some tonically active cells either increased or decreased their activity before vocalization. All cells were categorized on the basis of their discharge pattern, and it was found that cells of all types were found both in the PAG and medulla. The mean firing frequency of the medullary units (49 pps) was significantly greater ($t = 4.27$, $df = 61$, $p < 01$) than that of the PAG cells (31 pps).

In addition to their higher firing rates, the medullary cells often discharged with swallowing or respiratory activity. Many of the PAG cells also discharged at times other than vocalization, but in most cases this activity was not clearly related to any other behavior. A few PAG cells showed some rhythmic discharge loosely related to respiration, but these patterns were not as clear as those seen in the medulla.

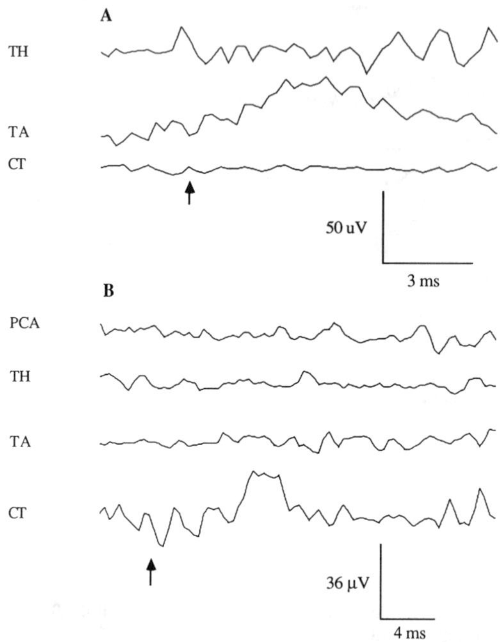

Fig. 3. Spike triggered averaging of rectified EMGs from two cells. Cell in A was from nucleus ambiguous (N= 1049) and in B was from reticular formation medial to the nucleus ambiguous (N = 727). Arrow indicates time of unit discharge. Abbreviations are the same as in Figure 2.

Although analysis of the ensemble averages indicates gross similarities between cells of the two groups, other analyses revealed important differences. Spike triggered averaging (STA; Fetz and Cheney, 1980) was done to try and relate muscle activity to unit discharge in the PAG and NA. STA generally was not successful with PAG cells, however, the example in Figure 3A shows facilitation of the TA muscle from an NA neuron. Figure 3B illustrates an example of CT EMG facilitation from triggering on a neuron about 2 mm medial to the nucleus ambiguus. In each case, there is only one muscle of those recorded showing marked facilitation. Such observations indicate the cells in question are either MNs or else they project to a very limited set of MNs. Considering that the cell in Figure 3B was recorded 2 mm medial to the NA, it is likely an interneuron.

Microstimulation results from the PAG and NA were also different. Stimulation with single stimulus pulses in the PAG was ineffective for facilitating muscles at low current levels, therefore, 20 ms trains of pulses (200 Hz) and averaging techniques were used to reveal effects on muscles. Figure 4A shows an example of facilitation of the PCA and TA muscles from stimulation in the PAG. In most cases where PAG stimulation led to EMG facilitation, effects were observed in more than one muscle. In a few cases of stimulation at low current (20 μA), effects in a single muscle were noted. The shortest latencies to muscle facilitation from PAG microstimulation were 12 ms for laryngeal muscles and 20-30 ms for respiratory muscles.

Figure 4B shows facilitation of the TA muscle with a latency of 5 ms from a single stimulus pulse of 8μA delivered to the NA. Also, the EMG potential was able to follow stimulus frequencies up to 60 Hz. The cell depicted in Figure 4B, the same as that in Figure 3A, also gave bursts of activity synchronously with bursts of EMG during swallowing. Stimulation of twenty two cells in the NA resulted in EMG following at

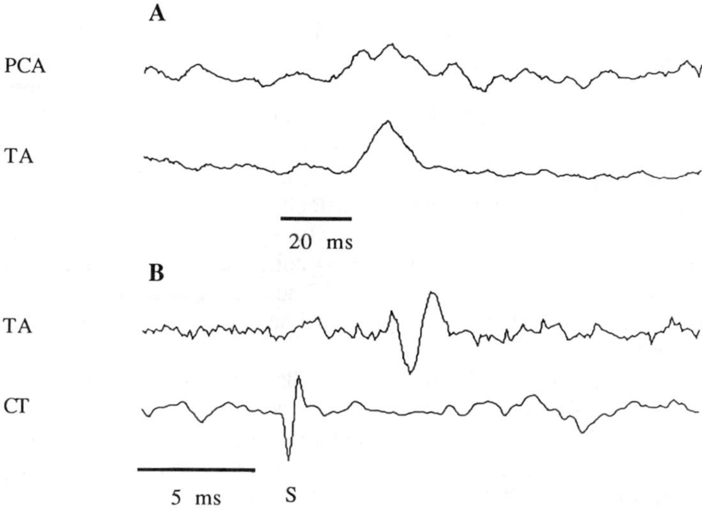

Fig. 4. Results of neuron microstimulation in the PAG and medulla. **A** shows results of PAG stimulation. Traces represent averages for 20 stimulus trains, each 20 ms long, delivered at time indicated by bar. EMGs were full-wave rectified. **B** shows results from a single stimulus pulse (8 μA) in the NA at a site from which a vocalization-related neuron was recorded. Trace CT shows stimulus artifact at time of stimulus presentation indicated by "S". Abbreviations are the same as in Figure 2.

frequencies above 60 Hz; many as high as 200 Hz. In the reticular formation surrounding the NA, 3 ms trains of pulses (1000 Hz) sometimes facilitated laryngeal muscles with 6 ms latencies and respiratory muscles at 8-12 ms.

Based on discharge properties, results from STA and microstimulation, 10 medullary cells were judged to be MNs, five for the TA, four for the TH, and one for the PCA muscle. For another twelve cells, STA results were not in agreement with those from microstimulation and hence they were not classified as MNs. Cells that produced longer latency responses from microstimulation were probably interneurons.

DISCUSSION

There are clearly some similarities and differences between the two populations of cells sampled in the present study, which are in part explained by their anatomical connections and locations. Located in the NA and surrounding reticular formation are laryngeal, pharyngeal and palatal MNs (Davis and Nail, 1984; Yoshida et al., 1981; Yoshida et al., 1985), respiratory related neurons (Long and Duffin, 1984), and cells involved in swallowing (Jean, 1984). Thus, the NA and surrounding reticular formation are involved in vocalization, swallowing and respiration.

The PAG, located in the midbrain, receives inputs from the limbic system and sends projections to lower brainstem motor nuclei including the NA, nucleus tractus solitarius, nucleus retro ambiguus and reticular formation (Jürgens and Pratt, 1979; Holstege, 1989;

Yoshida et al., 1987). The PAG may serve as a link between limbic system structures and the lower brainstem motor nuclei (Jürgens and Pratt, 1979), or it may coordinate several different cranial motor nuclei involved in vocalization and expression of affect (Lamandella, 1977; Larson, 1985). Regardless of its precise function, the PAG is widely regarded as an important structure in the neural control of vocalization.

Many of the neurons recorded in the medulla, such as that depicted in Figures 3 and 4 were probably MNs. This assertion is difficult to prove without their antidromic activation from the motor nerves (Yajima and Hayashi, 1983; Zealear and Larson, 1988). Nevertheless, the facts that ten cells were highly correlated with the timing and amplitude of EMG bursts, STA revealed time-locked EMG activity with a single muscle, and EMG potentials were able to follow microstimulation at low currents and high frequencies strongly suggest they were MNs.

Considering that some of the medullary cells were laryngeal MNs, others being interneurons, the similarity in discharge patterns between the PAG and medullary cells with respect to vocalization makes it apparent that there is little modification of neuronal discharge patterns from PAG cells to MNs. The higher mean firing rates of medullary cells is not regarded as a significant modulation of the patterns of unit discharge relative to vocalization. In other words, PAG cells, or cells at an even higher level of the neuraxis may be responsible for determining discharge patterns of laryngeal MNs for vocalization. The MNs receive inputs from other medullary sites for swallowing and respiration. While we cannot disprove at this time that the medullary cells and PAG cells receive common inputs from a third source, which influences discharge of both groups, the fact that PAG neurons are known to project to the NA region and PAG stimulation excites laryngeal muscles with longer latencies than does the NA, argues that PAG neurons affect the discharge of NA neurons. Hence, the PAG appears to be the highest site in the vocalization system, yet recorded in detail, where firing patterns of laryngeal MNs may be determined. Future studies aimed at limbic system sites should determine if they also fire like the PAG cells, or whether the latter are unique and hence responsible for determining discharge patterns of NA MNs during vocalization.

ACKNOWLEDGEMENTS

We would like to thank Mr. David Niemann for his assistance in running the experiments and data analysis. This project was funded by a grant from the NIH, NINCDS NS 19290.

REFERENCES

Adametz, J. and J. L. O'Leary. (1959). "Experimental mutism resulting from periaqueductal lesions in cats." *Neurol.* 9:636-642.

Bandler, R. and P. Carrive. (1988). Integrated defence reaction elicited by excitatory amino acid microinjection in the midbrain periaqueductal grey region of the unrestrained cat. *Brain Res.* 439:95-106.

Davis, P. J. and B. S. Nail. (1984). On the location and size of laryngeal motoneurons in the cat and rabbit. *J Comp Neurol.* 230:13-32.

Fetz, E. E. and P. D. Cheney. (1980). Postspike facilitation of forelimb muscle activity by primate corticomotoneuronal cells. *J Neurophysiol.* 44(4):751-772.

Holstege, G. (1989). An anatomical study on the final common pathway for vocalization in the cat. *J Comp Neurol.* 284:242-252.

Jean, A. (1984). Brainstem organization of the swallowing network. *Brain Behav Evol.* 25:109-116.

Jürgens , U. and D. Ploog. (1970). Cerebral representation of vocalization in the Squirrel monkey. *Exp Brain Res.* 10:532-554.

Jürgens, U. and R. Pratt. (1979). Role of the periaqueductal grey in vocal expression of emotion. *Brain Res.* 167:367-378.

Jürgens, U. and K. Richter. (1986). Glutamate-Induced vocalization in the Squirrel monkey. *Brain Res.* 373:349-358.

Lamandella, J. T. (1977). The limbic system in human communication. In: *Studies in Neurolinguistics,* edited by J. Whitaker and H.A. Whitaker, pp. 157-222. Academic Press, New York.

Larson, C. R. (1985). The midbrain periaqueductal gray: A brainstem structure involved in vocalization. *J Speech Hear Res.* 28:241-249.

Larson, C. R. and M. K. Kistler. (1986). The relationship of periaqueductal gray neurons to vocalization and laryngeal EMG in the behaving monkey. *Exp Brain Res.* 63:596-606.

Larson, C.R. and M.K.Kistler. (1987) Brainstem neuronal activity associated with vocalization in the monkey. In: *Vocal Fold Physiology: Laryngeal function in phonation and respiration*, edited by T. Baer, K.S. Harris, and C. Sasaki, pp. 154-167. Little, Brown and Co., Boston.

Long, S.E. and Duffin, J. (1984). The medullary respiratory neurons: a review. *Can J Physiol Pharmacol.* 62:161-182.

Magoun, H. W., D. Atlas, E. H. Ingersoll and S. W. Ranson. (1937). Associated facial, vocal and respiratory components of emotional expression: An experimental study. *J Neurol Psychopath.* 17:241-255.

Robinson, B., W. (1967). Vocalization evoked from forebrain in Macaca mulatta. *Psychol Behav.* 2:345-354.

Yajima, Y. and Y. Hayashi. (1983). Identification of motoneurons in the nucleus ambiguus by antidromic stimulation of the superior and the recurrent laryngeal nerves in rats. *Brain Res.* 288: 302-306.

Yoshida, Y., T. Mitsumasu, M. Hirano and T. Kanaseki. (1985). Somatotopic representation of the laryngeal motoneurons in the medulla of monkeys. *Acta Otolaryngol* (Stockh). 100:299-303.

Yoshida, Y., T. Mitsumasu, M. Hirano and T. Kanaseki. (1987). Afferent connections to the nucleus ambiguus in the brainstem of the cat: an HRP study. In: *4th International Conference on Vocal Fold Physiology,* edited by T. Baer, K.S. Harris, and C. Sasaki., pp. 45-61. Little, Brown Col., Boston.

Yoshida, Y., T. Miyazaki, M. Hirano, T. Shin, T. Totoki and T. Kanaseki. (1981). Localization of efferent neurons innervating the pharyngeal constrictor muscles and the cervical esophagus muscle in the cat by horseradish peroxidase. *Neurosci Lett.* 22:91-95.

Zealear, D. L. and C. R. Larson. (1988). A microelectrode study of laryngeal motoneurons in the nucleus ambiguus of the awake vocalizing monkey. In: *Vocal Physiology: Voice Production, Mechanisms and Functions*, edited by O. Fujimura, and S. Saito, pp. 29-38. Raven, New York.

22

Influence of Pitch and Intensity on Cricothyroid and Thyroarytenoid Activity in Singers and Nonsingers

Per-Åke Lindestad, Björn Fritzell, and *Anders Persson

*Department of Logopedics and Phoniatrics, * Department of Clinical Neurophysiology, Huddinge University Hospital, S-141 86 Huddinge, Sweden.*

Quantitative analysis of the EMG signal can enhance our knowledge of laryngeal muscle activity patterns during phonation, and EMG has been used in many studies to estimate laryngeal muscle activity levels (Faaborg-Andersen, 1957; Arnold, 1961; Yanagihara and von Leden, 1968; Hirano et al., 1969; Shipp and McGlone, 1971; Gay et al., 1972; Hirano et al., 1970; Shipp et al., 1979). The hooked wire technique, which was used in many of these studies, created new possibilities for easy and natural phonation during examinations (Hirano and Ohala, 1969). The methods used for quantification of the EMG signal were primarily the visual estimation of the amplitude and frequency of the interference pattern (Faaborg-Andersen, 1957; Arnold, 1961; Yanagihara and von Leden, 1968; Hirano et al., 1970) or analysis of the rectified and smoothed (integrated) EMG signal (Shipp and McGlone, 1971; Gay et al., 1972; Shipp et al., 1979). By using the latter method a semi-quantitative measure is obtained, that apart from the mean amplitude also reflects the "density" of the signal, which depends on the firing rate of motor units.

Most studies describe the phonatory behaviour of individuals, mostly males. A few studies include individuals of both sexes (Hirano, et al., 1969; Gay et al., 1972; Hirano et al., 1970; Hirano, 1981). However, we have not been able to find any studies comparing groups of subjects, such as males vs. females and singers vs. nonsingers. Very few statistical analyses have been presented (Shipp et al., 1979).

A method for quantitative analysis of the EMG interference pattern, called "turns/amplitude analysis" has previously been used in skeletal muscles, mainly for clinical purposes (Willison, 1964; Rose and Willison, 1967; Fuglsang-Fredrikssen and Månsson, 1975; Philipsson and Larsson, 1988). Concentric recording electrodes were used in all experiments. The method is different from those mentioned above in that it compares two independent measures of EMG signal characteristics, namely the amplitude and a measure of frequency (turns/s). We have recently tested the method in laryngeal muscles in an attempt to evaluate its clinical usefulness (Lindestad et al., 1990).

The purpose of the present investigation was to test the turns/amplitude analysis for quantification of laryngeal muscle activity during phonation, and to use it for comparison of muscle activity patterns between males and females and between singers and nonsingers. The use of a large number of electrode positions for each muscle allowed a powerful statistical analysis.

MATERIAL AND METHODS

Twelve normal, vocally healthy subjects, (six males and six females, three experienced amateur singers in each group), were tested. The mean age of the males was 38 years and 34 for the females.

The experiments took place in a soundproof booth with the subject placed in a supine position. EMG was recorded with a concentric needle electrode (outer diameter 0.65 mm) and standard EMG equipment (MS 6, Medelec Ltd). The intensity of each phonation was recorded by means of a sound pressure meter (Brüel & Kjær 2235), placed 30 cm from the mouth of the subject, and the audio and EMG signals were recorded on tape (TEAC XR-30H) and analyzed off line. The frequency response of the system was 3.2 Hz to 10 kHz.

The activity of the cricothyroid and thyroarytenoid muscles was studied during sustained phonations at low, medium and high pitch, and at three different levels of intensity for each pitch. Thus, for each electrode position, nine phonations were performed. Registrations were made from one muscle and one electrode position at a time. Each phonation was maintained for at least five seconds. The voice pitch (F0) levels were chosen by the experimenter to represent different parts of the subject's voice range, where he/she felt confident that the modal register was used (in the females modal or middle register, as defined by the subject). A previously prepared individual phonetogram indicated that the subject was able to produce substantially different intensity levels at these pitches. None of the singers had any difficulties in keeping the pitch constant while varying the intensity. One male and one female nonsinger had slight difficulties, but in no instance was the deviation from the intended pitch greater than one semitone. In five males the activity level during high pitched falsetto phonation was compared to modal phonation activity of the same pitch.

Principles of the turns/amplitude analysis

A computer program (designed by S. Stålberg, Uppsala, Sweden) adapted to a personal computer, (Apple IIC), was used. The two parameters turns/s (T) and mean amplitude (A) were calculated from the interference pattern. A turn is defined to occur when the amplitude difference between three successive peaks exceeds 100 µV. The mean amplitude is the average value of the amplitudes between turns in one 200 ms epoch. Each epoch is the sum of four 50 ms sweeps on the oscilloscope. The values were collected from four-second periods within each phonation. Care was taken to choose for analysis a part of the phonation that was sufficiently stable. Since the sound signal was available simultaneously, there was no risk of unintentionally including any prephonatory activity in the analysis. The starting point for the analysis period was selected manually and was consequently somewhat variable. However, in order to adjust for the variability of our method, five epochs were collected from each phonation, starting at the same part of the phonation each time, and the mean value was noted as the result. (No difference was found between the means of five and ten epochs from the same phonation, therefore we analyzed only five times). The SPL measurements were used to verify that the subject actually produced significant differences between the high, medium and low intensity phonations, while little attention was paid to the absolute values of SPL. However, the intensity level differences recorded were around 5 to 15 dB, in the total material within the range from 65 dB for low to 105 dB for high intensity.

Statistical analysis

The number of electrode positions from each muscle type varied between individuals from two to eight, but in most subjects the mean values were based on four electrode positions. Altogether there were recordings from 49 electrode positions from the cricothyroid and 48 from the thyroarytenoid muscles. The inter-individual variation was great, especially in the cricothyroid muscle and there was also considerable variation within individuals, between electrode positions. However, the effect of these variations was partly neutralized by using the arithmetic mean of all electrode positions for each subject in the analysis.

Two and three-factor analysis of variance was used to compare the turns and amplitude values for different pitch and intensity levels. Comparisons between males and females and between singers and nonsingers were made. For example when analysing data obtained from the males, A or T was assigned as the dependent variable and pitch (low, medium, high), intensity (low, medium, high) and singing ability (singer, nonsinger) as the independent variables. When analysis of variance is repeated many times in the same material there is always a risk to get a false positive result by chance. To avoid this, the level of acceptance for statistical significance was set at $p < 0.01$.

RESULTS

Cricothyroid

In the male singers there was an increase in both A and T with increasing pitch, although this was almost concealed by the effect of increasing intensity, which was larger than in the nonsinger group. The pitch effect as well as the intensity effect, were close to but did not reach significance.

In the male nonsinger group there was an increase in A and T with pitch, although this was significant only for T. No consistent effect of intensity variation was seen (Figure 1 a and b).

There was a significant difference between the female singers and nonsingers in the effect of pitch difference on A. Thus, while there was a slight decrease in A in the singer group, there was a marked increase in the nonsinger group. An increase in T was present in both groups, although this was significant only in the nonsinger group. No consistent effect of intensity variation was seen (Figure 1 c and d).

All twelve subjects were also tested "en block", looking for differences between singers and nonsingers regardless of sex. The general levels of T and A were higher in the singer group, but the most obvious finding was the difference in the effect of intensity control. Thus, in the singer group there was an increase in both A and T with increased intensity, while there was a slight decrease in A in the nonsinger group. The difference between the groups, which was statistically significant for A, is illustrated in Figure 4.

Thyroarytenoid

The increase in A and T with increasing pitch was evident for male singers and nonsingers and this increase was significant for A and T in the singer group, while it was only significant for T in the nonsinger group (Figure 2 a and b).

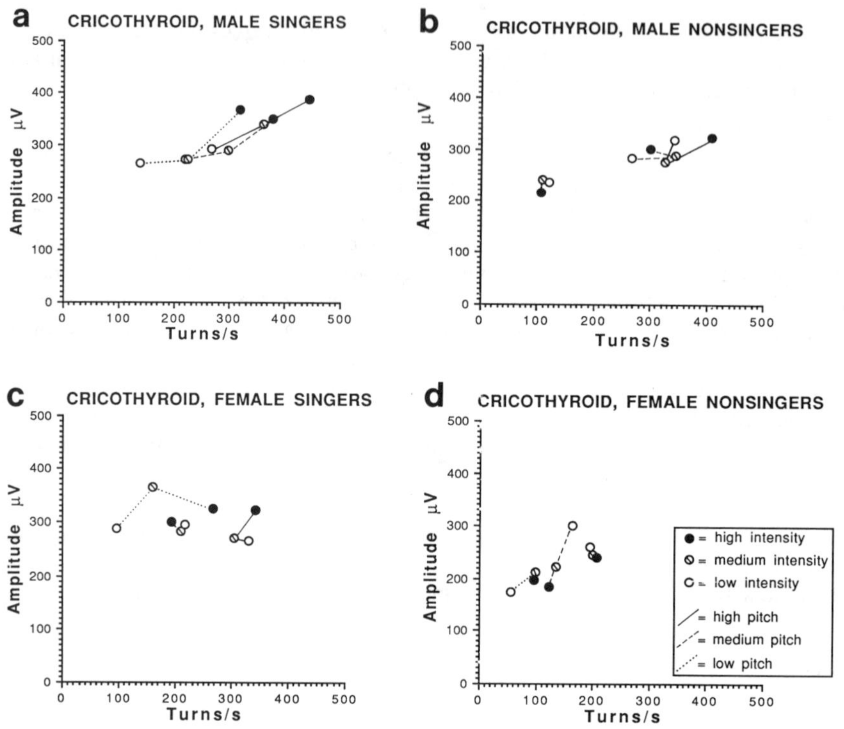

Fig 1. Mean values of cricothyroid activity. Note the consistent increase in both turns/s and amplitude during increased intensity at all pitches in the male singers. The same fenomenon was present in the female singers, but only at low pitch. In the nonsingers, pitch variation had much greater effect on activity level than did intensity changes.

The difference between male singers and nonsingers in activity in the thyroarytenoid with raised pitch was statistically significant. It is illustrated graphically in Figure 5.

The increase in A and T with increasing pitch was evident for female singers and nonsingers and this increase was significant for A and T in both groups. There was no consistent effect of intensity change. No significant differences between the groups were noted (Figure 2 c and d).

The mean A and T values for falsetto in the singer group are based on values from two subjects. These were approximately the same as those for medium pitch modal phonation. The falsetto A values in the male nonsinger group were somewhat higher than for high pitch modal register. Statistically, the mean A and T values for falsetto were significantly different from those for low pitch modal phonation in both groups, but not from medium and high pitch. The mean A and T levels were slightly lower in high than in low intensity falsetto phonation in the singers and lower for T, but unchanged for A in the nonsingers (Figure 3 a and b).

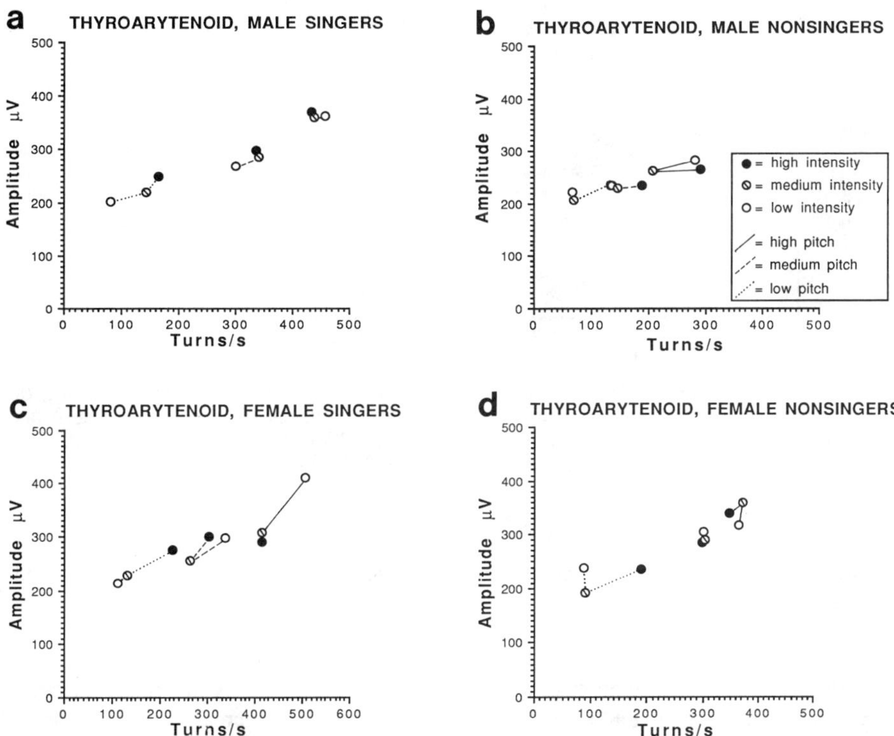

Fig 2. Mean values of thyroarytenoid activity. Note the similar pattern in all groups. Pitch changes had a significant ($p < 0.01$) effect on activity level, while intensity variation had no consistent effect, except at low pitch in all groups. Note also the significant ($p < 0.01$) difference between the activity levels at the different pitches in the male singers compared to the nonsingers.

DISCUSSION

The most important new development brought about by the turns/amplitude analysis was the possibility for improved quantification of EMG activity changes caused by pitch and intensity alterations and the opportunity for statistical analysis.

The increase in T and A with raised pitch as noted in the cricothyroid muscle was expected (Faaborg-Andersen, 1957; Arnold, 1961; Yanagihara and von Leden, 1968; Hirano et al., 1969; 1970; Shipp and Mc Glone, 1971; Gay et al., 1972; Hirano, 1981). This was significant for T in all groups but not for A, and present only for T among the female singers. Part of the explanation for this may be found in the inter-individual variations, which were greater in the cricothyroid than in the thyroarytenoid. However, when comparing our results with others, one must bear in mind the principal difference between our measure of absolute amplitude and the data obtained by using the smoothed and rectified signal, which partly depends on the frequency content. Evidently our T

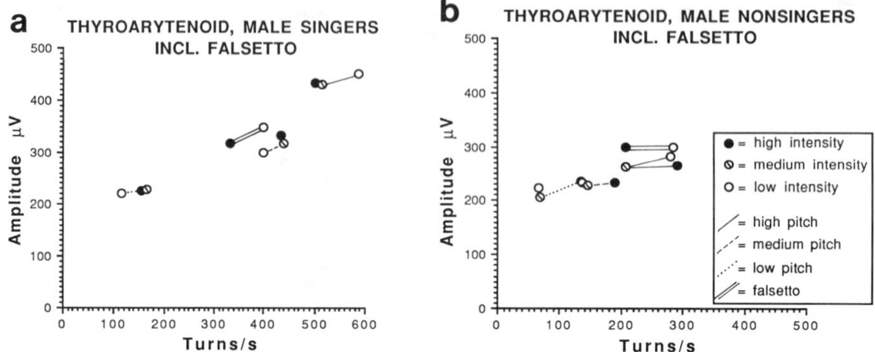

Fig 3. Mean values of thyroarytenoid activity in both groups of males, including during falsetto phonation. Note that activity during falsetto equaled that during medium pitch in the singers, while it was slightly higher than during high pitch in the nonsingers. The activity decreased somewhat with increasing intensity in both groups.

measure shows the best agreement with the results of studies where the smoothed and rectified signal was used.

We found a positive effect with increased intensity on the cricothyroid activity in the male singers. The reports in the literature on this matter vary. A decrease in amplitude with increased intensity on swell tone has been noted repeatedly in singers (Hirano et al 1969; 1970). Yanagihara and von Leden (1968) found an increase in amplitude at low pitch and a decrease at medium and high pitch. Arnold (1961) found an increase in activity with increasing intensity, while Gay et al. (1972) found an activity increase in some subjects and no change in others. These differences may partly be explained by different laryngeal behaviour in swell tone versus separate sustained phonations with different intensity. Higher cricothyroid activity during singing with an active than with an inactive diaphragm has recently been reported (Sundberg et al., 1988). From that study we know that at least one of our male singers, who participated in both studies, showed this activity pattern. One might hypothesize that in our experiments diaphragmatic activity increased with intensity, at least in the singer group. It should be emphasized again that the pitch (F0) level was not affected by intensity variation in our study.

The increase in activity in the thyroarytenoid muscle with raised pitch has been described by many others (Faaborg-Andersen, 1957; Shipp and Mc Glone, 1971; Gay et al., 1972; Hirano et al., 1970; Shipp et al., 1979).

We found no overall positive correlation between thyroarytenoid muscle activity and increase in intensity. The variability in T and A with intensity changes within the different pitches was in fact very little, except in low pitch phonation. The latter finding has previously been reported in singers (Hirano et al., 1977). Increased activity at all pitches (Hirano et al., 1969; Hirano, 1981) and unchanged activity levels with increased intensity (Faaborg-Andersen 1957; Gay et al 1972) have also been reported.

There were no sex differences in thyroarytenoid behaviour, which is quite in accordance with a previous study (Hirano et al., 1970). The difference between male singers and nonsingers is interesting. Shipp and Mc Glone (1971) reported that the

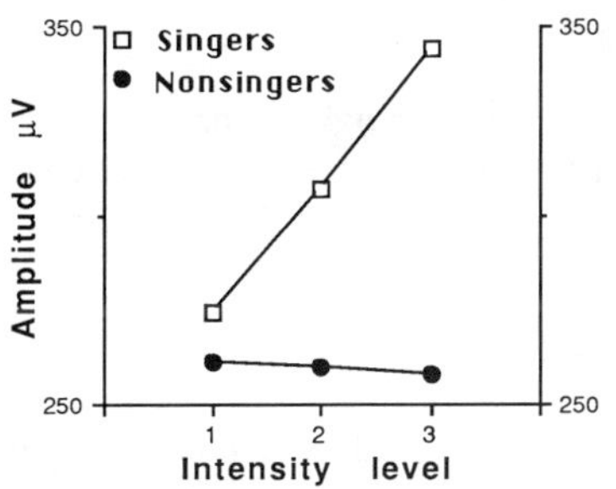

Fig 4. Cricothyroid: Mean amplitude levels for all singers and nonsingers at different intensity levels, regardless of pitch. This figure illustrates the significant ($p < 0.01$) differences in effect of variation in intensity , as described in Figure 1.

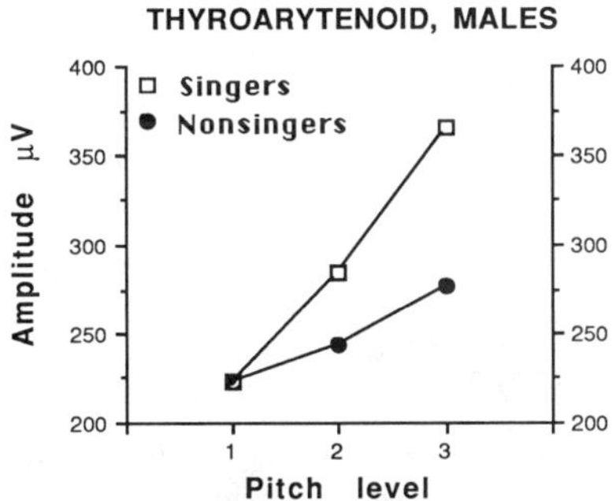

Fig 5. Thyroarytenoid: Mean amplitude levels in male singers and nonsingers at different pitch levels, regardless of intensity. This figure illustrates the significant ($p < 0.01$)difference in degree of increase in activity with increasing pitch, as described in Figure 2.

increase in thyroarytenoid activity with pitch in male nonsingers was greater at lower pitches, which is in accordance with our findings. Singers, on the other hand seem to have a specific ability to keep the thyroarytenoid active at high pitches, an ability that probably comes with training.

The high levels of thyroarytenoid activity in the falsetto of the male nonsingers is in accordance with the findings of Shipp and Mc Glone (1971). In the singers we found a decrease in activity compared to modal phonation at the same pitch, also described in several studies (Hirano et al., 1969; 1970; Hirano, 1981). However, the levels in our study were still higher than for low and medium pitch modal phonation. Our results indicate that the actual level of thyroarytenoid activity is of minor importance in register regulation. Furthermore, there appears to be differences between singers and nonsingers. Our finding of decreased activity with increased intensity during falsetto in singers is in accordance with previous studies (Hirano et al., 1969; 1970; Hirano, 1981). Gay et al (1972) however, found no effect with intensity change in nonsingers.

The increase in the number of turns/s has been shown to attenuate beyond 50% of maximum muscle force in big skeletal muscles (Fuglsang-Fredrikssen and Månsson, 1975; Philipsson and Larsson, 1988). No such effect was seen in our study. Although the highest activity levels of the laryngeal muscles during phonation probably is considerably less than 100% of maximum contraction force, it is likely to be well over 50%. Thus, laryngeal muscles seem to act differently than larger muscles do in this respect, most probably because the motor units are small and motor unit potential durations are short.

To sum up we can conclude that it is possible to detect differences in the levels of amplitude and turns/s in cricothyroid and thyroarytenoid muscles between males and females as well as between non-singers and amateur singers. In all groups the principle role of both the cricothyroid and the thyroarytenoid seems to be to take part in the regulation of F0. More activity changes with intensity variation were observed in the cricothyroid than in the thyroarytenoid, especially in the singers. The activity levels of male falsetto phonation were not significantly different from those for modal voice of the same high pitch.

ACKNOWLEDGEMENTS

The study was supported by Karolinska Institutet. Excellent technical support was given by Michael Gehlen. The authors also want to thank Zsuzsanna Wiesenfeld-Hallin for revising our English.

REFERENCES

Arnold, G. (1961). Physiology and pathology of the cricothyroid muscle. *Laryngoscope* 71:687-753.

Faaborg-Andersen, K. (1957). Electromyographic investigation of intrinsic laryngeal muscles in humans. *Acta Phys. Scand. Suppl.* 41.

Fuglsang-Fredriksen, A., and Månsson, A. (1975). Analysis of electrical activity of normal muscle in man at different degrees of voluntary effort. *J. Neurol. Neurosurg. Psychiat.* 38:683-694.

Gay, T., Hirose, H., Strome, M., and Sawashima, M. (1972). Electromyography of the intrinsic laryngeal muscles during phonation. *Ann. Otolaryngol.* 81: 401-409.

Hirano, M. (1981). The function of the intrinsic laryngeal muscles in singing. In: *Vocal Fold Physiology*, edited by K. Stevens, M. Hirano, pp.155-167. University of Tokyo Press, Tokyo, Japan.

Hirano, M. and Ohala, J. (1969). Use of hooked-wire electrodes for electromyography of the intrinsic laryngeal muscles. *J. Speech Hear. Res.* 12:362-373.

Hirano, M., Ohala, J., and Vennard, W. (1969). The function of laryngeal muscles in regulating fundamental frequency and intensity of phonation. *J. Speech Hear. Res.* 12:616-628.

Hirano, M., Vennard, W., and Ohala, J. (1970). Regulation of register, pitch and intensity of voice. *Folia Phoniatr.* 22:1-20.

Lindestad, P-Å., Fritzell, B., and Persson, A. (1990). Evaluation of laryngeal muscle function by quantitative analysis of the EMG interference pattern. *Acta Otolaryngol.* (Stockh) 109:467-472.

Philipsson, L. and Larsson, P. (1988). The electromyographical signal as a measure of muscular force: a comparison of detection and quantification techniques. *Electromyogr. Clin. Neurophys.* 28:141-150.

Rose, A. and Willison, R. (1967). Quantitative electromyography using automatic analysis: Studies in healthy subjects and patients with primary muscle disease. *J. Neurol. Neurosurg. Psychiat.* 30:403-410.

Shipp, T., Doherty, T., and Morrissey P. (1979). Predicting vocal frequency from selected physiologic measures. *J. Acoust. Soc. Am.* 66:678-684.

Shipp, T. and Mc Glone, R.E. (1971). Laryngeal dynamics associated with voice frequency change. *J. Speech Hear. Res.*14:761-768.

Sundberg, J., Leanderson, R., and von Euler, C. (1988). Activity relationship between diaphragm and cricothyroid muscles. *STL-QPSR*, 6:83-91. (Dept. of Speech Communication and Music Acoustics, Royal Institute of Technology, Stockholm).

Willison, R. (1964). Analysis of electrical activity in healthy and dystrophic muscle in man. *J. Neurol. Neurosurg. Psychiat.* 27:386-394.

Yanagihara, N. and von Leden, H. (1968). The cricothyroid muscle during phonation-electromyographic, aerodynamic and acoustic studies. *Ann. Otol. Rhinol. Laryngol.* 75:987-1006.

23

F0 Raising Role of the Sternothyroid Muscle - An Electromyographic Study of Two Tenors

Seiji Niimi, Satoshi Horiguchi, and *Noriko Kobayashi

*Research Institute of Logopedics and Phoniatrics, Faculty of Medicine, University of Tokyo, Hongo, Tokyo, 113 Japan, *ATR Auditory and Visual Perception Research Laboratories, Osaka, Japan*

The functions of the strap muscles in speech production have been studied by several researchers (Faaborg-Andersen and Sonninen, 1960; Simada and Hirose, 1970; Ohala and Hirose, 1970; Kunitake, 1971; Erickson et al., 1977; Atkinson, 1978). These workers agree that in general the strap muscles contribute to lower the fundamental frequency (F0), or at least they become active when the F0 becomes lower. On the other hand, there is little research concerning the functional differences among the strap muscles. Since the location of the origin and the insertion of each strap muscle are unique for each muscle, there should be some functional differences among the strap muscles.

Looking at the anatomical framework of the larynx, the F0 raising mechanism is explained as follows: the thyroid cartilage rotates downward around the cricothyroid joint, or the frontal part of the cricoid ring comes closer to the thyroid cartilage resulting in a longer distance between the inner front part of the thyroid cartilage and the arytenoid cartilage. This results in a higher tension of the vocal cord. It is well known that the approximation of these two cartilages is executed by the contraction of the cricothyroid muscle.

Anatomically, the same approximation could be performed by the contraction of the sternothyroid muscle as well as by the cricothyroid muscle, since the attachment of the sternothyroid muscle is anterior to the center of the rotation (cricothyroid joint). It is natural to hypothesize that the sternothyroid muscle might act as an F0 raiser (Figure 1).

To test such a hypothesis, EMG signals from the sternothyroid muscle and the cricothyroid muscle were analyzed.

METHOD

Two professional tenor singers (M.Y. 57 years old and T.M. 59 years old) served as the subjects. Electromyograms (EMG) were recorded from the cricothyroid muscle (CT) and the sternothyroid muscle (ST) using bipolar hooked-wire electrodes inserted percutaneously (Hirose, 1971). The locations of the electrodes were verified by various non-singing tasks as below:

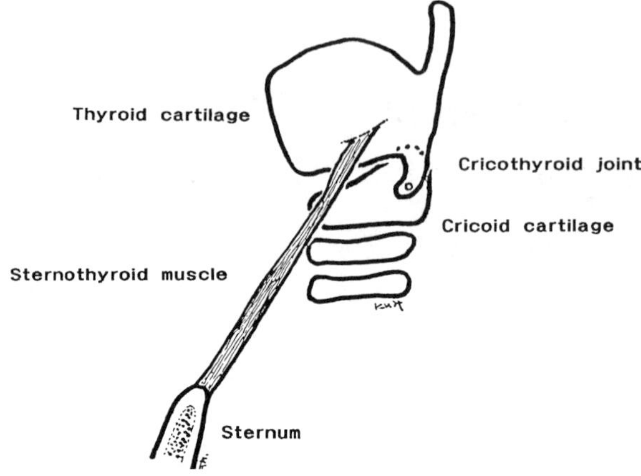

Fig. 1. Schematic drawing of the anatomical relationship between the sternothyroid muscle and the cricothyroid joint.

swallowing
jaw open/close
flexion of the neck
lowering the larynx

These verification manoeuvres were performed several times during the recording session to make sure the electrodes stayed in the target muscles.

The subjects were asked to phonate a sustained vowel /a/ at a comfortable pitch, a higher pitch (C4), and a lower pitch (C3) with "normal vibrato", "rapid vibrato" and "trill". These tasks were performed in a sitting position. Since the terminology has not been in general agreement, these terms were interpreted by each subject.

As the result, in the present study, the trill meant two ranges of pitch alternation: 2-semitones and 4-semitones. Voice intensity was not controlled.

Modulation frequencies of F0 perturbation were approximately 4.5 Hz, 5 Hz, and 5 Hz for normal vibrato, rapid vibrato, and trill, respectively.

Electromyographic signals were rectified and integrated for the interval of 5 ms. Those preprocessed signals were aligned with a reference point. In this study, the reference point was chosen by visual inspection at the moment when the acoustic signal began to increase in amplitude during each manoeuvre. These aligned EMG signals were averaged over 6 to 9 samples to improve the signal-to-noise ratio.

RESULTS

Non-singing manoeuvres

Swallowing: For both subjects, the activity of CT was suppressed during deglutition. The slight activity of ST after swallowing action was observed in both subjects. For subject M.Y., ST became active just before swallowing.

Jaw opening and closing: As expected, ST became active for jaw opening. Greater activity was observed for /a/ production than for /i/ production, since for /a/ production, a

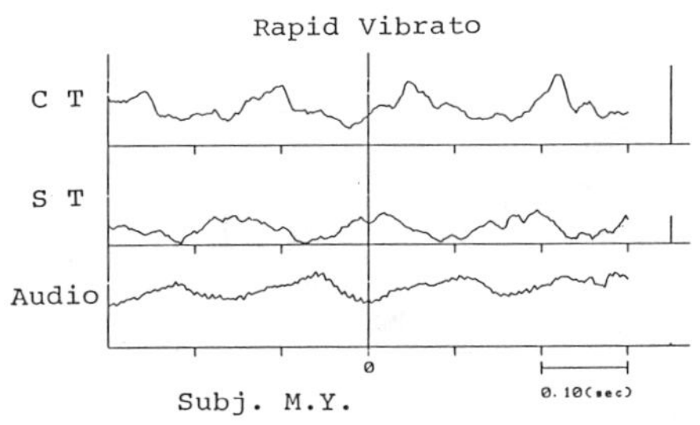

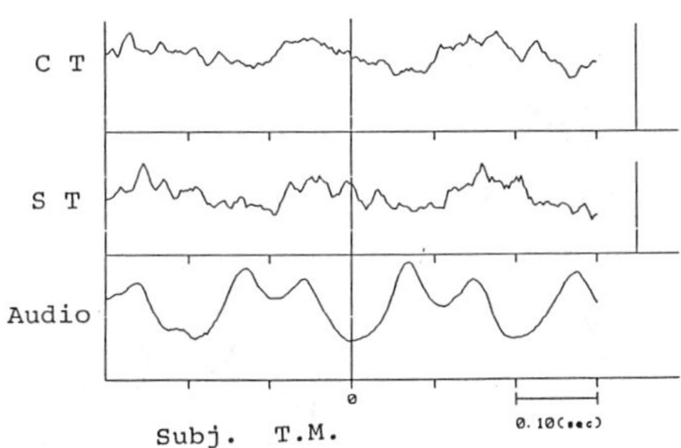

Fig. 2. Electromyographic activities of the cricothyroid (CT) and the sternothyroid (ST) muscles in rapid vibrato. The vertical line on the right of each figure indicates 0.3 mV as the calibration.

wider jaw opening is required. On the other hand, CT showed continuous activity through out the period of phonation.

Flexion of the neck: In both subjects, there was little or no activity in both channels.

Lowering the larynx: When the subjects were asked to shift the larynx downward volitionally, the sternothyroid muscle became active.

Singing tasks

Scale: Interestingly, for scale singing, both CT and ST were more active in higher pitches.

1) Normal vibrato:

CT: As expected, this muscle was more active in high pitch in both subjects. There was no modulation pattern observable at any pitch in subject M.Y. On the other hand, in subject T.M., this muscle showed a modulation pattern which corresponded to the acoustic modulation.

ST: This muscle was less active in low pitch than in high pitch in both subjects. In subject M.Y., no modulation pattern was observed at any pitch. In contrast, in subject T.M., a modulation pattern was clearly seen even at low pitch, where the muscle activity became smaller. Modulation patterns of CT and ST observed in subject T.M. were in the same phase.

2) Rapid vibrato:

Comparing with "normal vibrato", F0 perturbation is greater and modulation was faster in this manoeuvre. It could be assumed that rapid vibrato would be the exaggerated performance of the normal vibrato.

In both subjects, both the cricothyroid muscle and the sternothyroid muscle showed modulation patterns for the rapid vibrato. It can be assumed that these two muscles were recruited for a greater degree of F0 modulation.

For subject M.Y., these two muscles showed reciprocity in their patterns. When one increased in activity, the other decreased. But for subject T.M., these two muscles showed activity patterns in phase (Figure 2a).

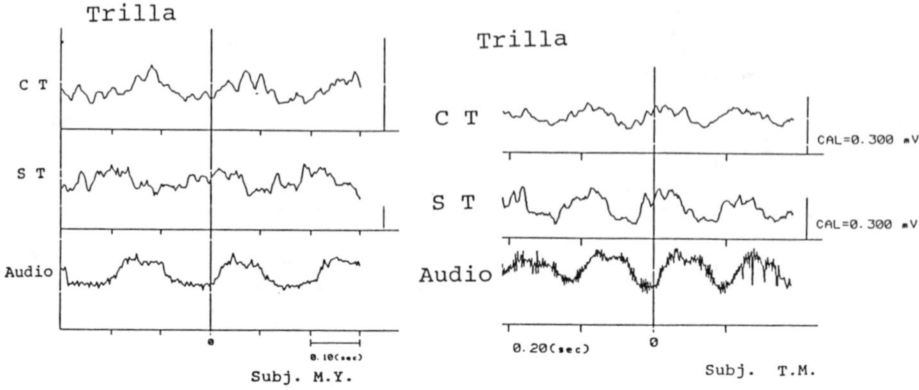

Fig. 3. Electromyographic activities of the cricothyroid (CT) and the sternothyroid (ST) muscles in Trilla. In subject M.Y., the reciprocal pattern of the muscle activity was observed, although not in subject T.M. The vertical line on the right of each figure indicates 0.3 mV as the calibration.

3) Trill:

CT: Modulation patterns were present in all tasks. However, they were clearly seen in the low pitch, presumably, because of the small background EMG activity. The overall activity of this muscle depended on the pitch level, as expected.

ST: Modulation patterns were observed in all manoeuvres. In subject M.Y., a reciprocal relationship was again observed between the sternothyroid muscle and the cricothyroid muscle. In other words, the sternothyroid muscle became active immediately after the cessation of the cricothyroid muscle activity (Figure 3a).

In subject T.M., the reciprocity between the ST and the CT was not observed (Figure 3b).

DISCUSSION

Since the function of the strap muscles has not been clearly understood, whether the electrodes were in the target muscle or not is always an intriguing question. In this study, to observe the sternothyroid activities, the electrode was inserted near the level of the lower border of the thyroid cartilage and about 1 cm laterally from the midline. Since the hooked-wire electrode was inserted at this point deep enough to touch the surface of the thyroid cartilage, and since the distance between the needle tip and actual active site of the electrode was about 2 mm, the active part of the electrode must have been in the sternothyroid muscle.

In this study, since the activity patterns obtained from the "ST" channel were distinctly different from those from the "CT" channel for several non-singing tasks as stated above, we believe that there was little possibility of the contamination from CT activity.

Another possible source of contamination is the sternohyoid muscle. If the insertion site is lower than the level of the lower border of the thyroid cartilage, the electrode could be in the sternohyoid muscle, because the lower portion of the sternothyroid muscle is closely covered by the sternohyoid muscle. While it has been reported that the sternohyoid muscle becomes active in neck flexion, the EMG activity from our "ST" channel showed little or no activity for that manoeuvre and it showed a marked activity for the downward shift of the larynx in this study. Judging from these unique activity patterns, it can be concluded that the location of our electrode was in the ST.

For scale singing, ST showed greater activity in higher F0 than lower F0 in both subjects. This observation suggests that this muscle plays a physiological role in raising F0 in singing.

There could be another argument regarding the observed greater activity of the sternothyroid muscle for higher F0 production, however. In operatic singing, which was used in this study, the singer tries to maintain the larynx in a low position to produce the so-called "covered voice". For the production of high-pitched covered voice, it is necessary to stabilize the larynx in a lower position and prevent its rising, opposing the natural tendency. Considering the anatomical relationships and the observed marked sternothyroid muscle activity for pulling the larynx down, the contraction of the sternothyroid muscle can serve as a stabilizing force for the whole framework of the larynx. Therefore, it may be suspected that this use of ST in higher F0 is characteristic of singer's manoeuvres and may not be commonly used in speech mode. However, even for the smaller pitch perturbation in the vibrato, for which the excursion of the larynx in the vertical dimension is smaller, the ST modulation pattern was maintained. This observation suggests that ST muscle activity during vibrato is not for the stabilization of the larynx but for the regulation of the F0 in singing voice.

There are some remaining questions. In subject M.Y., there was an observable reciprocity between CT and ST. For normal vibrato, in subject M.Y., modulation patterns could not be observed in ST. This means that the sternothyroid muscle plays not so great a role of F0 raising in subject M.Y. as it does in subject T.M.

In subject T.M., CT and ST showed an in-phase activity. It is possible to speculate that ST and CT play the same physiological role in some of the manoeuvres in this experiment, i.e., in vibrato.

CONCLUSION

Although the data were taken from a small number of subjects, it was suggested that, at least for professional singers in singing, the sternothyroid muscle can serve as one of the pitch raisers. The mechanism of pitch raising by the sternothyroid muscle was speculated as follows. When the muscle contracts, the anterior part of the thyroid cartilage tilts down to approach to the cricoid cartilage, resulting in a higher tension of the vocal cord.

REFERENCES

Atkinson, J.E. (1978). Correlation analysis of the physiological factors controlling fundamental voice frequency. *J. Acoust. Soc. Am.* 63:211-222.

Erickson, D., Liberman, M., and Niimi, S. (1977). The geniohyoid and the role of the strap muscles. *Status Report on Speech Research* 49:103-110. (Haskins Labs., New Haven, CT.)

Faaborg-Anderson, K. and Sonninen, A. (1960). Function of the extrinsic laryngeal muscles at different pitches. *Acta Otolaryngol.* 51:89-93.

Hirose, H. (1971). Electromyography of the articulatory muscles: Current instrumentation and techniques. *Status Report on Speech Research* 25/26:73-86. (Haskins Labs., New Haven, CT.)

Kunitake, H. (1971). Function of the extrinsic laryngeal muscles - An electromyographic study (in Japanese). *Jpn. J. Otolaryngol.* 74:1156-1201.

Ohala, J. and Hirose, H. (1970). The function of the sternohyoid muscle in speech. *Ann. Bull. RILP.* 4:41-44. (Research Inst. of Logopedics and Phoniatrics, University of Tokyo).

Simada, Z. and Hirose, H. (1970). The function of the laryngeal muscles in respect to the word accent distinction. *Ann. Bull. RILP.* 4:27-40. ((Research Inst. of Logopedics and Phoniatrics, University of Tokyo).

24

The Postganglionic Sympathetic Innervation of the Larynx in Cats

Yoshikazu Yoshida, Tatsuya Saito, Yasumasa Tanaka, Minoru Hirano, *Masatoshi Morimoto, and *Takeshi Kanaseki

*Dept. of Otorhinolaryngology and Head and Neck Surgery, School of Medicine, Kurume University, Kurume City, 830 Japan, *Saga Medical College, Saga City, 840-01 Japan*

It has been accepted in general that in the larynx the sympathetic nerve supplies chiefly the vessels and glands, and regulates blood flow volume and laryngeal glandular secretion. There have been several anatomical investigations regarding the sympathetic nerve supply in the larynx. Sasaki (1943) investigated the terminations of the sympathetic nerve fibres in the laryngeal mucosa. Itoh (1929) observed changes of the intrinsic laryngeal muscles after sectioning the cervical sympathetic trunk, and resectioning the cervical sympathetic ganglia. He also identified the existence of the sympathetic nerve fibres in the recurrent laryngeal nerve (RLN). Lemere (1932) also identified the existence of the unmyelinated fibres in the ramus anastomoticus. The pathways of the laryngeal sympathetic nerve fibres to the larynx were examined by Sugano (1929) and Suzuki (1935) using silver impregnation. The fluorescence histochemistry for demonstrating catecholamines was introduced by Falck et al. (1962). Nielsen (1969), using the fluorescence histochemical technique, identified the postganglionic fibres originating from the superior cervical ganglion (SCG) in the vagus.

However, these investigations do not provide a detailed explanation of the pathways and distribution of the postganglionic sympathetic nerve. In 1982, Hisa reported, for the first time, the origin and course of noradrenergic nerve fibres contained in laryngeal nerves and their destinations in the larynx using the same technique as Nielsen's investigation. The fluorescence histochemistry is useful to label all nerve fibres containing catecholamines morphologically in the larynx. This technique is, however, unable to trace the postganglionic fibres from the cells of origin in the cervical sympathetic ganglia individually. Recently, Marfurt et al. (1986) found that a horseradish peroxidase (HRP) labels peripheral sympathetic fibres and axonal terminals in a variety of orofacial and cerebral tissues after wheat germ agglutinin (WGA)-HRP injection into SCG. They also indicated the advantages of high visibility and specificity, applicability to the study of tissue and situations where other anatomical methods are neither appropriate nor feasible. Therefore, in order to clarify systematically, not only the pathways from each cervical sympathetic ganglion and peripheral distribution of the postganglionic sympathetic nerve fibres, but also the areas of innervation for each laryngeal nerve, we attempted WGA-HRP studies.

The present paper describes our current results. This is one of a series of studies of the neural system related to the functions of the larynx.

METHOD AND MATERIALS

The experimental studies were carried out on 33 cats weighing 0.5-2.0 kg. The experiments were divided into six groups (Table 1). The superior laryngeal nerve (SLN) and RLN were intact in groups 1 to 3. Under these conditions, WGA-HRP reaches the larynx via both SLN and RLN from each cervical ganglion. In groups 4 to 6, SLN at the level 1.0 cm rostral to the thyroid foramen and RLN at the level of the caudal end of the thyroid gland, were sectioned. The cut ends were tied. Under these conditions, WGA-HRP is carried to the larynx via other routes besides SLN and RLN. Each animal was anaesthetized with intramuscular injections of Ketamine (30-40 mg/kg) and Xylazine hydrochloride (0.5-1.0 mg/kg). The cervical sympathetic ganglion: the superior cervical ganglion (SCG), the middle cervical ganglion (MCG) or stellate ganglion (SG) of the right side was exposed and prepared for injection after a middle cervical skin incision. 4.5-6.0 µl of 2% WGA-HRP conjugate using a 10 µl glass misconstruing coupled to a micropipette was injected by pressure into SCG, MCG or SG in each case. The surgery was performed under an operating microscope. For a complete description of the method, see Yoshida et al. (1988).

RESULTS

Labelling in the brain stem and spinal cord

In the present experiments of groups 1 to 6, following WGA-HRP injection into SCG, MCG or SG, no labelled cell bodies, fibres and terminals were recognized in the nucleus tractus solitarii or other nuclei. But in the spinal cord, numerous HRP labelled neurons were found in the ipsilateral intermediolateral nucleus. They extended from Th 1 to Th 4 in groups 1, 2, 4, and 5, and from Th 1 to Th 8 in groups 3 and 6. This shows that some of the injected WGA-HRP was taken up internally by preganglionic fibres within each cervical sympathetic ganglion and transported retrogradely to their cell bodies of origin in the spinal cord segments.

Labelling in the larynx

The results are summarized in Table 1.

Group 1: After WGA-HRP injection into SCG, on the outside of the laryngeal framework, labelled fibres were observed along the internal branch of SLN (Int-SLN) (Figure 3A), the external branch of SLN (Ext-SLN) (Figure 3B), RLN, and on the wall of the superior laryngeal artery (SLA), ipsilaterally, as a perivascular network formation (Figure 3C). Labelled sympathetic nerve fibres in the rostral part of SLA were more numerous in number than in the peripheral part. We could not trace labelled nerve fibres of the SLA to the larynx.

Inside of the laryngeal framework, HRP labelled sympathetic nerve fibres were identified in the arytenoid region (Figures 1A, 1C, Figure 3D), the mucosa of the posterior glottis (Figure 1C), ipsilaterally, and in the walls of the hypopharynx bilaterally with an ipsilateral predominance (Figures 1C, 1D, 1E, 1F, 1G, Figure 3F). In particular, in the posterior wall of the hypopharynx, a small number of fibres crossed over the

Table 1: *Summary of results. See text for abbreviations of laryngeal postganglionic sympathetic nerve fibres in the cat.*

Experimental group	Number of animals	Site of HRP injection	SLN and RLN	Side	HRP labeled sympathetic nerve fibres				
					Nerve	Vessel	Distribution in larynx		
							Rostral end	Caudal end	Regions of appearance
1	8	SCG	Intact	Ipsilat.	Int-SLN Ext-SLN	SLA	Rostral to arytenoid	Caudal end of thyroid	Arytenoid emin., post. glottis, mucosa covering PCA, lat. and post. walls of hypopharynx
2	12	MCG			Int-SLN Ext-SLN RLN	-	Glottis	IV tracheal ring	Vocal fold caudal aspect., subglottis, mucosa covering. PCA, lat. and post. walls of hypopharynx, mucosa of trachea
3	4	SG			RLN	-	I tracheal ring	?	Mucosa of trachea
4	3	SCG	Sectioned	No HRP labelled fibres					
5	3	MCG							
6	3	SG							

midline to the contralateral side (Figure 1C). Labelled sympathetic nerve fibres appeared chiefly around the laryngeal glands, on the wall of vessels and in the connective tissue surrounding them. In a rostrocaudal direction, they were distributed from the level rostral to the arytenoid eminence to the level of the caudal end of the thyroid cartilage (Figure 2). Labelled fibres in the posterior glottis were smaller than those in the hypopharynx in number. Figures 1 and 2 schematically depict the distribution of HRP labelled sympathetic nerve fibres originating from each of the cervical ganglion in the larynx.

Group 2: Outside of the larynx, following WGA-HRP injection into MCG, labelled nerve fibres were recognized along Int-SLN, Ext-SLN and RLN ipsilaterally. Inside of the laryngeal framework, HRP reacted fibres were recognized ipsilaterally in the caudal aspect of the vocal fold (Figure 1D), the subglottis (Figures 1E, 1F, 1G, Figure 3E), the mucosa covering the posterior cricoarytenoid muscle (Figure 1F), the lateral and posterior walls of the hypopharynx (Figures 1F, 1G) and the tracheal mucosa (Figure 1H). The number of labelled nerve fibres in the subglottis were larger than in the hypopharynx. In groups 1 and 2, HRP labelled nerve fibres were identified on the walls of the blood vessels measuring from 10 m to 100 m in diameter. Those in the laryngeal glands were seen at the terminal part exclusively. In addition their number was greatest in the subglottis, the posterior glottis and the arytenoid region, in that order. When viewed dorsoventrally, the dorsal part exhibited a fuller distribution of labelled fibres than the ventral part.

Group 3: Following WGA-HRP injection into SG, labelled sympathetic nerve fibres were found along RLN (Figure 3G) and around the glands of the trachea in the level caudal to the first tracheal ring (Figure 1H, Figure 2). They disappeared along Int-SLN, Ext-SLN, and on the wall of the laryngeal arteries.

Groups 4, 5, and 6: In the experiments of groups 4, 5, and 6, SLN and RLN were cut and tied before WGA-HRP injection. Following WGA-HRP injection into the cervical sympathetic ganglion individually, no labelled nerve fibres were seen in the larynx in any of the cases. From the findings of the experiments of group 4 to 6, it seems that the

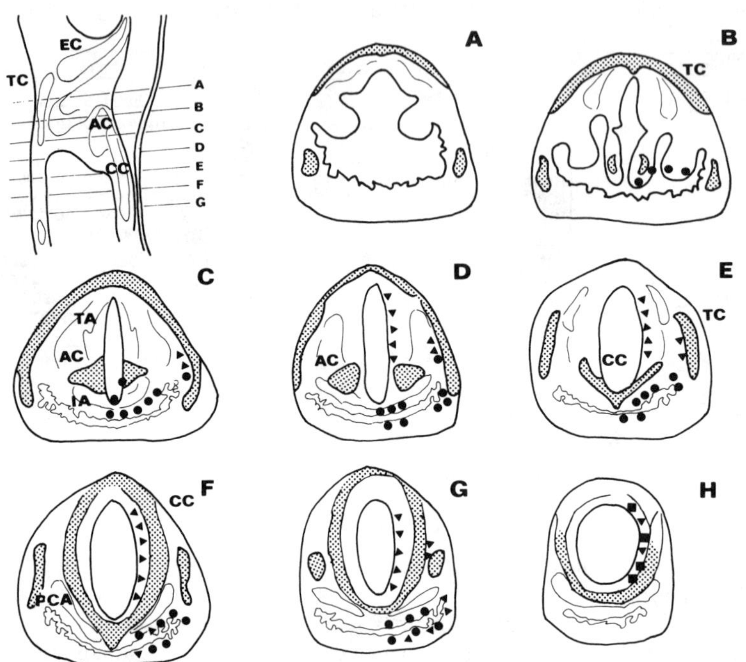

Fig. 1. Schematic depictions of peripheral distribution of HRP labelled sympathetic nerve fibres originating from SCG (solid circles), MCG (solid triangles) and SG (solid squares) in cross sections of the larynx after injection of WGA-HRP into each cervical sympathetic ganglion. In the top left of this figures is an illustration showing the location in the larynx of each serial section. EC, epiglottic cartilage; TC, thyroid cartilage; AC, arytenoid cartilage; CC, cricoid cartilage; TA, thyroarytenoid muscle; IA, interarytenoid muscle; PCA, posterior cricoarytenoid muscle.

postganglionic sympathetic nerve fibres enter the larynx exclusively through SLN and RLN.

DISCUSSION

Pathways of the sympathetic nerve fibres to the larynx

Regarding the pathways of the postganglionic sympathetic nerve fibres originating from the SCG in humans, Mitchell (1954) stated that sympathetic fibres reach the larynx joined with SLN directly, but more often they pass through the pharyngeal plexus and so indirectly to the larynx. In the HRP study using cats, Lucier et al. (1986) observed that reaction product was localized in the posterior portion of the cervical sympathetic ganglion after HRP application to Int-SLN. It is generally accepted that the laryngeal nerves contain many unmyelinated fibres. Suzuki (1935) reported that following resection of SCG in dogs, unmyelinated fibres in SLN degenerated, while those in RLN remained unchanged. This observation means that unmyelinated postganglionic

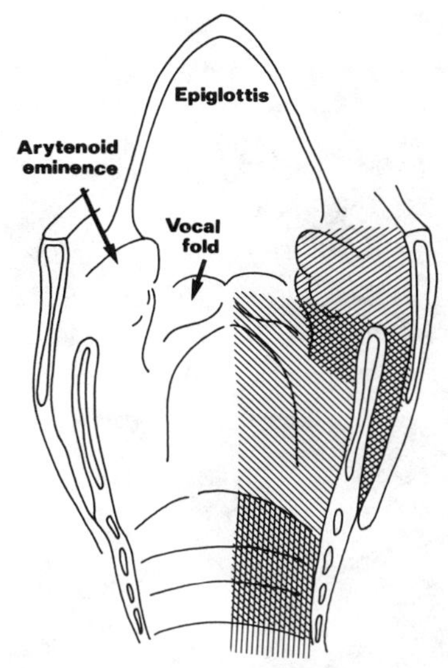

Fig. 2. Outline representation of a ventral view of the cat's larynx opened along the posterior ventral midline. Distribution of sympathetic nerve fibres originating from SCG (oblique lines to left), MCG (oblique lines to right) and SG (straight lines).

sympathetic nerves originating from SCG enter the larynx through SLN. On the other hand, in the dog, Hisa (1982) stated that noradrenergic fibres originating from SCG were considered to enter SLN and RLN. In the cat, numerous adrenergic fibres originated from SCG were found in the cervical vagus proper by direct fluorescence microscopic method (Nielsen et al., 1969). The present study demonstrates that SLN and RLN received the sympathetic nerve fibres from SCG. Our results support Hisa's findings, but not Suzuki's finding. These inconsistencies are assumed to be due to technical differences.

Information concerning the course of postganglionic fibres originating from MCG, Suzuki (1935) confirmed degeneration of the unmyelinated sympathetic nerve fibres in RLN after resection of MCG of the dog. In addition, Hisa (1982) concluded from his observation that RLN received noradrenergic nerve fibres not only from SCG but also from MCG directly. According to Mitchell (1954), the human's filaments from MCG accompanied the laryngeal branches of the inferior thyroid artery. The present study clarified that the sympathetic innervation pathway from MCG to the larynx was via Int-SLN and Ext-SLN and RLN in the cat. Our results agree with previous descriptions except Mitchell's report.

Concerning SG, in an HRP study, Kalia and Mesulam (1980) stated that the cat's larynx received fibres from the rostral part of this ganglion. A pathway from SG to the larynx, however, was not mentioned. The canine RLN contained unmyelinated fibres originating from MCG and SG (Itoh, 1929). Following removal of SG in the dog, no definite change of the unmyelinated fibres was recognized in SLN. However, unmyelinated fibres in RLN degenerated (Suzuki, 1935). We also observed labelled sympathetic nerve fibres (after WGA-HRP injection into SG), in RLN, but not in SLN. Furthermore the number of labelled fibres in RLN were much smaller in the cases of SCG (Group 1) and MCG (Group 2), than in the case of SG (Group 3). The present findings suggest that the sympathetic nerve fibres contained in RLN are distributed chiefly to the trachea and the outside of the larynx.

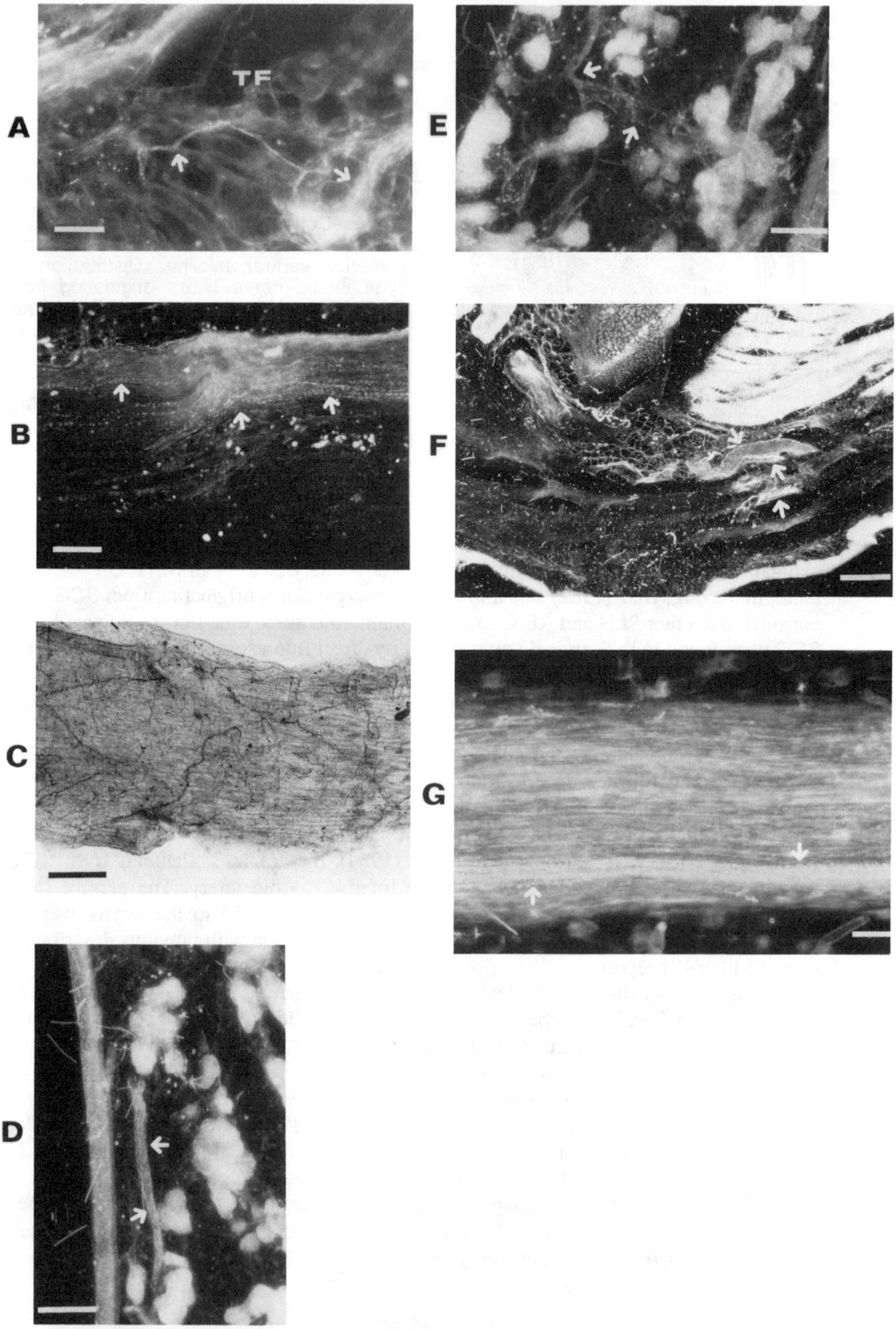

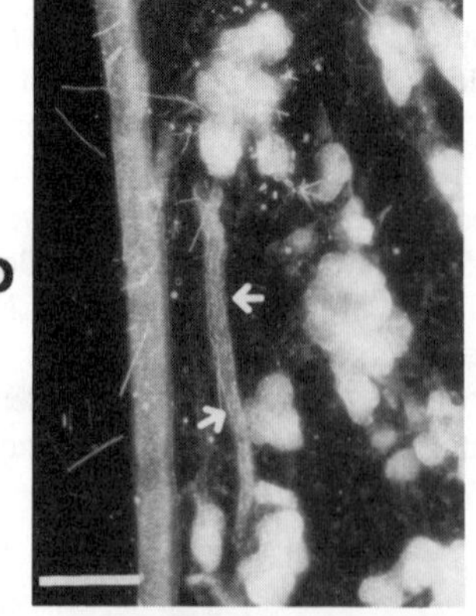

Fig. 3. Photomicrographs displaying seven sections of the larynx. **A**, **B**, **C**, and **D** are samples of WGA-HRP injection into SCG. **E** and **F** are of MCG. **G** is of SG. Arrows indicate labelled sympathetic nerve fibres. **A**. Cross section of the right thyroid foramen (TF). Calibration bar, 100 µm. **B**. Horizontal section of the right Ext-SLN. Sympathetic nerve fibres ran along Ext- SLN. Calibration bar, 50 µm. **C**. Transmitted view of the right superior laryngeal artery after being opened and spread out. Labelled sympathetic nerve fibres formed a network of perivascular innervation. Calibration bar, 100 µm. **D**. Cross section of the right arytenoid eminence. Labelled sympathetic nerve fibres were around the glands. Calibration bar, 500 µm. **E**. Cross section of the right subglottis. Labelled sympathetic nerve fibres appeared around the glands. Calibration bar, 100 µm. **F**. Cross section of the right anterior wall of the hypopharynx. Labelled fibres were observed on wall of the vessel. PCA, posterior cricoarytenoid muscle. Calibration bar, 100 µm. **G**. Horizontal section of the right RLN. Many labelled fibres ran together with RLN. Calibration bar, 50 µm..

Some investigators found that the sympathetic fibres innervating the larynx ran together with the arteries. Mitchell (1954) stated that in the human, sympathetic fibres derived from the parent external carotid perivascular plexus accompanied the superior thyroid arteries, and filaments from the corresponding plexus on the subclavian artery. These latter were invariably reinforced by filamentous contributions from MCG. In contrast, Hisa's findings indicated that the laryngeal nerves are the only source of sympathetic nerve supply to the canine larynx and that they are distributed on the ipsilateral side. According to Kimoto (1960) the arteries supplying the cat's larynx are SLA branching from the carotis communis, the inferior laryngeal artery branching from the inferior thyroid artery and the branch of the superior thyroid artery. Following WGA-HRP injection into SCG, we observed labelled fibres only on the SLA. However, after cutting both SLN and RLN, no labelled sympathetic fibres were found in the larynx. The present study shows that laryngeal nerves are the exclusive pathways of sympathetic fibres originating from the cervical sympathetic ganglia, in cats.

Distribution of the sympathetic nerve fibres in the larynx

Descriptions concerning distribution of the sympathetic nerve fibres originating from each of the cervical ganglion in the larynx could not be found in past literature. The present study indicates that ganglionic innervation occurs rostrocaudally in the larynx. That is, SCG innervates in the rostral part, MCG in the middle part, and SG in the caudal part and trachea in that order. It seems that the larynx is the boundary in distribution of the sympathetic nerve fibres originating from the cervical ganglia in the upper respiratory tract. As mentioned before, the laryngeal sympathetic nerves regulate laryngeal blood flow volume and glandular secretion. Silver impregnation in the human showed the terminations of autonomic nerves in the adventitia and media of laryngeal small arteries (Sasaki, 1943). Hisa et al. (1982) observed abundant fluorescent nerve fibres surrounding the blood vessels in the laryngeal muscles. He also pointed out that they may be evidence for the existence of sympathetic innervation to regulate the blood flow volume of the larynx. In the present investigation, labelled sympathetic nerve fibres were identified on the wall of small blood vessels. However, it was difficult to differentiate whether the vessel was an artery or a vein, or to determine to which layer of the vessel the fibres reached in the present WGA-HRP technique. Pressman and Kelemen (1955) reported that laryngeal secretions are under the control of the sympathetic nervous system. Electron microscopic observation clarified the existence of the adrenergic terminals near gland cells and myoepithelial cells (Hisa et al., 1982). While we observed the sympathetic fibres in the terminal part of laryngeal glands, we were unable to identify whether the fibres supply the myoepithelial cell or not.

As regards the sympathetic innervation to the intrinsic laryngeal muscles, Itoh (1929) concluded that the intrinsic laryngeal muscles receive the sympathetic nerve fibres for maintenance. Arnold (1959) also described that the perivascular sympathetic supply assists in the maintenance of the intrinsic muscular tonus. In addition, Hisa (1982) reported that, in the intrinsic laryngeal muscles, many noradrenergic nerve fibres were observed to run parallel with the muscle fibres and separate from the blood vessels. No obvious evidence for the existence of direct innervation has been obtained. On the other hand, Nomoto (1989) observed that after transection RLN, the sympathetic nerves around the vessels entered into the Schwann tubes and reached the denervated neuromuscular junctions, instead of the motor nerve. Our WGA-HRP experiment could not trace into the muscle, because the muscle has its own intramuscular enzyme. Further work is needed to solve these problems.

REFERENCES

Arnold, G.E. (1959). Vocal rehabilitation of paralytic dysphonia. *Arch. Otolaryngol.* 70:444-453.

Falck, B., Hillarp, N.A., Thieme, G., and Torp, A. (1962). Fluorescence of catechol amines and related compounds condensed with formaldehyde. *J. Histochem. Cytochem.* 10:348-354.

Hisa, Y. (1982). Fluorescence histochemical studies on the noradrenergic innervation of the canine larynx. *Acta Anat.* 113:15-25.

Hisa, Y., Matsui, T., Fukui, K., Ibata, Y., and Mizukoshi, O. (1982). Ultrastructural and fluorescence histochemical studies on the sympathetic innervation of the canine laryngeal glands. *Acta Otolaryngol.* 93:119-122.

Itoh, C. (1929). Sympathetic innervation of the intrinsic laryngeal muscles. *J. Otolaryngol. Jpn.* 34:1207-1230.

Kalia, M. and Mesulam, M-M.(1980). Brain stem projection of sensory and motor components of the vagus complex in the cat: II laryngeal, tracheobronchial, pulmonary, cardiac, and gastrointestinal branches, *J. Comp. Neurol.* 193:467-508.

Kimoto, R. (1960). Über den Blutversorgungsplan des Kehlkopfes und der Luftrohen von Katze. *Kurume Med. J.* 23:2178-2197.

Lemere, F. (1932). Innervation of the larynx II. Ramus anastomoticus and ganglion cells of the superior laryngeal nerve. *Anato. Rec.* 54:389-407.

Lucier, G.E., Egizii, R., and Dostrovsky, J.O. (1986). Projections of the internal branch of the superior laryngeal nerve of the cat. *Brain Res. Bull.* 16:713-721.

Marfurt, C.F., Zaleski, E.M., Adams, C.E., and Welther, C.L. (1986). Sympathetic nerve fibers in rat orofacial and cerebral tissues as revealed by the HRP-WGA tracing technique: A light and electron microscopic study. *Brain Res.* 366:373-378.

Mitchell, G.A.G. (1954). The autonomic nerve supply of the throat, nose and ear. *J. Laryng.* 68:495-516.

Nielsen, K.C., Owman, C.H., and Santini, M. (1969). Anastomosing adrenergic nerves from the sympathetic trunk to the vagus at the cervical level in the cat. *Brain Res.* 12:1-9.

Nomoto, M. (1989). An ultrastructural study of the neuromuscular junctions of the cat intrinsic laryngeal muscles. II. Synapse formation by autonomic nerves. *J. Otolaryngol. Jpn.* 92:875-885.

Pressman, J.J. and Kelemen, G. (1955). Physiology of the larynx. *Physiol. Rev.* 35:506-554.

Sasaki, Y. (1943). Distribution of nerve fibers in the human larynx. *Tohoku Med. J.* 32:569-594.

Sugano, M. (1929). Über die Kehlkopfnerven, experimentelle Untersuchungen über die Innervation des Kehlkopfes. *J. Otolaryngol. Jpn.* 35:1338-1361.

Suzuki, S. (1935). Über die Beziehungen zwischen dem Vagus und dem Sympathicus. *Tokyo Igakkai Zassi* 49:1659-1675.

25

Neurophysiological Control of Vocal Fold Adduction and Abduction for Phonation Onset and Offset During Speech

Christy L. Ludlow, Susan E. Sedory and Mihoko Fujita

National Institute on Deafness and Other Communication Disorders, Bethesda, MD 20892, USA

The purpose of this study was to examine the relationship between vocal fold movement and laryngeal muscle activation during speech. Several investigators have described the activation patterns of the laryngeal muscles during speech articulation (Sawashima and Hirose, 1983; Löfqvist et al., 1989). In such studies, muscle activation signals were lined up on the basis of an event in the speech signal, such as voice onset following an obstruent. Such results do not provide information on the relationship between movement and muscle action. For example, increases in the cricothyroid muscle during voiceless sounds (Löfqvist et al., 1989) could aid vocal fold abduction with phonation offset or might be contributing to vocal fold adduction for phonation onset after the consonant. Further, phonation onset and offset may depend on factors other than vocal fold position such as changes in subglottic air pressure and supraglottal valving (Hirose and Niimi, 1987) changes in the speech signal may not be a good indicator of vocal fold movement.

Therefore to determine the role of the laryngeal muscles for different speech gestures, the relationship between muscle activation changes and vocal fold movement should be examined. By measuring laryngeal muscle activation prior to different vocal fold movements, such as adduction and abduction, it can be determined how voicing changes are dependent upon laryngeal muscle activation.

Further, since laryngeal muscle actions are most likely highly interdependent (Sonesson, 1982), correlations between activations of different muscles should be examined to determine the relationship between the laryngeal muscles for achieving voicing changes during speech.

METHODS

Three normal subjects, (48/F, 30/F, and 51/M), naive to the purpose of the study, participated after informed consent. Following a subcutaneous injection of Lidocaine to reduce discomfort, the location of each muscle, the right thyroarytenoid (RTA), the left thyroarytenoid (LTA), the right cricothyroid (RCT), and the left cricothyroid (LCT) was determined using a bipolar needle electrode. Verification gestures for the RTA and LTA included increased activation during phonation and effort closure without prominent phonatory onset and offset bursts indicative of lateral cricoarytenoid placement (Hirano and Ohala, 1969). For verification of the LCT and RCT, a pitch glide and phonation at different pitch levels confirmed placements without activation on head turning or elevation indicative of strap muscle interference. Once the muscle position was determined, bipolar hooked wire electrodes were inserted into the same position with 27 gauge 30 mm needles. The needle containing the wires was moved within the muscle until maximal activation was achieved and the pattern was correct for the target muscle. Once the correct placement was achieved, the needle was removed leaving the bipolar hooked wires in place. A surface recording of the posterior cricoarytenoid (PCA) was made using a pharyngeal electrode inserted through the nasal passage into the hypopharynx which recorded muscle activity through the hypopharyngeal mucosa (Fujita et al., 1989). Verification included increased activity with deep inhalation, and decreased activity during effort closure and phonation. Recordings were obtained in all five muscles simultaneously with signal amplification and band pass filtering between 100 and 5000 Hz for the bipolar hooked wires and between 50 to 1000 Hz for the surface electrode.

Five minutes after electrode placement the lights were dimmed, the room quietened and the subject relaxed before recording one minute of quiet respiration. The subject was then moved to a sitting position, the nasal cavity and posterior oropharynx sprayed with Lidocaine and a nasopharyngoscope was inserted with the fiberoptic tip placed below the epiglottis and centered above the vocal folds. Placement was constantly monitored throughout the experiment.

To record changes in glottal opening, the amount of light passing through the glottis was detected with a photoglottographic (PGG) light detector held against the skin below the cricoid cartilage. The PGG signal was fed through a current to voltage converter with a pre-amp of 1 ma to 10 volts gain. The amplified signal was passed through a 500 Hz low pass filter then sent to two separate outputs, one to a DC amplifier with an adjustable gain resulting in a DC signal from 0 to 500 Hz. The other was passed through a high pass filter of 30 Hz to extract out the DC component resulting in an AC signal from 30 to 500 Hz with an adjustable gain. The AC PGG, DC PGG and the five EMG signals were recorded simultaneously while the subjects repeated [isi] and then [siʔi] between 10 and 20 times each at a comfortable speaking rate. Both speech items were produced with stress on the first vowel. Maximum muscle activation gestures were then recorded including, quick deep inhalation (PCA), effort closure (RTA and LTA) and quick exhalation (PCA), high pitch [i] during ascending and descending glides (RCT and LCT) and dry and liquid swallows (RCT and LCT).

The PGG and EMG signals were digitized at 5000 samples per second (sps) with anti-aliasing filtering at 2000 Hz and the EMG signals converted to microvolts. To maximize and standardize the signal to noise level for each EMG signal, following full wave rectification, the minimum noise level between motor unit firings was measured in microvolts and subtracted to extract background noise from each EMG channel. The maximum peak amplitude was measured from the EMG signals during the maximum gestures recordings and used to convert each EMG signal into the percent of maximum activation for that muscle.

A 500 Hz single pole recursive low pass digital filter was used to smooth each EMG signal prior to downsampling to 2500 sps and automatic measurement. To identify

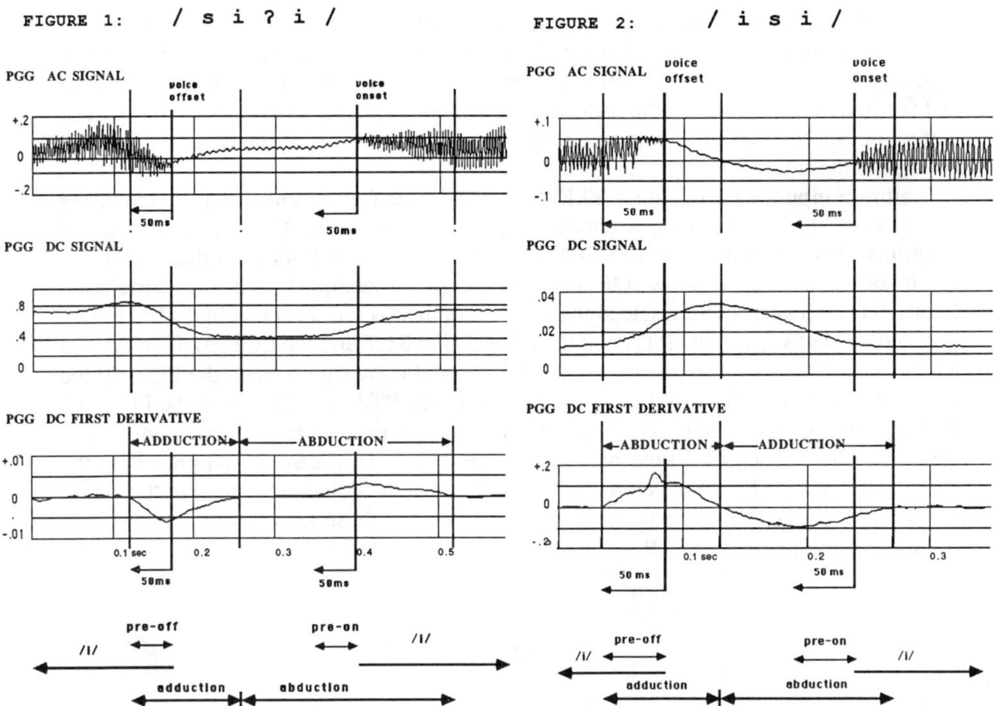

Figs.1 and 2. Tracings of the AC photoglottographic signal (PGG AC) on the top, the DC photoglottographic signal (PGG DC), middle, and the first time derivative of the DC photoglottographic signal (PGG DC First Derivative) during production of the speech token [si?i] in Figure 1 and [isi] in Figure 2. The 6 measurement intervals are illustrated at the bottom of the figure in line with the points in the signal which were used to mark each of the intervals: the initial [i], 50 ms prior to voice offset (pre-off), the adduction period, the abduction period, 50 ms prior to voice onset and the final [i].

different phases in glottic movement for the production of [?] in [si?i], the onset of vocal fold adduction was identified as the point where the first time derivative of the PGG DC signal first went below the zero line while the onset of abduction was where the signal first returned to the zero line (Figure 1). Similarly, for [s] in [isi] the onset of vocal fold abduction was the point where the first time derivative of the PGG DC signal went above the zero line and adduction onset was defined as the point when the signal first returned to zero (Figure 2). These points bounded the periods of vocal fold adduction and abduction during which the mean EMG activity was computed by summing the points and dividing by the number of points in the period. This approach included all EMG activity during the movement period. Since the onset of EMG activity prior to movement was variable it was decided to include only that during movement. To measure EMG activity in relation to changes in the speech signal, voice offset and onset times were identified from visual inspection of the PGG AC signal and muscle activity was averaged for a fixed time period of 50 ms prior to voice offset and onset. These two 50 ms periods usually fell during the first part of the vocal fold adduction or abduction phases, that is, the early part of each movement phase, during [ʔ] and [s] respectively. As illustrated in Figures 1 and 2, muscle activation was measured during 6 time intervals for each [iʔi] and [isi] token: the initial [i], the adduction or abduction phase, 50 ms at the early part of that phase, the following abduction or adduction phase, 50 ms at the early part of that phase, and the final [i].

Before computing correlations, all EMG signals were further smoothed by computing the mean of 125 points with a continuously sliding window. This eliminated signal amplitude changes resulting from individual motor unit firings. Following that, a 50 point continuously sliding window (20 ms) was used to compute Pearson Correlation Coefficients between two muscle signals. The output was a time series plot of r (Figure 3) computed between 1) the RTA and the LTA, 2) the RCT and the LCT, 3) the RTA and RCT, 4) the LTA and LCT, 5) the summed RTA and LTA signals with the PCA, 6) the summed RCT and LCT with the PCA, 7) the summed RTA and RCT with the PCA and 8) the summed LTA and LCT with the PCA. The maximum r was automatically identified during each of 3 time periods (Figure 3) in each token: the [i] preceding the consonant; the time from the beginning of vocal fold adduction or abduction to the end of vocal fold abduction or adduction, the entire movement phase for [ʔ] or [s] respectively (Figure 1 and 2); and the [i] following the consonant.

RESULTS

To compare the mean percent of maximum muscle activation occurring during the [iʔi] and [isi] productions within each of the 6 time intervals repeated ANOVAs were computed for each muscle while blocking on subjects. The six time intervals were: the initial [i], 50 ms prior to phonation offset (pre), the adduction (for ʔ) to abduction (for s) period (close/open), the abduction (for ʔ) to adduction (for s) period (open/close), the 50 ms prior to phonation onset (post) and the final [i]. The results for the comparisons within each of the five muscles studied are presented in Figures 4, 5, and 6. The probability of the F ratio obtained for the main factor is listed above each time interval using a criterion alpha level of <0.009 to maintain an experimentwise error rate of less than 10%. If the subject blocking factor had a significant ($p<0.009$) interaction with the main factor then an "S" is listed for that comparison.

PCA activation (Figure 4) increased 50 ms prior to phonation offset for [s] (pre), during vocal fold opening for the [s], and during phonation onset (post) and vocal fold abduction following the glottal stop. Therefore, the PCA was active for both abduction gestures; when the glottis was going from a phonatory position to open, and when it was going from a closed position to a phonatory position. The greatest differences in PCA activation between abduction and adduction were seen when a 50 ms time window was used to average muscle activity only during the early part of both abduction gestures. There were no significant subject by main effect interactions demonstrating that similar results occurred in all 3 subjects.

Similar patterns were seen in the right and left TAs which were very different from the PCA (Figure 5). Significant increases occurred prior to the glottal stop during phonation offset (pre) for the glottal stop as well as vocal fold adduction . Activation was also greater during vocal fold closure after the [s] than during vocal fold opening

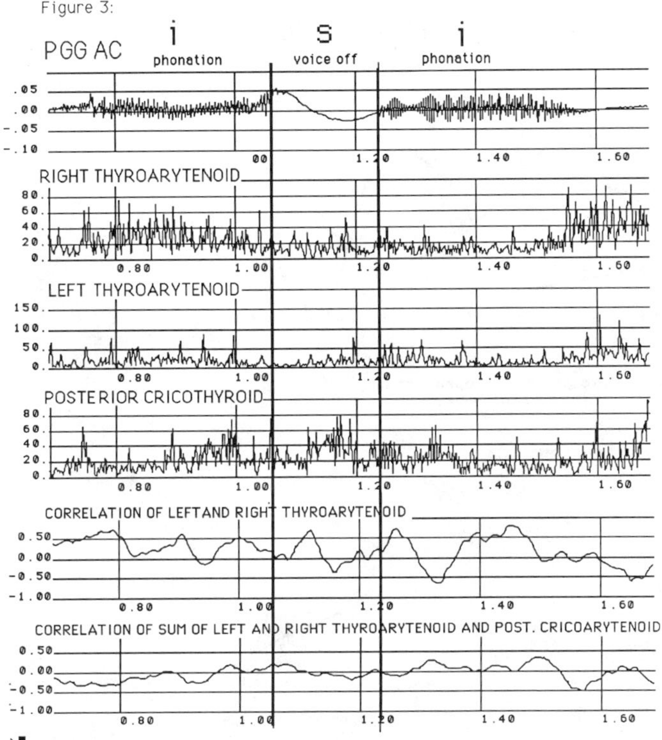

Fig. 3. Tracings of the AC photoglottographic signal (PGG AC) on the top, and the rectified and smoothed electromyographic recordings of the Right Thyroarytenoid, the Left Thyroarytenoid and the Posterior Cricoarytenoid displayed in Percent of Maximum Activation. The Pearson Correlation Coefficients for the same signals are displayed below for the correlation of the right and left thyroarytenoid muscles and at the bottom for the correlation between the sum of the two thyroarytenoid signals with the posterior cricoarytenoid.

following [ʔ]. This was significant in the RTA and a similar trend was seen on the left. However, this difference for [s] was more due to activity depression during vocal fold opening after the glottal stop than due activation increasing during vocal fold adduction following [s]. Further, the LTA showed a linear decrease from the initial to the final [i] possibly due to stress changes between the initial and the final vowel. Therefore, the TA muscles were activated for glottal closure from the phonatory position but not during adduction from the open to the phonatory position. As with the PCA however, the greatest differences were seen during the 50 ms time period preceding phonation offset which was the first part of the adductory gesture (Figure 1).

Different patterns were seen in the two CT muscles (Figure 6). In the RCT, activation decreased during vocal fold adduction following the [s] in comparisons with activation for [ʔ]. In the LCT, activation decreased between the initial stressed and the final unstressed [i], for both the [iʔi] and [isi]. Significant differences in LCT activation between [iʔi] and [isi] occurred 50 ms prior to phonation onset (post) as well as during vocal fold adduction at the end of [s]. This suggests that the LCT was more active during the initial part of vocal fold adduction than for abduction. Activity did not increase during vocal fold adduction for the glottal stop since [isi] and [iʔi] activation levels were similar in both CTs.

To determine the degree of subject variation which might be responsible for the differences between the two CT muscles, we plotted the mean values for the two types of utterances for all 3 subjects (Figure 7). Generally, the subjects showed similar patterns except subject 1 whose RCT increased in activation for both tokens from the initial to the final vowel in the opposite direction from changes in stress. For the LCT subjects 1 and 3

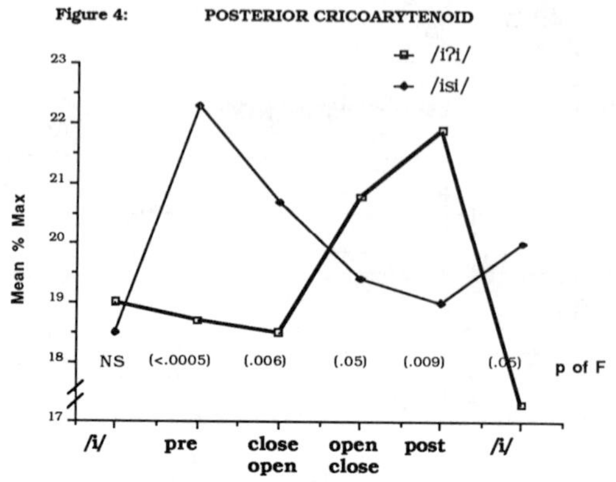

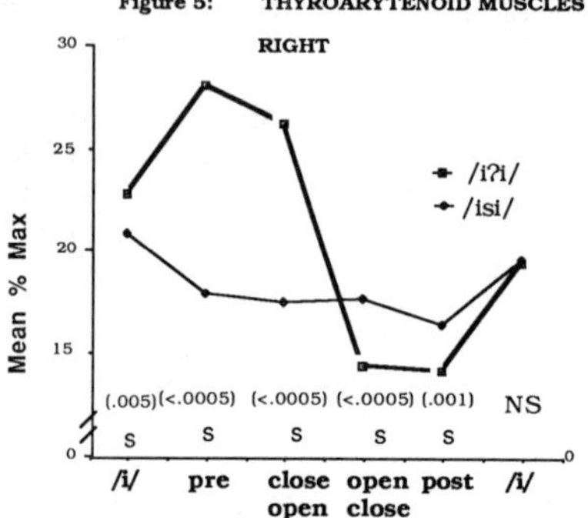

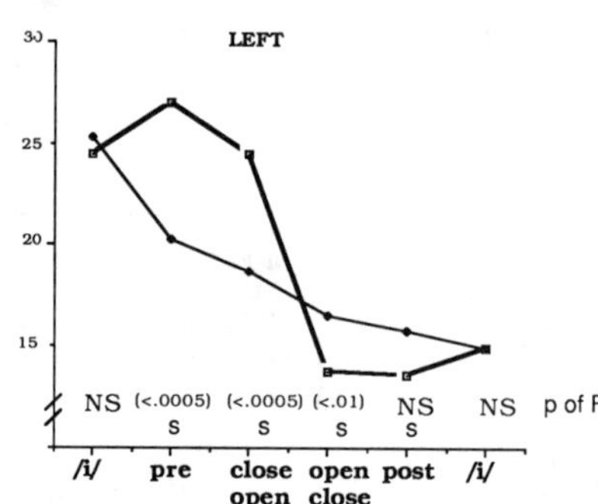

Figure 6: CRICOTHYROID GROUP RESULTS

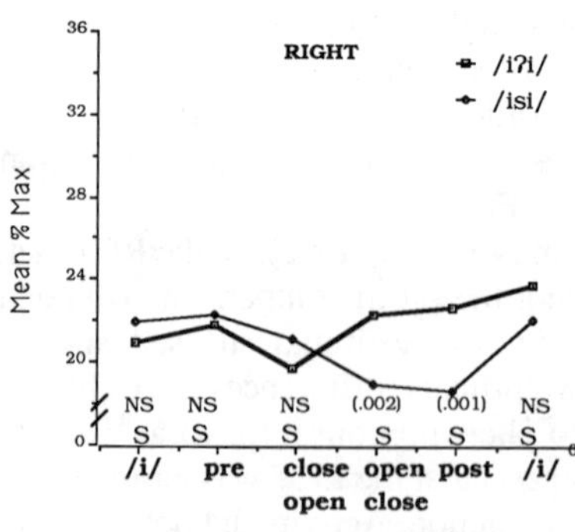

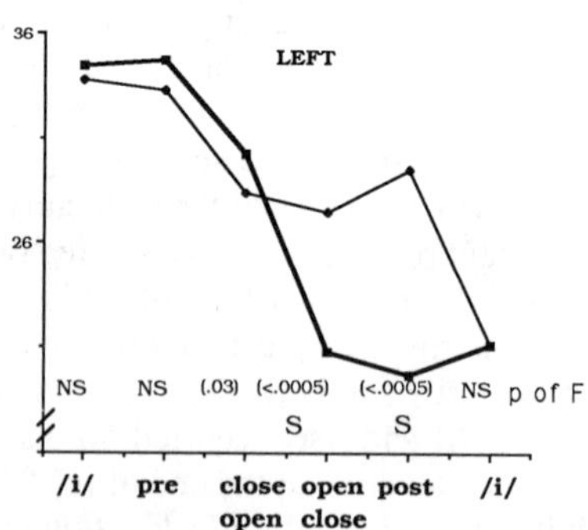

Figs. 4, 5 and 6. A line graph plotting the mean percent of maximum activation of the Posterior Cricoarytenoid muscle (Figure 4), the Right and Left Thyroarytenoid (Figure 5) the Right and Left Cricothyroid (Figure 6) for 23 tokens from 3 subjects during 6 intervals for the speech items [iʔi] and [isi]. The intervals are: the initial [i]; 50 ms prior to voice offset (pre); the closing period for [ʔ] and the opening period for [s] (close/open); the opening period for [ʔ] and the closing period for [s] (open/close); 50 ms prior to voice onset (post); and the final [i].

Figure 7: CRICOTHYROID INDIVIDUAL RESULTS

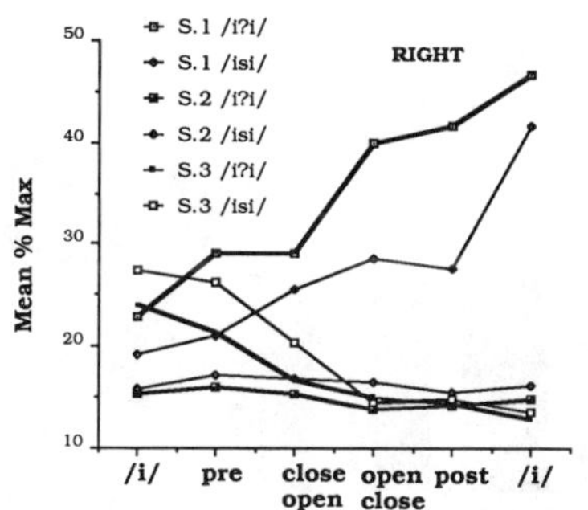

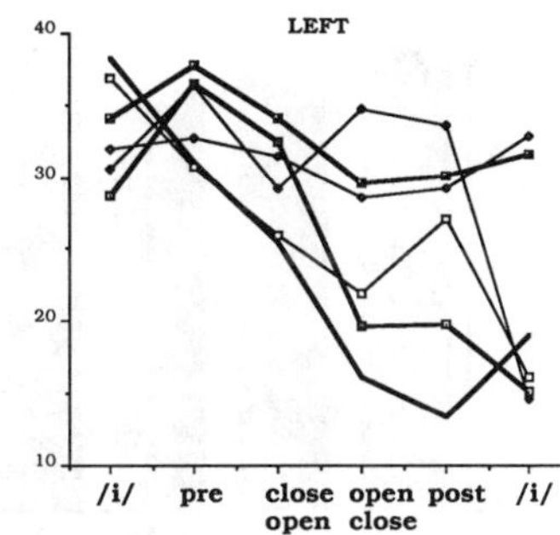

Fig. 7. A line graph plotting the mean percent of maximum activation of the Right and Left Cricothyroid muscles for between 6 and 10 tokens from each of 3 subjects during 6 time intervals for the speech items [i?i] and [isi].

decreased in activity from the initial to the final vowel during [i?i] and [isi] except for an increase during vocal fold adduction following [s]. Subject 2 had a flat curve for [isi] with a significant increase during 50 ms prior to phonation offset prior to the glottal stop, indicating activation for vocal fold adduction from the phonatory position. Therefore, the CT demonstrated both a relationship with stress and with vocal fold adduction for speech.

To compare maximum Pearson Correlation Coefficients during three intervals, the initial [i], the voice offset intervals for either the [?] or the [s], and the final [i], F ratios were computed for 1) task differences between [?] and [s]); 2) muscle differences between TAs and CTs; 3) side differences between RTA with RCT versus LTA with LCT; 4) agonists versus antagonists (differences between correlations between agonist pairs such as the 2 CTs, the two TAs, the RTA and RCT and the LTA and LCT, versus those between antagonists such as the summed TAs with the PCA and the summed CTs with the PCA; and, 5) differences between muscles of the same type versus two different muscle types on the same side (correlations between the two TAs and the two CTs versus correlations between the RTA with RCT and the LTA with LCT). No task effects were found, and only one significant difference between muscles, during the initial [i] ($p \leq 0.02$). Right to left differences occurred during the two vowels but not on the consonant ($p \leq 0.02$). Significant differences in correlations were found between agonists or antagonists ($p < 0.0005$) for all three intervals (Figure 8). The side versus muscle type factor was also significant ($p < 0.0005$) for all three intervals although this seemed to be chiefly due to higher correlations occurring between the LTA and LCT than between the two TAs and the two CTs or the RTA and RCT (Figure 8).

DISCUSSION

Different muscle activation patterns were found among the three laryngeal muscles studied. The PCA was active for both vocal fold opening gestures studied; opening from

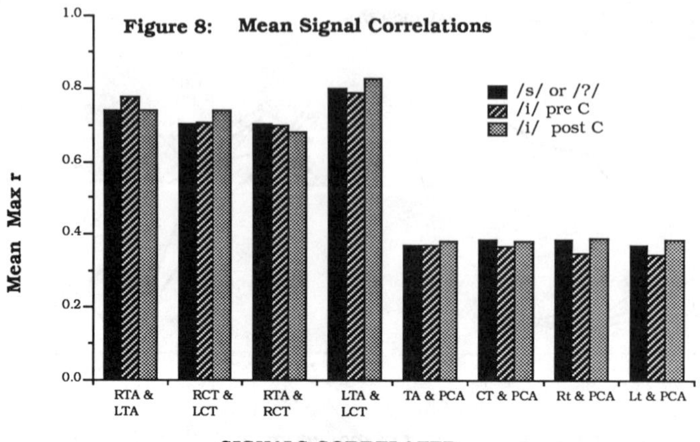

Fig. 8. A histogram of the group mean maximum Pearson Correlation Coefficients during the initial [i], the voice offset interval for the consonant, and the final [i] for all 23 tokens of 3 subjects. The muscle signals with were cross-correlated are listed below each bar graph. For the four right bar graphs, two muscle signals were added before being correlated with the PCA: the right and left thyroarytenoid (TA) (TA & PCA); the right and left cricothyroid (CT) (CT & PCA); the right TA and CT (Rt. & PCA); the left TA and CT (Lt & PCA).

the closed position following the glottal stop and opening from the phonatory position for the production of [s]. These results are similar to those previously reported with hooked wire PCA recordings (Sawashima and Hirose, 1983). The increases in activation for abduction were greater when muscle activity was averaged over a shorter time window during 50 ms at the beginning of the closing cycle for either [isi] or [iʔi]. Therefore, the muscle activation patterns were very rapid and discrete in this muscle. This timing aspect is somewhat more rapid for speech than during respiration where the muscle is tonically active throughout the cycle and increases during inhalation (Payne et al., 1981; Fujita et al., 1989).

The right and left TA muscles had very similar activation patterns but differed from the PCA (Figure 5). These muscles were active only during one of the two adductory phases studied: vocal fold closing from the phonatory position for production of a glottal stop. They were not active for vocal fold adduction following [s]. This suggests that the TA is not used for all vocal fold adductory gestures during speech and may only be consistently employed for glottal stops. Therefore, although the TA was found to have a role in vocal fold adduction, it is used selectively. The linear trend for decreasing activation in the TA on the [isi] token also suggested some contribution of the TA during stress. This is in agreement with the findings of Titze et al. (1989) that the TA combined with the CT to regulate fundamental frequency.

The activation patterns of the two CTs were less similar and had greater subject variation. An increasing pattern of activation over the entire segment from the initial to the final [i] was seen only in one subject only in the RCT. The most common pattern was that of decreasing activation from the initial to the final [i] which occurred in 8 of the 12 muscle patterns. There were a few instances of adductory actions. In two subjects, significant increases were found during vocal fold adduction following [s] and in subject 1 an increase in LCT activation occurred during vocal fold adduction for the glottal stop. Therefore, the most consistent actions of the CT muscles were related to stress changes while adductory actions were less consistent and seemed to compliment those of the TA. No instances of abductory actions were found for speech which differs from respiration when this muscle is most active during vocal fold abduction (Mathew et al., 1988).

The correlations suggested that the TA and CT muscles were highly related. The degree of correlation between these two muscles on the same side of the larynx was as high or greater than those between the same muscle on opposite sides of the larynx. This was particularly evident on the left side. These results replicated to some degree those of an earlier study (Ludlow et al., in press) which found higher correlations between the TA and CT on the same side of the larynx than between the same muscle, either the TA and CT, on opposite sides of the larynx. These two studies then emphasize the high degree of coordination between the TA and CT muscles both for stress and articulatory changes during speech.

Previous studies have not reported on differences in muscle activation patterns between the right and left sides. Often only one side is recorded and assumed to be representative of the two sides. However, asymmetries of the laryngeal framework are usually present (Hirano et al., 1989). Therefore asymmetries in muscle activation patterns between the two sides may be needed to compensate for these anatomical asymmetries to keep the vocal folds relatively symmetric during vibration.

REFERENCES

Fujita, M., Ludlow, C.L., Woodson, G.E., Naunton, R.F. (1989) A new surface electrode for recording from the posterior cricoarytenoid muscle. *Laryngoscope* 99:316-320.

Hirano, M., Kurita, S., Yukizane, K., and Hibi,S. (1989). Asymmetry of the laryngeal framework: a morphologic study of cadaver larynges. *Ann. Otol. Rhinol. Laryngol.* 98:135-140.

Hirano, M., and Ohala, J. (1969) Use of hooked-wire electrodes for electromyography of the intrinsic laryngeal muscles. *J. Speech Hear. Res.* 12:362-373.

Hirose, H. and Niimi, S. (1987) The relationship between glottal opening and transglottal pressure differences during consonant production. In: *Laryngeal Function in Phonation and Respiration*, edited by T. Baer, C. Sasaki and K.S. Harris. pp 381-390. College-Hill Press, Boston, USA.

Löfqvist, A., Baer, R.S., McGarr, N.S. and Story, R.S. (1989) The cricothyroid muscle in voicing control. *J. Acous. Soc. Am.* 85:1314-1321.

Ludlow, C.L., Sedory, S.E. and Fujita, M. (in press) Correlations between intrinsic laryngeal muscles during different speech gestures. In: *Festschrift for Osamu Fujimura*, edited by S. Kiritani, H. Hirose and H. Fujisaki. Ohmsha Publishers, Tokyo, Japan

Mathew, O.P., Sant 'Ambrogio, F., Woodson, G.E. and Sant 'Ambrogio, G. (1988) Respiratory activity of the cricothyroid muscle. *Ann. Otol. Rhinol. Laryngol.* 97:680-687.

Payne, J., Higgenbottam, T. and Guidi, G. (1981) Respiratory activity of the vocal cords in normal subjects and patients with airflow obstruction: An electromyographic study. *Clin. Sci.* 61:163-167.

Sawashima, M and Hirose, H. (1983) Laryngeal gestures in speech production. In: *The Production of Speech*, edited by P. MacNeilage, pp 11-38. Springer, New York.

Sonesson, B. (1982) Vocal fold kinesiology. In: *Speech Motor Control*, edited by S. Grillner, B. Lindblom, J. Lubker and A. Persson, pp 113-117. Pergamon Press, Oxford.

Titze, I., Luschei, E.S. and Hirano, M. (1989) The role of the thyroarytenoid muscle in regulation of fundamental frequency. *J Voice* 3:213-224.

26

Laryngeal Manual Compression in the Evaluation of Patients for Laryngeal Framework Surgery

Stanley M. Blaugrund, *Tatsuzo Taira, and *Nobuhiko Isshiki

*Dept. of Otolaryngology, Lenox Hill Hospital, New York City, New York 10021-1883, USA, * School of Medicine, Kyoto University, Kyoto, Japan*

Suspended within the larynx as if they were elastic bands, the shape, position and tension of the vocal folds are readily influenced by laryngeal compression and cricothyroid approximation. This is the fundamental basis for laryngeal framework surgery (LFS), an indirect surgical means of correcting alterations in voice due to incomplete glottic closure; as in unilateral paralysis, vocal fold atrophy, and sulcus vocalis. LFS has also been successful in the correction of intractable pitch disorders and in androphonia in the female. Forceful manual compression of the thyroid and cricoid cartilages, modifies the position, shape and tension of the vocal folds. This is the basis for the Laryngeal Manual Compression Tests (LMCTs), which gives valuable adjunctive examinations in the preoperative assessment of patients under consideration for laryngeal framework surgery. The LMCTs are simple to perform and non-invasive. Subjective improvement of voice on compression is documented objectively by well attested methods of aerodynamic, acoustic and stroboscopic analysis. Pressure applied to the anterior aspect of the thyroid cartilage results in the lowering of vocal pitch. This was first described as a diagnostic test of phonasthenia by Gutzmann (1910). He observed in normal persons, when asked to produce a singing tone, that pressure exerted on the thyroid cartilage and then immediately released, produced momentary pitch elevation with prompt resumption to normal. Whereas in phonasthenic voices, original pitch is resumed following a longer delay. In severely pathological voices there was no return to normal pitch.

Brodnitz (1955) described a patient with a functional voice disorder, in whom to his surprise, had a lowering of pitch in response to anterior-posterior pressure. This was a complete reversal of the findings as reported by Gutzmann. Brodnitz interpreted this to mean that lowering of vocal fold tension by pressure on the thyroid cartilage is over ridden in functional voice disorders by the patients "unconscious urge" to speak in an abnormally high pitched voice. He described a series of 24 males with postmutational voice problems of which 20 patients exhibited paradoxical initial pitch elevation as opposed to pitch lowering on application of anterior-posterior compression (Brodnitz, 1958). Brodnitz advocated the routine application of the thyroid pressure test as a means of differentiating mutational from functional voice disorders. With the addition of lateral

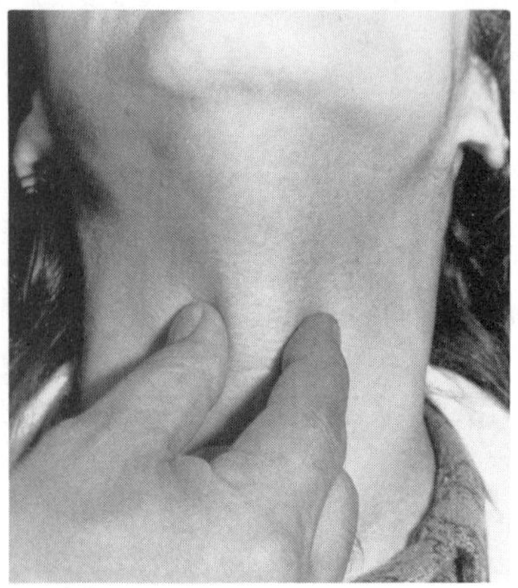

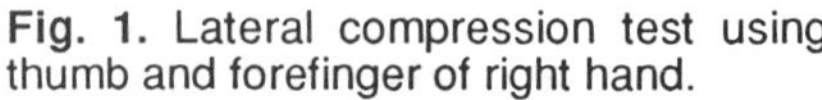

Fig. 1. Lateral compression test using thumb and forefinger of right hand.

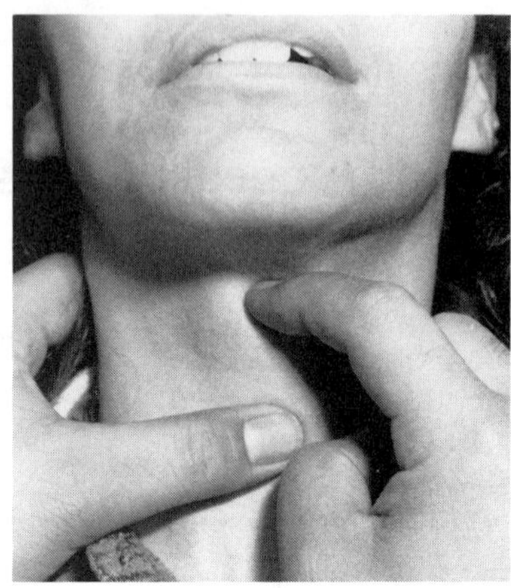

Fig. 2. Cricothyroid approximation test using forefinger of right hand and thumb of left hand.

compression and cricothyroid approximation, these techniques are valuable in the assessment of patients for LFS.

LARYNGEAL MANUAL COMPRESSION TESTS

The LMCTs are simple to apply and require no special instrumentation. Results defined subjectively and verified by aerodynamic, acoustic and videostroboscopic analysis give pertinent information in estimating the probability of success of LFS. There are four compression tests.

1. Lateral compression test

This test is most valuable in patients with incomplete glottic closure, such as symptomatic unilateral recurrent nerve paralysis, vocal fold atrophy and sulcus vocalis. The thumb and forefinger are used (Figure 1). The thyroid ala is identified using the superior notch as a landmark. The thumb and forefinger slide laterally to define a point approximately over the center of the cartilage on both sides. The patient is asked to sustain phonation using /a/ while precise lateral to medial pressure is applied. Compression should be repeated in several positions on the thyroid ala until maximum improvement of voice is attained. Findings are corroborated using stroboscopic, aerodynamic and acoustic tests and compared with objective findings without compression.

If voice quality is not significantly improved, pathology other than glottal gap may be present. Foremost consideration must be given to the possibility of calcification of the thyroid cartilage which is relatively more common in men than in women, and when present, is frequently encountered at the site where compression is most desirable. In young women and in patients with short thick necks, there may be difficulty in finding the thyroid notch and the inferior margin of the thyroid ala.

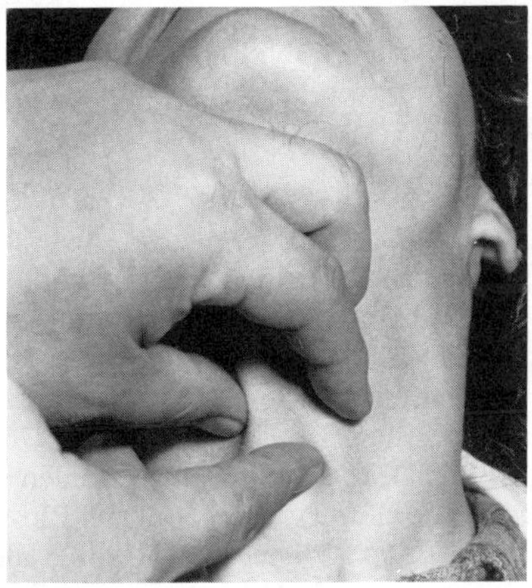

Fig 3. Combined lateral compression and cricothyroid approximation test using thumb and forefinger of left hand forefinger of right hand.

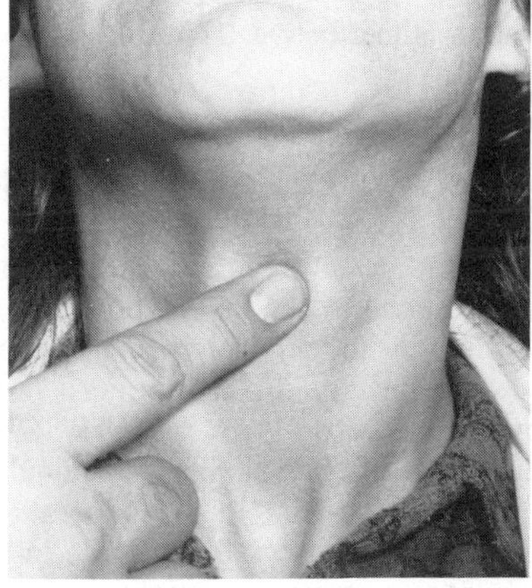

Fig. 4. Anterior-posterior compression test using forefinger of right hand.

2. Cricothyroid approximation

This is an important examination in the evaluation of pitch disorders because of the role played in regulation of cordal tension by the cricothyroid muscle. The forefinger is positioned above the thyroid notch with the thumb below the mid-portion of the cricoid cartilage (Figure 2). The thyroid and cricoid cartilages are approximated while the patient sustains /a/ in phonation. Pitch increases due to heightened vocal fold tension. Approximation of the folds is improved and there is less air loss and more efficient glottic closure. If this occurs, surgical correction by cricothyroid approximation (Thyroplasty type IV) may be indicated.

3. Combined lateral compression and cricothyroid approximation

In this examination, tests 1 and 2 are performed simultaneously. This test is effective in evaluating patients in whom there is imperfect glottic closure due to atrophic vocal fold with concomitant decrease in tension and stiffness. For example, unilateral paralysis with vocalis muscle atrophy and in age induced cordal bowing (presbylaryngis).

The index finger is positioned in the thyroid notch while thumb and middle finger are placed on the mid portion of the thyroid ala. The thumb or forefinger of the opposite hand is positioned beneath the cricoid cartilage and pressure is applied in four dimensions while the patient is asked to phonate (Figure 3). If pitch is increased and the glottal gap closed, combined Thyroplasty type I and Thyroplasty type IV may be indicated.

4. Antero-posterior compression test (Brodnitz test)

Relaxation of the vocal fold by direct anterior compression on the thyroid cartilage during sustained /a/ phonation relieves stiffness and tension (Figure 4). This results in lowering of pitch and is elicited in male patients with high pitched mutational voice. Speech therapy is the treatment of choice in this situation. However, when speech rehabilitation is ineffective, Thyroplasty type III may be indicated(Isshiki, 1980a; Isshiki et al., 1983).

DISCUSSION

In recent years LFS has gained wide acceptance as an alternative form of phonosurgery. Phonosurgery, a term coined in the early 1960's by von Leden (pers. comm.), is by definition surgery "solely and primarily" concerned with improvement of the voice. Procedures include excision of mass lesions of the vocal folds by direct microlaryngoscopy, (Jako, 1970; Kleinsasser, 1964; Saito et al., 1966; Scalco et al., 1960; Strong, 1970) injection of Teflon in paralytic dysphonia, (Arnold, 1962; Dedo et al., 1973; von Leden et al., 1967; Lewy, 1963) injection of collagen in other types of dysphonia (Ford and Bless, 1986), injection of botulinum toxin in hyperfunctional states (Blitzer et al., 1988), and such other procedures as laryngeal reinnervation (Berendes et al., 1968; Boles and Fritzell, 1969; Crumley, 1985) and laryngeal framework surgery (Isshiki, 1980 a and b; Isshiki et al., 1975; Isshiki et al., 1978). The latter comprises a group of techniques that modify vocal fold characteristics by indirect means. These techniques all fall under the broad category of phonosurgery.

Laryngeal framework surgery as defined by Isshiki (1980b) consists of four techniques: type I, lateral compression: type II, lateral expansion: type III, relaxation (shortening) of the vocal fold; and type IV, stretching (lengthening) of the vocal fold. Arytenoid adduction was described by Isshiki et al. (1978), and modifications of all these procedures have been reported by others (LeJeune et al., 1983; Koufman, 1986). Laryngeal framework surgery seems destined to provide an acceptable alternative in the management of a host of voice disorders. Thyroplasty type I is gaining wide acceptance as an alternative procedure to Teflon injection for dysphonias due to a widened glottic gap.

Teflon injection has been successful in the vocal rehabilitation of many hundreds of patients. It is the procedure of choice of most laryngologists in the management of these disorders. However, it is not without its problems. Teflon's propensity to migrate, the difficulties involved in its removal when necessary, and the stiffness caused by its presence, are adverse factors in its appropriateness for this type of surgery. Thyroplasty type I is likely to prove an acceptable alternative since it is precise, reversible when indicated, and there is little likelihood of migration of the silicone plug.

Questions that arise in the preoperative and postoperative evaluation of these patients include the following: 1. what measurable amount of medial displacement of the vocal fold is necessary for optimum medialization? 2. what is the actual change in voice following LFS as determined by quantitative measurement? 3. which of the various thyroplasties should be selected in order to achieve optimum results? These questions can only be answered through the utilization of objective criteria prior to and following surgery.

LMCT is helpful in answering these questions in most instances. When there is objective improvement in voice with lateral compression, Thyroplasty type I and/or Arytenoid adduction is indicated. If combined lateral compression and cricothyroid approximation enhance the findings, Thyroplasty type IV should be added. If these tests reveal improvement in voice preoperatively, one can be reasonably confident that surgery will be successful. If the LMCTs result in no improvement, measures should be undertaken to elicit the reasons why.

Reasons for failure could be: 1, ineffectively applied pressure, 2, wrong position on the thyroid ala, 3, excessive calcification of the thyroid cartilage, 4, splinting of the strap muscles, or 5, patient intolerance to pressure.

It must be emphasized that LFS may be successful in improving voice even though the LMCTs result in equivocal or negative results.

Preoperative and postoperative evaluation of patients with correctable voice disorders utilizing objective measurements is essential in order to accurately document the results of surgery. (These examinations are too numerous to mention here). Some include, direct and indirect laryngoscopy, acoustic and aerodynamic analysis, stroboscopic analysis of the vocal fold, hot wire flow metering (vocal efficiency index), neurophysiological examinations, audiometry, pulmonary function testing, psychiatric evaluation and computerized tomography (CT) and magnetic resonance imaging (MRI).

Laryngeal manual compression tests applied in tandem with objective evaluations offer valuable information in the preoperative investigation of patients with dysphonia. LFS is usually successful when results of these tests are positive. The utilization of LMCT, therefore, is suggested for use as a standard preoperative examination in patients under consideration for LFS.

CONCLUSION

Laryngeal Maual Compression Tests, LMCTs, are described and the indications and reasons for failure of the tests are elucidated. Salient features of the preoperative manual compression tests are summarized as follows:

1. Manual force applied to the laryngeal framework results not only in the modification of position, tension and shape of the vocal folds, but also in laryngeal behaviour.
2. Tests are easily performed in an out-patient setting and require no special instrumentation.
3. The decision as to which type of Thyroplasty might be most effective in restoring voice is facilitated.
4. The results of Laryngeal Framework Surgery, LFS, can be predicted with reasonable accuracy utilizing the manual compression tests in tandem with videostroboscopic, aerodynamic and acoustic analysis.

LMCTs are recommended as standard adjunctive tests in the preoperative assessment of patients being considered for LFS.

REFERENCES

Arnold, G.E. (1962). Vocal rehabilitation of paralytic dysphonia. *Arch. Otolaryngol.*, 76:358-368.

Berendes, J. and Miehlke, A. (1968). Repair of the recurrent laryngeal nerve and phonation: Basic consideration and techniques. *Int. Surg.* 49:319-329.

Blitzer, A., Brin, M.F., Fahn, S., and Lovelace, R.E. (1988): Localized injection of botulinum for the treatment of focal laryngeal dystonia (spastic dysphonia). *Laryngoscope*, 98:193-197.

Boles, R. and Fritzell, B. (1969). Injury and repair of recurrent laryngeal nerve in dogs. *Laryngoscope*, 79:1405-1418.

Brodnitz, F.S. (1955). Minutes NY Society for speech and voice therapy. *Folia Phoniat.*, 7:115.

Brodnitz, F.S. (1958). The pressure test in mutational voice disturbance. *Ann. Otolaryngol.*, 67:235-240.

Crumley, R.L. (1985). Update of laryngeal reinnervation concepts and otions. In: *Surgery of the Larynx*, edited by R. Bailey and H. Biller, pp 135-147. WB Saunders Company, Philadelphia, PA.

Dedo, H.H., Urrea, R.D., and Lawson, L. (1973): Intracordal injection of Teflon in the treatment of 135 patients with dysphonia. *Laryngoscope*, 83:1293-1299.

Ford, C.N. and Bless, D.M. (1986). Clinical experience with injectable collagen for vocal fold augmentation. *Laryngoscope*, 96:863-869.

Gutzmann, H. (1910). Diagnostik und Therapie der Funktionellen Stimmstoerungen. *Mediz.-Pädag. Monatsschr. f. d. ges. Sprachheilkunde*, 20:55.

Isshiki, N. (1980a). Phonosurgery to change vocal pitch. *HNO-Praxis* (Leipzig) 6:179-180.

Isshiki, N. (1980b). Recent advances in phonosurgery. *Folia Phoniatr.*, 32:119-154.

Isshiki, N., Okamura, H., and Ishikawa, T. (1975). Thyroplasty type I (lateral compression for dysphonia due to vocal cord paralysis or atrophy). *Acta Otolaryngol.*, 80:465-473.

Isshiki, N., Taira, T., and Tanabe, M. (1983). Surgical alteration of the vocal pitch. *J. Otolaryngol.* 12:335-340.

Isshiki, N., Tanabe, M., and Sawada, M. (1978). Arytenoid adduction for unilateral vocal fold paralysis. *Arch. Otolaryngol.*, 104:555-558.

Jako, G.J. (1970). Laryngoscope for microscopic observation, surgery and photography. *Arch. Otolaryngol.* 91:196-199.

Kleinsasser, O. (1964). Mikrochirurgie im Kehlkopf. *Arch. Ohrenheilk.*, 183:428-433.

Koufman, J.A. (1986). Laryngoplasty for vocal cord medialization: An alternative to Teflon. *Laryngoscope*, 96:726-731.

von Leden, H., Yanigahara, N., and Werner-Kukuk, E. (1967). Teflon in unilateral vocal paralysis: Preoperative and postoperative function studies. *Arch. Otolaryngol.*, 85:666-674.

LeJeune, F.E., Guice, C.E., and Samuels, P.M. (1983). Early experiences with vocal ligament tightening. *Ann. Otol. Rhinol. Laryngol.* 92:475-477.

Lewy, R.B. (1963). Glottic reformation with rehabilitation in vocal cord paralysis: The injection of Teflon and Tantalum. *Laryngoscope*, 73:547-555.

Saito, S., Ogino, M., Ishikura, M., Shinno, Y., and Fukuda, H. (1966). Microsurgery under direct laryngoscopy. *J. Jap. Bronco-esoph. Soc.* (In Japanese), 17:253-266.

Scalco, A.N., Shipman, W.F., and Tabb, H.G. (1960): Microscopic suspension laryngoscopy. *Ann. Otol. Rhinol. Lar.*, 69:1134-1138.

Strong, M.S.(1970): Microscopic laryngoscopy. *Laryngoscope* 80:1540-1552.

27

Clinical Application of High-speed Digital Imaging of Vocal Fold Vibration

Hajime Hirose, Shigeru Kiritani, and Hiroshi Imagawa

Research Institute of Logopedics and Phoniatrics, Faculty of Medicine, University of Tokyo, Tokyo, 113 Japan

Observation of vocal fold vibration is highly important for a study of the physiology and pathology of voice production. The observation and measurement of vocal fold vibration have generally been made by means of an ultra-high-speed cinematography or a stroboscope. Ultra-high-speed movie system can provide accurate images of the vibrating vocal folds with good resolution. However, this system is usually massive and costly, and it is always very time-consuming to obtain final results from a frame-by-frame analysis of the exposed film.

In addition, for the simultaneous recording of voice signals, special considerations are necessary for reducing the mechanical noises from the high-speed camera that are picked up by the microphone.

Stroboscopy is a very useful technique for observing vocal fold vibration in a clinical situation. However, stroboscopy cannot provide a precise cycle-by-cycle analysis of vocal fold vibration. Moreover, it is impossible to make a direct and exact comparison between the stroboscopic image and the acoustic signal.

In recent years, a new method of digitally imaging vocal fold vibration has been developed in the authors' institute using a solid-state image sensor attached to a conventional camera system. This system is relatively free from the mechanical noises and suitable for simultaneous recordings of voice signals. Since the entire system is compact and easy to handle, the application for clinical practice is very promising. In the present report, preliminary results of the analysis of pathological vocal fold vibration in dysphonic cases are reported with special reference to abnormal voice quality (Hirose, 1988; Hirose et al., 1988; Kiritani et al., 1986; 1988).

METHOD

High-speed imaging of vocal fold vibration was performed using our newly developed system. In the present system, a specially designed lateral-viewing laryngeal tele-endoscope is attached to a single-lens reflex camera. A MOS-type solid-state image sensor consisting of 100 x 100 picture elements is attached to the back-lid of the camera at the position of the film plate. When the shutter is released, an image scan is made under computer control, and image signals are stored in an image memory through a high-speed

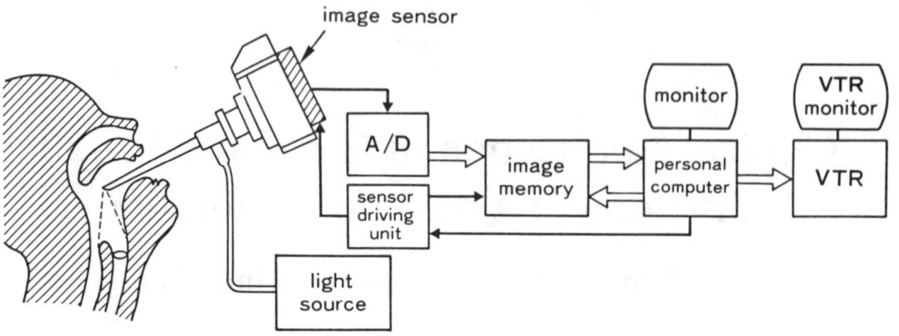

Fig. 1. Block diagram of the present system.

A/D converter. After the data storage, the images can be reproduced and displayed on a monitor CRT screen or recorded on an ordinary video recorder. By reducing the number of horizontal scan lines, it is possible to obtain image data with a maximum rate of 4,000 frame per second.

Figure 1 shows a block diagram of the system. The image memory has a 2-megabyte memory and a high-speed, 8-bit A/D converter. As a light source, a pair of 250 W halogen lamps are used.

Data recording is made in the same manner as in still photography of the larynx. The larynx is visualized through a view finder with the tip of the scope in the pharynx. The camera shutter is released so as to start data acquisition. During the shutter opening of approximately 150 msec, 200 to 400 data frames are stored in the memory. Other physio-

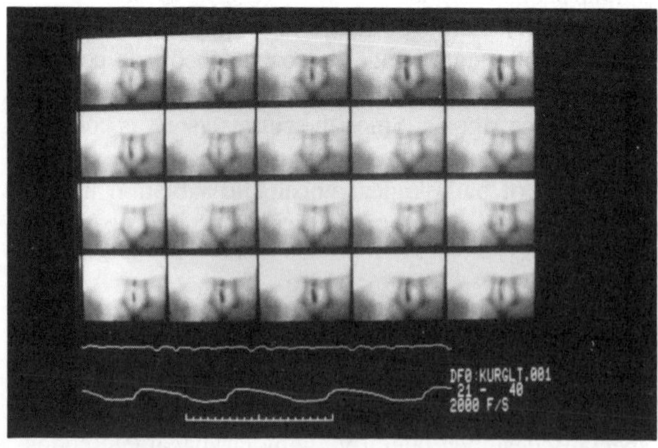

Fig. 2. An array of images obtained from Case 1. The present sequence runs from left top toward right. Simultaneously recorded audio (upper) and EGG (lower) signals are displayed in the lower column. Frame rate: 2000 fps.

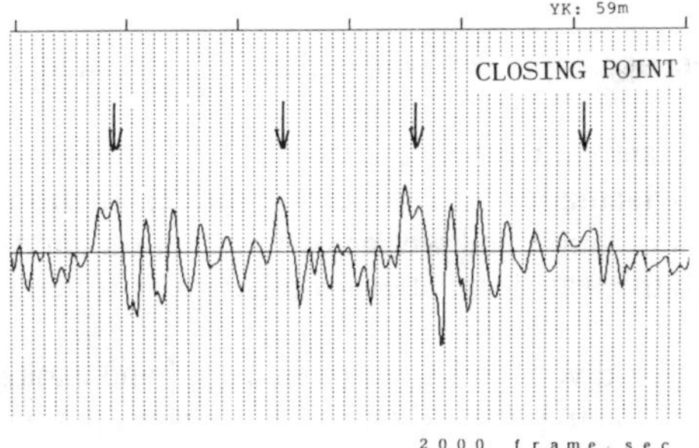

Fig. 3. Acoustic waveforms of a voice sample obtained from Case 1 (vocal fold cyst (R), same as in Figure 2).

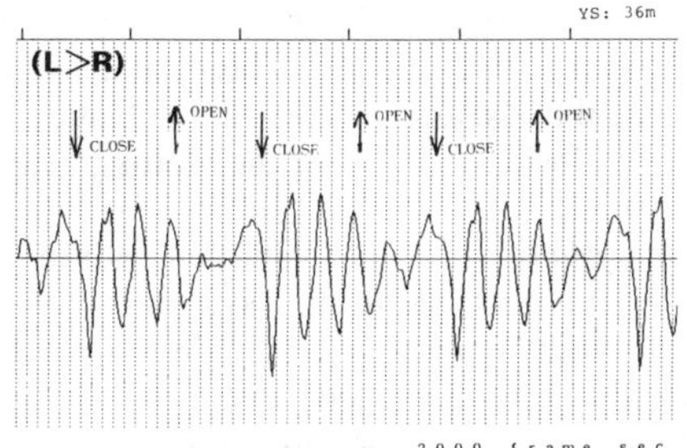

Fig. 4. Acoustic waveforms of a voice sample obtained from Case 2 (male, polypoid vocal fold).

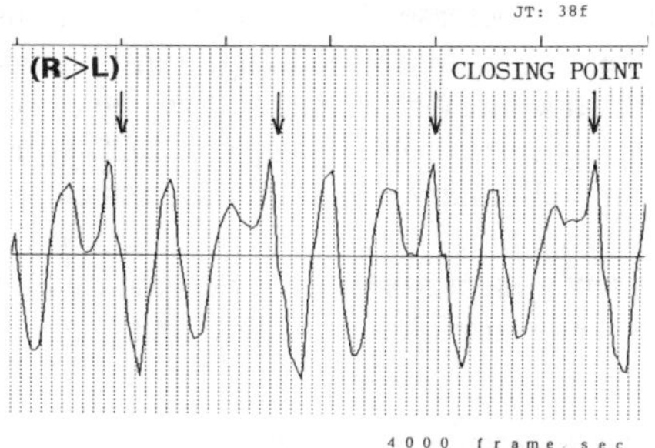

Fig. 5. Acoustic waveforms of a voice sample obtained from Case 3 (female, polypoid vocal fold).

logical data, such as voice and electroglottographic (EGG) signals, can also be recorded simultaneously.

For the purpose of clinical application of the present system, recordings were made in those cases with organic changes in the vocal fold associated with "rough" quality of voice. Consecutive picture frames were compared to the acoustic wave forms simultaneously recorded.

RESULTS AND COMMENTS

An application of the present system for the analysis of pathological larynx has proved promising. Incomplete glottal closure and asymmetrical or irregular vibratory patterns were easily identified in cases with recurrent laryngeal nerve paralysis, vocal fold polyp, polypoid vocal fold or sulcus vocalis. Further, it was confirmed that, in most cases, pathological vibratory patterns were accompanied by irregularity in simultaneously recorded acoustic signals.

For example, in case 1, a 59 year-old male with cyst of the right vocal fold, the amplitude of vibration of the right fold was much smaller than the left (Figure 2). In this case, two distinct periods of strong and clear excitation and weak noisy excitation alternated with each other resulting in fluctuation in the waveform at every other pitch period (Figure 3).

In case 2, a 36 year-old male with polypoid vocal fold, the pitch period and excitation at the closing moment were both stable, although polypoid change was more dominant in the left fold. Fluctuation was principally due to noisy excitation observed at the open period of the glottis (Figure 4).

In case 3, a 38 year-old female with polypoid vocal fold, the vibratory movement of the right vocal fold appeared to be much smaller than the left. This resulted in marked asymmetry in the vibratory pattern of the vocal folds, associated with fluctuation in pitch period, although the excitation pattern at the closing moment of the glottis in each pitch period was strong and stable (Figure 5).

The procedure for the recording and analysis of vocal fold vibration with the present system is simple compared to the conventional high-speed filming system. While the system is useful for practical purposes, a few technical improvements in the system's performance, particularly in the maximum frame rate, are still needed.

The maximum frame rate is basically restricted by the brightness of the image on the sensor produced by the optic system and the maximum sampling rate of the sensor. It is expected that the brightness of the image can be increased by further modifications to the endoscope, the light source and the image sensor. Since the image sensor used in the present system does not seem to have optimal sensitivity characteristics, the use of a different type of sensor in the future is being considered. For example, a CCD-type sensor combined with fiberoptic system is now in preliminary use for the assessment of vibratory patterns of the vocal fold during running speech.

For clinical purposes, however, the present system has sufficient capability for the observation of pathological vibratory patterns and is useful as a practical unit.

REFERENCES

Hirose, H. (1988). High-speed digital imaging of vocal fold vibration. *Acta Otolaryngol.*, (Stockholm), Suppl. 458:151-153.

Hirose, H., Kiritani, S., and Imagawa, H. (1988). High-speed digital image analysis of laryngeal behaviour in running speech. In: *Vocal Physiology: Voice Production, Mechanisms and Functions*, edited by O. Fujimura, pp. 335-345. Raven Press, New York.

Kiritani, S., Honda, K., Imagawa, H., and Hirose, H. (1986). Simultaneous high-speed digital recordings of vocal fold vibration and speech signal. *Proc. ICASSP 86, Tokyo*, Vol. 3:1633-1636.

Kiritani, S., Imagawa, H., and Hirose, H. (1988). High speed digital image recording for the observation of vocal cord vibration. In: *Vocal Physiology: Voice Production, Mechanisms and Functions, edited by O. Fujimura*, pp. 261-268. Raven Press, New York.

28

Vocal Fold Closure, Perceived Breathiness, and Acoustic Characteristics in Normal Adult Speakers

Maria Södersten, Per-Åke Lindestad, and Britta Hammarberg

Karolinska Institute, Dept. of Logopedics and Phoniatrics, Huddinge Hospital, Sweden

It is well known that incomplete vocal fold closure often corresponds to a breathy voice quality (e.g., Laver, 1980; Fritzell et al., 1986), but the relationship is complex. One acoustic correlate of breathiness in normal speakers is a higher amplitude level of the fundamental compared to the second partial (Bickley, 1982; Henton and Bladon, 1985). The relative amplitude level of the fundamental vs. the first formant has also been shown to correspond well to breathiness for normal voices (Ladefoged et al., 1988) and for paralytic dysphonic voices (Hammarberg et al., 1984). Hammarberg et al. (1984) also found that the vocal behaviour hypofunction and hyperfunction are important to take into consideration when investigating the acoustics of breathiness. A physiological definition of a hypofunctional (lax) voice is that it is produced with low laryngeal effort as opposed to a hyperfunctional (tense) voice produced with a greater laryngeal effort (Laver, 1980). In the Hammarberg at al. study of pathological voices (1984), a breathy/hypofunctional voice was characterized as having relatively high spectral energy for the fundamental as compared to the first formant. In a breathy/hyperfunctional voice, the fundamental had less spectral energy.

In a previous investigation, we studied glottal closure patterns during fiberscopy and evaluated the degree of breathiness in sustained vowels, under different pitch and loudness conditions, in normal Swedish-speaking subjects (Södersten and Lindestad, 1990). Among the findings, ratings for incomplete glottal closure as well as perceived breathiness were significantly higher for the women than for the men. We were interested in adding acoustic data to our previous physiological and perceptual findings.

The purposes of the study were (a) to establish the relative level of the fundamental (L0) to the first formant (L1) in audio-taped /i:/ and /ae:/ vowels in normal speakers, (b) to compare the difference L0-L1 to perceived breathiness, and (c) to compare the findings of perceived hypo- and hyperfunction to perceived breathiness in the same material. Further, (d) to compare the acoustic and perceptual data from the audio-taped vowels to our previous findings of glottal closure and perceived breathiness in audio-video-fiberscopic recordings, elicited from the same subjects. The information presented below about glottal closure and perceived breathiness during fiberscopy is given in more detail in Södersten and Lindestad (1990) which we refer to as "our previous study".

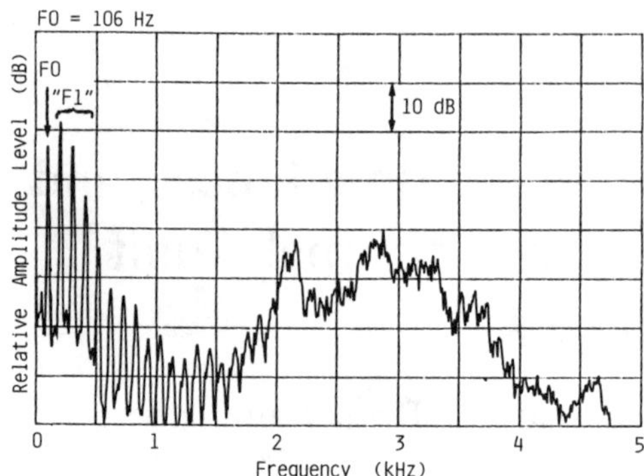

Fig. 1. Harmonic spectrum of the long Swedish vowel /i:/ with F0 and the estimated "F1" indicated for one male subject phonating at normal loudness.

SUBJECTS AND MATERIAL

Nine women and nine men, ranging in age from 20 to 35 years, served as subjects. They were Swedish-speaking logopedics and medical students, vocally healthy according to a clinical examination, and non-smokers. Some of the subjects had had some voice training and experience in choir singing, but none could be regarded as having a professionally trained voice.

In our previous study, the subjects produced the long Swedish vowel /i:/ during audio-video-fiberstroboscopy at three pitch and three loudness levels. The vowel /i:/ was chosen since it gives the best view of the glottis. Only the data of habitual pitch at soft, normal, and loud voice were used in the present paper. Habitual pitch, defined as the semitone closest to the mean fundamental frequency, ranged from 185 to 233 Hz for the women and from 104 to 131 Hz for the men. Thus, the audio-video-taped material consisted of 54 /i:/-vowels (18 subjects x 3 loudness levels) which had been analyzed previously as to glottal closure and perceived breathiness.

For the perceptual and acoustic analyses, 54 /i:/-vowels and 54 /ae:/-vowels (the same 18 subjects x 3 loudness levels) were recorded immediately before the fiberscopy in a sound-proof booth according to a standardized recording procedure (Hammarberg, 1986). The duration of the vowels was 2 s to 8 s with a mean of 4 s. The vowel /i:/ was chosen since it was used during the fiberscopy, and the open vowel /ae:/ for its separation of F0 and F1, which was important for the acoustic analysis. The /i:/ and /ae:/ vowels were randomly copied onto two listening tapes for the perceptual evaluation. Ten of the 54 audio-taped /i:/-vowels, and 10 of the 54 /ae:/-vowels were duplicated for calculation of intrajudge reliability.

METHODS

In our previous study, six speech clinicians had judged glottal closure patterns from a demonstration tape on which the audio-video sequences had been copied in random order. A 1 to 6-point scale was used for judging the degree of incomplete closure (1 corresponding to complete closure all along the folds, and 6 corresponding to incomplete closure all along the folds) and four categories A to D when other incomplete closure patterns occurred, such as a spindle or an hour-glass shape (see Södersten and Lindestad,

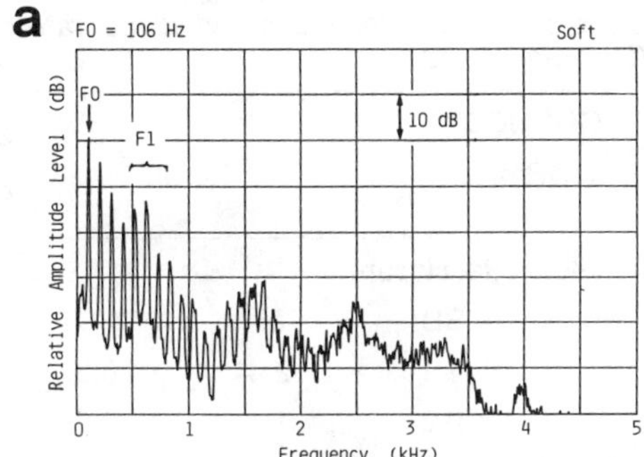

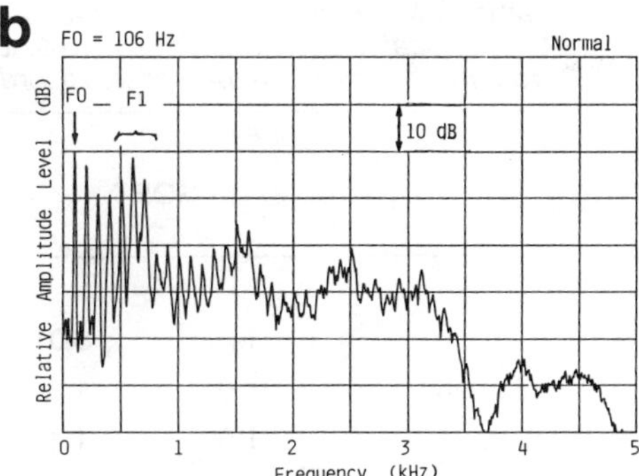

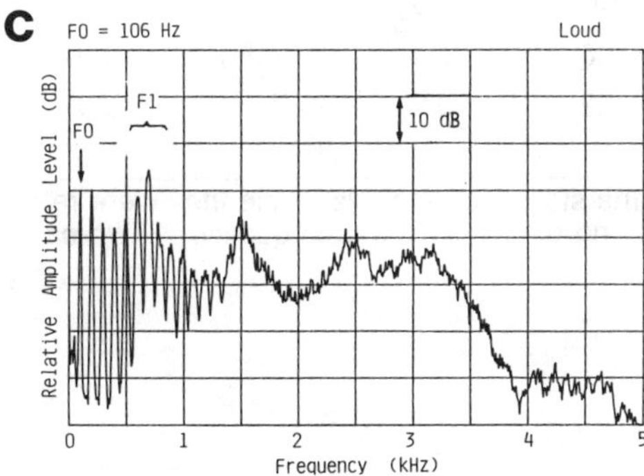

Fig. 2. Harmonic spectra of the long Swedish vowel /ae:/ with F0 and F1 indicated for one male subject phonating in (**a**) soft, (**b**) normal, and (**c**) loud voice.

1990). The judges listened to the voices while evaluating glottal closure. (These ratings were later compared to those obtained when the judges rated the material without sound. The ratings did not differ significantly.)

The perceptual analyses were performed by five speech clinicians who had participated in the glottal closure evaluation. They judged the degree of perceived breathiness, hypofunction, and hyperfunction using a 7-point rating scale. The audio-video-taped /i:/-vowels during fiberscopy had been analyzed in our previous study. The audio-taped /i:/ and /ae:/-vowels were evaluated by the same speech clinicians on two separate occasions within a week.

The acoustic analysis was performed using the facility "Average spectrum analysis" of a Dynamic Signal Analyser (Hewlett & Packard, 3562A). We measured the difference L0-L1 in both vowels /i:/ and /ae:/. In order to arrive at an estimation of L1 ("L1") in /i:/, with its low first formant frequency, we decided to measure the spectral level of the partials Nos. 2, 3, and 4 for all subjects (Figure 1). This was automatically done by the Analyser after manual marking of the relevant spectral region. Thus "L1" for /i:/ was defined as the spectral energy of these three partials.

In the open vowel /ae:/, which has a more evident separation of F0 and F1, the level of the first formant was derived from the three partials forming the resonance peak (Figure 2a to 2c).

Table 1. *Mean degree (M) and standard deviation (SD) of incomplete glottal closure (1 to 6-point scale) and breathiness (0 to 6-point scale) for three loudness conditions, rated from the audio-video-fiberscopic recordings (9 women, 9 men)*

	LOUDNESS					
	SOFT		NORMAL		LOUD	
	Incomplete glottal closure					
	M	SD	M	SD	M	SD
Women[a]	4.0	1.3	2.9	1.1	2.4	0.9
Men	1.9	1.1	1.5	0.8	1.1	0.2
	Breathiness					
	M	SD	M	SD	M	SD
Women	1.8[b]	0.5	1.0	0.4	0.8	0.6
Men	0.6[c]	0.3	0.2	0.2	0.1	0.2

[a] One subject's data were not included in the statistical analysis, since they were rated as categories C and D. [b] One sample missing due to poor sound quality. [c] Two samples missing due to poor sound quality.

RESULTS

Reliability

Intra- and interjudge reliabilities for rating glottal closure and perceived breathiness during fiberscopy were satisfactory and have been reported in our previous study.

Intrajudge reliability for ratings of breathiness in the audio-taped vowels varied between 80 and 100% according to one half scale point or less (or r=0.88 to 0.99). For hypofunction, intrajudge agreement ranged between 80 and 100% according to the same criterion (or r=0.48 to 0.89) and for hyperfunction between 80 and 90% (or r=0.43 to 0.92).

Interjudge reliability for breathiness rated from the audio-taped vowels varied between r=0.64 and 0.89. Interjudge agreement on hypofunction was r=0.40 to 0.92, and for hyperfunction r=0.47 to 0.85.

Glottal closure

The previous findings of glottal closure showed that the degree of incomplete closure increased significantly with decreased loudness ($p<0.01$) according to a two-way analysis of variance (ANOVA) (Table 1).

Estimated breathiness in the vowel /i:/ during fiberscopy

The ratings of breathiness were in general low and varied between 0 and 3 on the 7-point scale. Although the variation was small, the degree of breathiness decreased significantly ($p<0.001$) when loudness increased (Table 1).

Table 2. *Mean degree (M) and standard deviation (SD) of breathiness, hypofunction, and hyperfunction (0 to 6-point scale) in /i:/ and /ae:/ for three loudness conditions, rated from the audio-taped recordings (9 women, 9 men)*

	LOUDNESS											
	SOFT				NORMAL				LOUD			
	/i:/		/ae:/		/i:/		/ae:/		/i:/		/ae:/	
Sex	Breathiness											
	M	SD	M	SD	M	SD	M	SD	M	SD	M	SD
W	1.9	0.5	2.1	0.7	0.9	0.4	1.4	0.6	0.3	0.4	0.3	0.3
M	1.2[a]	0.5	0.6	0.5	0.2	0.2	0.1	0.2	0.0	0.1	0.0	0.0
	Hypofunction											
	M	SD	M	SD	M	SD	M	SD	M	SD	M	SD
W	1.2	0.4	1.3	0.6	0.5	0.4	0.7	0.5	0.0	0.0	0.2	0.1
M	1.0	0.6	0.6	0.3	0.1	0.1	0.1	0.1	0.0	0.0	0.0	0.0
	Hyperfunction											
	M	SD	M	SD	M	SD	M	SD	M	SD	M	SD
W	0.0	0.0	0.0	0.0	0.0	0.0	0.0	0.0	0.3	0.3	0.1	0.3
M	0.0	0.0	0.0	0.0	0.0	0.0	0.0	0.0	0.5	0.3	0.4	0.5

[a] One sample missing due to poor sound quality.

Estimated breathiness, hypofunction and hyperfunction in the audio-taped vowels /i:/ and /ae:/

No significant difference in degree of perceived breathiness was found between the two vowels as shown by a three-way ANOVA. Both audio-taped vowels were perceived significantly more breathy for the women than for the men ($p<0.001$). The degree of breathiness decreased significantly ($p<0.001$) with increase in loudness (Table 2).

The degree of breathiness and hypofunction correlated significantly for both vowels, i.e., there was an increased degree of perceived breathiness with an increase in degree of perceived hypofunction. The correlation coefficients for degree of breathiness and hypofunction varied between $r=0.70$ and $r=0.85$ ($p<0.01$) for the three loudness levels with a mean of $r=0.80$. There was a tendency for the degree of hypofunction to be more common in soft and normal voice for the women as compared to the men (Table 2), while the degree of hyperfunction was slightly higher for the men than for the women in loud voice.

Acoustic analyses of the audio-taped vowels /i:/ and /ae:/

For both vowels, the difference L0-L1 decreased significantly ($p<0.001$) when loudness increased, but to a smaller extent in /i:/ than in /ae:/ (Figure 3, 4). For the women, the difference L0-"L1" was found to be larger in /i:/ at all loudness levels compared to the L0-L1 difference in /ae:/. For both vowels the difference L0-L1 was significantly larger for the women compared to the men ($p<0.01$).

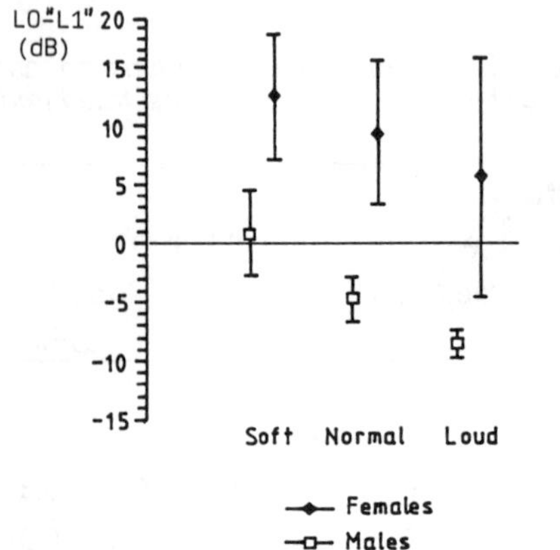

Fig. 3. Average level difference (dB) (±1 SD) between the fundamental (L0) and the first formant ("L1") in the vowel /i:/ in soft, normal, and loud voice for 9 women and 9 men.

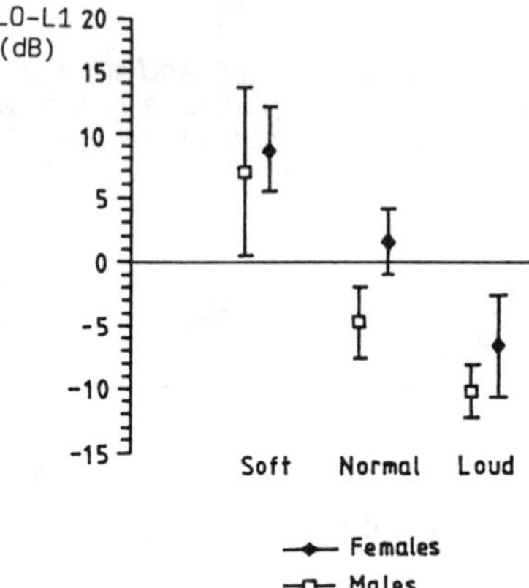

Fig. 4. Average level difference (dB) (±1 SD)between the fundamental (L0) and the first formant (L1) in the vowel /ae:/ in soft, normal, and loud voice for 9 women and 9 men.

For the vowel /i:/, the variability of the difference L0-"L1" for the women was large. In soft phonation, all 9 women and 5 of the 9 men showed a higher level of the fundamental as compared to "L1" (Figure 3). Also in normal and loud voice, a majority of the female subjects (8 and 7 respectively) showed a higher L0 compared to "L1", whereas all males had a higher "L1" than L0.

For the vowel /ae:/, in soft phonation, all women and all except one of the men showed a higher L0 as compared to L1 (Figure 4). For normal loudness, L0 dominated the spectrum for 6 women, while L1 dominated the spectrum for 8 men. For loud phonation, all female and male subjects had higher L1 than L0. An example of the changes in spectra for one male subject is shown in Figure 2 a, b, and c. The fundamental dominated the spectrum in soft phonation, whereas in normal and loud voice the first formant level was higher than the level of the fundamental.

Comparison of physiological, perceptual, and acoustic data

Correlations were calculated for (a) the degree of closure and the degree of perceived breathiness for the audio-video-taped phonations, and (b) the degree of perceived breathiness and the difference between L0 and L1 for both audio-taped vowels, using Pearson product-moment correlations. The correlations were made for each loudness level for the women and men together. Significant correlations ($p<0.01$) between glottal closure and perceived breathiness were found for soft ($r=0.71$), normal ($r=0.71$) and loud ($r=0.78$) phonation. For the vowel /i:/ significant correlations ($p<0.01$) between breathiness and the difference L0-"L1" were found for soft ($r=0.72$) and normal ($r=0.75$) but not for loud voice ($r=0.44$). For the vowel /ae:/ significant correlations ($p<0.01$) were found for normal ($r=0.69$) and loud ($r=0.60$) but not for soft phonation ($r=0.42$).

DISCUSSION

Results from the present study support the clinical experience that an increased degree of incomplete vocal fold closure corresponds to a higher degree of perceived breathiness, shown by the significant correlations between the two variables. Findings from our previous study, that incomplete posterior closure is the most common closure pattern in women and less common in men, are in agreement with results of others (Bless et al., 1986; Peppard et al., 1988). The degree of incomplete closure increased significantly with decreased loudness. Also the degree of perceived breathiness increased significantly as a function of decrease in loudness, a result also shown by Ptaçek and Sander (1963).

When we started the acoustic part of the study, we were primarily interested in analysing the vowel /i:/, since that vowel had been used in the clinical fiberscopic examination of vocal fold closure. However, when a first formant frequency is close to the fundamental, it is hard to distinguish the contribution from filter vs. source, i.e., the level of the fundamental is strongly dependent on the position of the first formant (Fant, 1959). The first formant frequency of the long vowel /i:/ in Swedish is about 280 Hz in female voices, and 260 Hz in male voices (Fant, 1959). Well aware of the proximity of F0 and F1 that causes problems in measuring L0 and L1 of high vowels, especially in high-pitched female voices, we tried to find a way of estimating "L1" in /i:/. Since the subjects kept the pitch satisfactorily stable during the three loudness conditions we decided to estimate "L1" as the spectral energy of partials Nos. 2, 3, and 4. Because of the expected difficulties with the acoustics of /i:/ we included the vowel /ae:/ in the present study. Typical values for the first formant frequency of the long Swedish vowel /ae:/ are about 790 Hz for women and 610 Hz for men (Fant, 1959). The degree of perceived breathiness did not differ significantly between the two vowels; therefore, acoustic measurements of /ae:/ ought to be satisfactory.

An interesting finding was that the fundamental was the highest partial in the spectrum, not only in soft but also in normal voice for a majority of the women, whereas the first formant was the highest part of the spectrum for the men in normal loudness, as expected. However, it should be remembered that the analyses were made on sustained vowels only, and it would be interesting to do spectrum analyses of running speech in future studies.

A comparison of the degree of perceived breathiness to the difference L0-L1, showed significant correlations (for /i:/ in soft and normal voice and for /ae:/ in normal and loud voice). These correlations confirmed a relationship between perceived breathiness and the difference L0-L1, i.e., a higher L0 in relation to L1 with increased degree of breathiness. Significant correlations were not found for the vowel /i:/ in loud voice or for /ae:/ in soft voice, however. It should be remembered that only the scale interval 0 to 3 was actually in usage for rating breathiness. This limited variation might be a fact that affected the correlations. A problem in perceptually analyzing normal data is the limited variation of some voice quality parameters, e.g., breathiness, which makes the rating difficult.

In the present study of normal voices, the degree of breathiness correlated significantly with perceived hypofunction. This finding is in agreement with the physiological finding of incomplete glottal closure for many of the women. A perceived hypofunctional voice corresponds to low laryngeal effort that can be realized by incomplete glottal closure, resulting in a breathy voice quality. This finding emphasizes the importance of including evaluation of perceived hypofunction and hyperfunction in further studies on breathiness and its acoustic correlates. Additional studies of noise components in breathy phonation are also needed to fully understand the acoustics of the voice quality. It might be that the relative level of the fundamental is the most important feature in hypofunctional/breathy voices, and that high frequency noise is a more important feature in hyperfunctional/breathy voices.

ACKNOWLEDGEMENTS

We thank the subjects who participated in the experiment and our colleagues who helped us with all evaluations. We are also indebted to Lennart Nord, Dept of Speech Communication & Music Acoustics, Royal Institute of Technology, Stockholm for help with the acoustic analyses, and to Barbara Wall for improving our English.

REFERENCES

Bickley, C. (1982). Acoustic analysis and perception of breathy vowels. *MIT Working Papers*, Vol. 1:71-81.

Bless, D., Biever, D., and Shaik, A. (1986). Comparisons of vibratory characteristics of young adult males and females. In: *Proceedings of International Conference on Voice*, edited by S. Hibi, M. Hirano, & D. Bless. Vol. 2, pp.46-54. Kurume, Japan.

Fant, G. (1959). *Acoustic Analysis and Synthesis of Speech with Applications to Swedish*. Ericsson Technics No. 1.

Fritzell, B., Hammarberg, B., Gauffin, J., Karlsson, I., and Sundberg, J. (1986). Breathiness and insufficient vocal fold closure. *J. of Phonetics*, 14:549-553.

Hammarberg, B., Fritzell, B., and Schiratzki, H. (1984). Teflon injection in 16 patients with paralytic dysphonia: Perceptual and acoustic evaluations. *J. of Speech and Hear. Dis.*, 49:72-82.

Hammarberg, B. (1986). *Perceptual and Acoustic Analysis of Dysphonia*. Doctoral dissertation, Karolinska Institute, Dept of Logopedics and Phoniatrics, Huddinge hospital, Sweden.

Henton, C.G. & Bladon, R.A.W. (1985). Breathiness in normal female speech: Inefficiency versus desirability. *Language & Communication*, 5:221-227.

Ladefoged, P., Maddieson, I., and Jackson, M. (1988). Investigating phonation types in different languages. In: *Vocal Fold Physiology, Vol. 2. Vocal physiology: Voice production, Mechanisms and Functions*, edited by O. Fujimura, pp. 297-317. Raven Press, New York.

Laver, J. (1980). *The Phonetic Description of Voice Quality*. Cambridge University Press, London.

Peppard, R., Bless, D., and Milenkovic, P. (1988). Comparison of young adult singers and nonsingers with vocal nodules. *J. of Voice*, 2:250-260.

Ptaçek, P., and Sander, E. (1963). Breathiness and phonation length. *J. of Speech and Hear. Dis.*, 28:267-272.

Södersten, M., and Lindestad P.-Å. (1990). Glottal closure and perceived breathiness during phonation in normally speaking subjects. *J. of Speech and Hear. Res.*, 33:601-611.

29

Perceptual Evaluation of a Glottal Source Model for Voice Quality Control

Satoshi Imaizumi, Shigeru Kiritani, and *Shuzo Saito

*Research Institute of Logopedics and Phoniatrics, University of Tokyo, Bunkyo-ku, Tokyo, 113 Japan, *Department of Electronics, Kogakuin University, Tokyo, 192 Japan*

Synthesis of natural sounding speech with various voice qualities still remains as a seemingly unattainable goal. Many researchers have been trying to reach this goal by developing voice source models by which intra- and inter-speaker variability in voice quality can be controlled.

For instance, Fant and Lin (1989) and Fant et al. (1986) have introduced a four-parameter model describing the time derivative of the glottal volume velocity waveform and tried to synthesize male and female voice quality with high fidelity. Fujisaki and Ljungqvist (1985) have proposed a seven parameter model which might have wider flexibility than other glottal source models. On the other hand, Klatt (1987) and Hasegawa et al. (1987) have insisted that an additive noise component must be included into the glottal source model to synthesize female voice quality with sufficient naturality. Although these studies provide a fruitful discussion on advanced techniques of high fidelity speech synthesis, there are few results reported on how natural voice quality can be reproduced for individual speakers by these glottal source models.

In this paper, we have examined how a seven-parameter polynomial model of the glottal source can reproduce the naturalness and personal characteristics of sustained vowels and VCVCV words uttered by five male and two female speakers.

MATERIALS AND METHODS

The following speech materials were recorded and analyzed:

1) Sustained vowels and vowel sequences: /a/, /i/, /u/, /e/, /o/, /aiueo/, /uoaei/.

2) $V_1CV_2CV_1$/ trisyllable nonsense words with C being /b, d, g, p, t, k, r/ and V_1, V_2 being /a, i, u/, embedded in the frame sentence /korewa - - - desu/ (This is - - -).

The materials 1) were taken from recordings of five male speakers, M_1, M_2, ... M_5, and two female speakers, F_1 and F_2, who had no laryngeal pathology. Each speaker uttered each item three times at three loudness levels and at three pitch levels.

The materials 2) were taken from recordings of two male speakers, M_1, M_2. Recordings were made at two different speaking rates, slow (S) and fast (F). The subjects were instructed to avoid unnaturalness. Each subject determined his own fast or slow rate. The subjects uttered each sentence five times.

The speech signal, the electroglottographic (EEG) signal, and for the materials in 2), the intra-oral pressure were recorded on a PCM Data Recorder. A high quality condenser microphone (B&K 2234) was used for the speech signal. The intra-oral pressure was used to detect the closed interval of the plosive consonants, and the EGG signal was used to detect the closed phase of the glottis for a fundamental frequency synchronous covariance LPC analysis (Childers and Larar, 1984). The formant frequencies derived by the LPC analysis were used to estimate the glottal volume velocity waveform by inverse filtering and also for the resynthesis of the speech sounds.

The glottal closure intervals were determined to begin at one positive peak in the EGG time derivative and end at the following negative peak. The beginning of the actual analysis frame was shifted in order to compensate for the time delay for the sound wave to propagate from the glottis to the microphone positioned 15 cm away from the lips.

The formant frequencies and bandwidths were modified manually through an interactive program in order to smooth out cycle-to-cycle fluctuations which occurred especially in the female voices. For the inverse filtering, the optimal formant frequencies and bandwidths were adjusted manually so as to minimize ripples in the glottal closure intervals and also formant-like peaks in their power spectrum.

For the sustained vowels, the time derivative of the glottal volume velocity waveform was estimated. In the inverse filtering, only one set of the lower five formant frequencies and bandwidths selected from a steady portion of each utterance was used. In other words, the cycle-by-cycle variation in formant trajectories was ignored for the sustained vowels.

For the VCVCV utterances, the time derivative of the glottal volume velocity waveform was estimated for each glottal cycle via a pitch synchronous inverse filtering. After that, not only the time derivative of the glottal volume velocity waveform but also the formant trajectories were represented by the functional models as described below.

Inverse filtered waveform, or time derivative of the glottal volume velocity waveform, was approximated in each cycle by the following polynomial function $g(t)$,

$$\begin{aligned} g(t) &= a(t-t_1)^2 + b && 0 < t \leq t_1 \\ g(t) &= b && t_1 < t \leq t_2 \\ g(t) &= c(t-t_1)^3 + d(t-t_1)^2 + e(t-t_1) + b && t_2 < t \leq T \end{aligned} \qquad (1)$$

where t=0 is the negative peak in the inverse filtered waveform, and t=T is the duration of one pitch. The parameters t_1, t_2, a, b, c, d, and e were determined based on the least square error criterion between the actual inverse filtered waveform $gi(t)$ and the model $g(t)$. One example from a female speaker is shown in Figure 1.

The trajectories of the formant frequencies for VCVCV utterances were modelled as the sum of three temporal functions (Imaizumi and Kiritani, 1989): a second order critical delay function which describes vowel-to-vowel transitions, and two first order delay functions which describe consonant-to-vowel and vowel-to-consonant transitions. The trajectories of formant bandwidth were represented by piece-wise linear approximation.

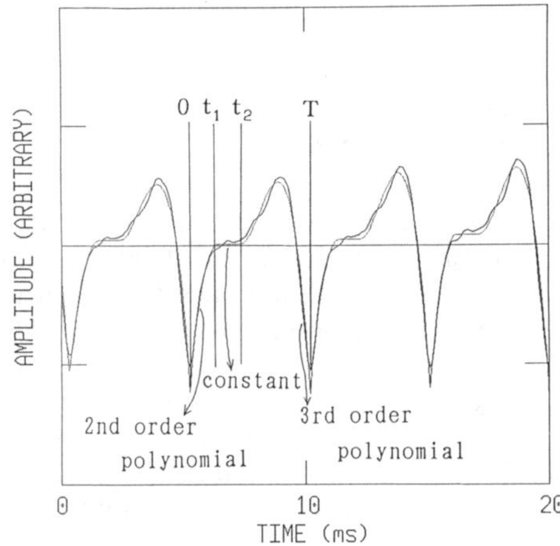

Fig. 1.The polynomial model of the glottal source adapted to a glottal source waveform obtained by inverse filtering /a/ uttered by subject F_2.

Three perceptual experiments were performed to examine how naturally and how flexibly voice quality could be reproduced by the polynomial model of the glottal source. Subjects were six students with normal-hearing capacity.

Experiment I was carried out to examine how closely the voice quality of the original vowel was reproduced by the polynomial model of the glottal source. The subjects rated the degree of similarity of the original vowel and the vowel synthesized using the polynomial model. For the sake of comparison, they also rated the resemblance between the original vowel and the vowel synthesized using Rosenberg's Type B model of the glottal source (Rosenberg, 1971). The rating was performed in a paired comparison method using a scale with seven successive categories, "1 completely different", "2 very different", "3 different", "4 neutral", "5 similar", "6 very similar", "7 perfectly the same".

Experiment II was carried out to examine how well the voice quality of vowels uttered by the five male speakers, M_1, ..., M_5, was reproduced by the glottal model using a multidimensional scaling method (Kruskal, 1964; Takane et al., 1977).

In this experiment five vowel samples of 0.5 s in length, O_1, O_2, ... , O_5, corresponding to the five male speakers M_1, M_2, ... , M_5, were resynthesized using one pitch interval extracted from the inverse filtered waveform. Then, using one pitch interval from the polynomial model of the glottal source adapted to each vowel, five vowels G_1, G_2, ... , G_5 having a length of 0.5 s were synthesized. The pitch and its fluctuation were the same for all samples as those observed from /a/ uttered by M_1. The intervals corresponding to the glottal closure periods were lengthened or shortened to adjust the fundamental frequency for all samples.

The listening subjects rated the dissimilarity in voice quality for each of all possible pairs of O_1, O_2, ... , and G_1, G_2, ... , G_5. The ratings on dissimilarity were then analyzed by the multidimensional scaling method INDSCAL included in the ALSCAL program (Takane et al. 1977), and the similarity among these ten vowel samples was represented by mutual distance in a two-dimensional space.

Experiment III was carried out to examine how closely the voice quality of the VCVCV utterances was reproduced by the polynomial model of the glottal source. The subjects rated the similarity between the original VCVCV utterances and the synthesized words. For comparison, they also rated the similarity of the original utterances and the resynthesized ones using formant trajectories obtained by the pitch synchronous analysis excited by the glottal source obtained by the inverse filtering. The rating was performed in a similar way as in Experiment I.

RESULTS AND DISCUSSION

The results of the perceptual judgments on the similarity of the original vowels and the synthetic vowels are shown in Figure 2. The samples used were /a/ uttered by the five male speakers and the two female speakers. The symbol G indicates the vowel synthesized using the polynomial model, and R represents the one synthesized with Rosenberg's glottal source model.

As shown in Figure 2, for all speakers the ratings for the synthetic vowels with the polynomial model of the glottal source (G) are higher than those for the vowels synthesized with Rosenberg's model (R). This result shows that the polynomial model of the glottal source is better than Rosenberg's model at reproducing the voice quality of the vowels for which glottal source models are adapted.

For the vowels uttered by the male speakers, M_1, M_2, ... , M_5, the medians of the ratings for the polynomial model scatter between "5 similar" and "7 perfectly the same". Those for Rosenberg's model lie between "3 different" and "5 similar". This result indicates that the polynomial model of the glottal source can reproduce the voice quality of the male speakers analyzed here.

For the female speaker, F_1, the median of the rating scores for the polynomial model is "6 very similar", although the median of the ratings for Rosenberg's model is "2 very different". On the other hand, for the female speaker, F_2, the median of the ratings for the polynomial model is "4 neutral", and the median for Rosenberg's model is "3 different". These results indicate that the polynomial model of the glottal source can reproduce some female voice qualities.

Figures 3a and 4a show the inverse filtered waveform and its model representation for subjects F_1 and F_2, respectively. Figures 3b and 4b show their power spectra. The poly-

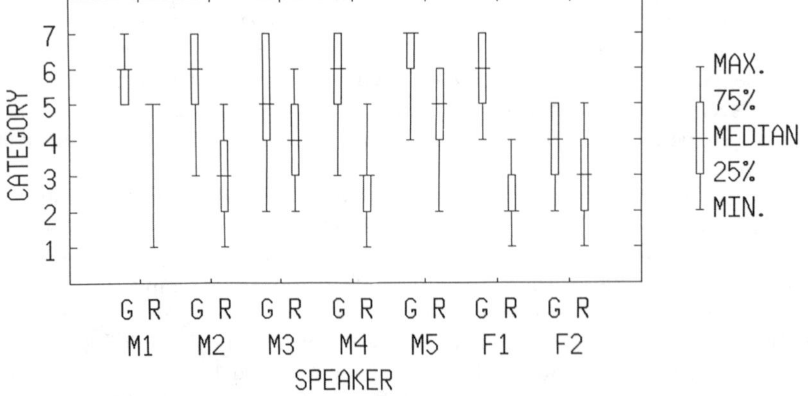

Fig. 2. The results of perceptual judgments on the degree of resemblance between original vowels and synthetic vowels with the polynomial model of the glottal source (G), and that between original vowels and synthetic vowels with Rosenberg's voice source (R). Category 7 represents the greatest possible resemblance.

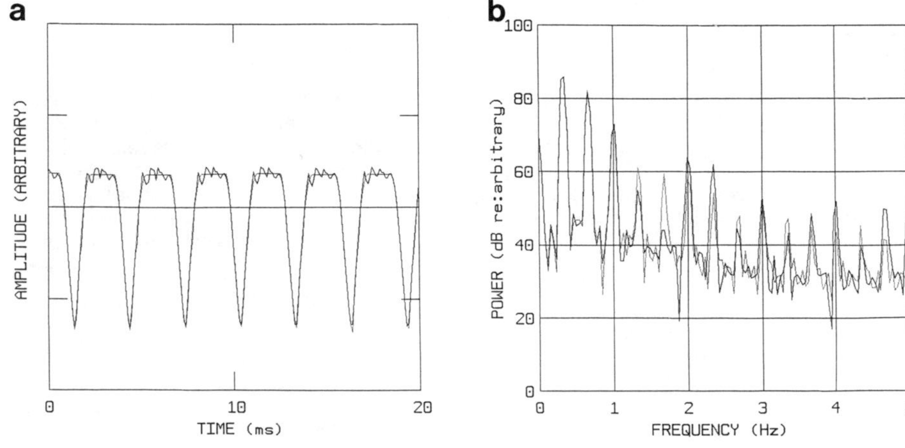

Fig. 3.The measured glottal source waveform and its model representation (**a**), and their power spectra (**b**). Female speaker F_1.

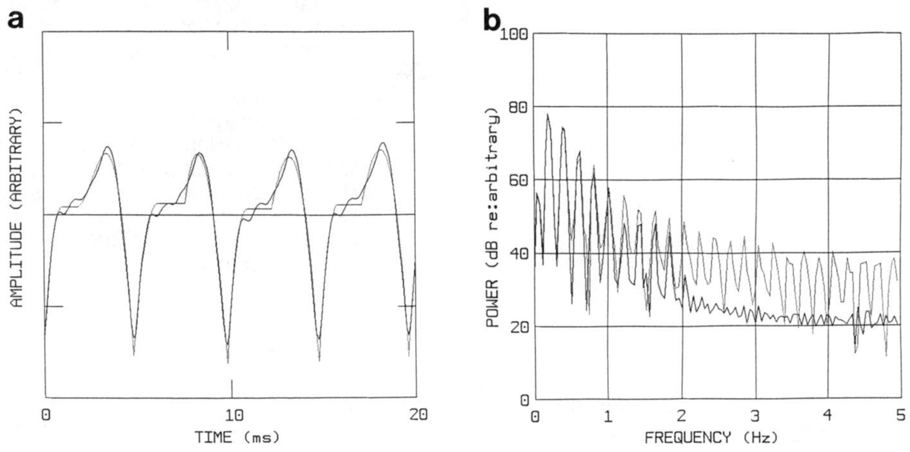

Fig. 4. Same as in Fig. 3, but for female speaker F_2.

nomial model of the glottal source for subject F_1 reproduces the voice quality of the original vowel very well, while that for F_2 does not.

In Figure 4a, the inverse filtered waveform or the measured glottal source have positive main lobes which skew right, and this characteristic is not represented well with the presented model. The intervals which are approximated by the constant b in the model contain waveform fluctuation in the measured glottal source. The negative peaks in the model source are too sharp compared to those of the measured glottal source. In Figure 4b, harmonics higher than 2 kHz are not visible in the power spectrum of the measured glottal source while the model source shows clear harmonics in this range. On the other hand, both source waveform and spectrum could be modelled fairly well in subject F_1, as

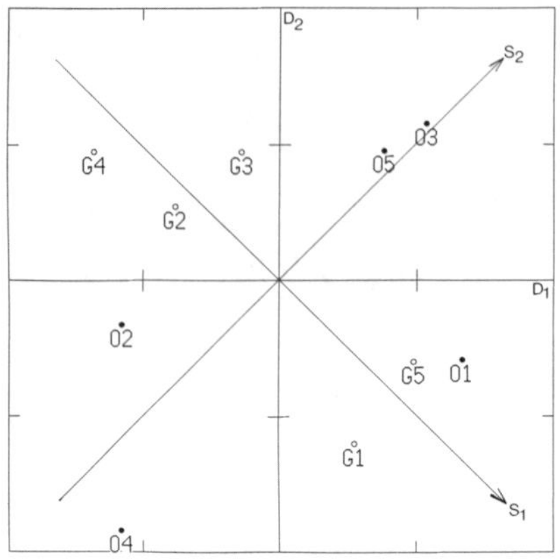

Fig. 5. Two dimensional representation of the similarity among vowels resynthesized from the inverse filtered waveform O_n and those from the polynomial model G_n. Here, n indicates the speaker number M_n. D_1 and D_2 are the dimensions extracted by the INDSCAL analysis, while S_1 and S_2 are their rotated version.

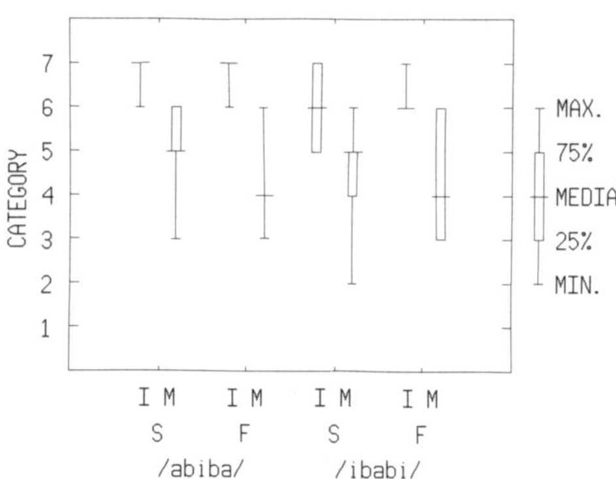

Fig. 6. The results of perceptual judgments on the degree of resemblance between the original VCVCV utterances of M_1 and the synthetic ones with the polynomial model of the glottal source (M), and that between the original utterances and the synthetic ones with the glottal source obtained by the inverse filtering (I). The letters on the second line of the abscissa indicate the instruction given to the speakers; S: slow and clearly; F: fast and clearly. Category 7 represents the greatest possible resemblance.

shown in Figure 3, although the waveform fluctuation in the intervals which are approximated by the constant b in the model are not approximated well.

The skewing and waveform fluctuation observed in Figure 4a might be caused by the source-tract interaction (Ananthapadmanabha and Fant, 1982; Koizumi et al., 1987; Rothenberg, 1981). The disappearance of harmonics higher than 2 kHz in subject F_2 is probably caused by the less sharp negative peak in the derivative of the glottal volume velocity waveform as compared to the model. The higher frequency range in the real voice is thus dominated by noise. These effects cannot be approximated with the present polynomial model of the glottal source.

The result of Experiment II is shown in Figure 5. In this figure, the similarity among the ten synthetic samples were represented by mutual distance in a two-dimensional space.

Figure 5 suggests three aspects of similarity between vowels synthesized from the inverse filtered waveform, O_n, and vowels synthesized from the model, G_n. Here, n indicates the speaker number M_n. Aspect 1: for M_1, O and G are relatively close on. Aspect 2: for M_2, M_4, and M_5, O and G are close on Dimension D_1, but distant on D_2. Aspect 3: for M_3, O and G are distant on D_1, but close on D_2. These facts indicate that the voice quality of each speaker has various aspects, some of which can be reproduced by the polynomial model of the glottal source, and some of which can not.

Figure 5 also shows that the voice samples On resynthesized from the inverse filtered waveform scatter in a two-dimensional space, while G_n resynthesized from the model scatter in a one-dimensional manner on the line S_1 and separate into two groups G_2, G_3, and G_4 versus G_1 and G_5. In other words, the two-dimensional variability of the voice quality is maintained in O_n, but is reduced to one dimension in G_n.

These results must be interpreted through an examination of the acoustical and perceptual meanings of dimensions D_1 and D_2, or S_1 and S_2 (Imaizumi, 1986). According to our preliminary examination, S_1 may indicate the contrast between "strained" versus "asthenic" voice quality, or in another definition (Hammarberg et al., 1980), a "hyperfunctional/tense" versus "hypofunctional/lax" quality. G_1 and G_5 have stronger harmonics in the high frequency range than the others. On the other hand, S_2 may indicate a "breathy/noisy" quality. These results indicate that the polynomial model of the glottal source can reproduce the voice quality represented by S_1, but not that represented by S_2.

Figure 6 shows the results of Experiment III, which was carried out to examine how closely the voice quality of the VCVCV utterances was reproduced by the polynomial model of the glottal source. In this figure, the medians of the ratings for the synthetic VCVCV words with the polynomial model of the glottal source (M) are 1 to 3 points lower than those for the synthetic ones with the glottal source obtained by the inverse filtering (I). There are, however, some high ratings such as "6 very similar" or "5 similar" for the synthetic VCVCV with the polynomial model.

The ratings for the synthetic VCVCV words with the polynomial model of the glottal source might be lowered partially due to unnaturalness of the modelled formant trajectories. It is encouraging for us that there were some high ratings, such as "6 very similar" or "5 similar", for the speech synthesized by rule with the polynomial glottal model, although there seems to be several aspects on the polynomial model which should be improved upon to simulate voice source dynamics in running speech.

CONCLUSIONS

The present study obtained the following results:

1. For male voices, the polynomial model of the glottal source can to some extent reproduce the voice quality of original vowels for which the model parameters are adapted. In a simple paired comparison based on a successive category method, Experiment I, the degree of similarity of an original vowel and a synthetic vowel using the source model was quite high. However, a detailed examination of the voice quality based on the multidimensional scaling method, Experiment II, showed that some aspects of voice quality are not reproduced by the model.

2. For voices which contain turbulence noise in the high frequency range, and those which contain waveform perturbation and skewing possibly caused by source-tract interaction, the polynomial model fails to reproduce good voice quality.

3. For the speech synthesized by rule with the polynomial glottal model, there were some high ratings such as "6 very similar" or "5 similar" to the original speech for which the model parameters were adapted.

ACKNOWLEDGEMENT

This work was supported by a Grant-in-Aid for Scientific Research on Priority Areas, the Ministry of Education, Science and Culture, Japan.

REFERENCES

Ananthapadmanabha, T.V. and Fant, G. (1982). Calculation of true glottal flew and its components. *STL-QPSR*, 1:1-30. (Dept. of Speech Communication and Music Acoustics, Royal Institute of Technology, Stockholm),

Childers, D. and Larar, J. (1984). Electroglottography for laryngeal function assessment and speech analysis. *IEEE Trans. BME-31*, 12:807-817.

Fant, G. and Lin, Q. (1989). Frequency domain interpretation and derivation of glottal flow parameters. *STL-QPSR* 2-3:1-21. (Dept. of Speech Communication and Music Acoustics, Royal Institute of Technology, Stockholm).

Fant, G., Liljencrants, J., and Lin, Q. (1986). A four-parameter model of glottal flow. *STL-QPSR* 4:1-13 (Dept. of Speech Communication and Music Acoustics, Royal Institute of Technology, Stockholm).

Fujisaki, H. and Ljungqvist, M. (1985). A comparative study of glottal waveform models. *IEICE Technical Report* (EA85-58):23-29.

Hammarberg, B., Fritzell, B., Gauffin, J., Sundberg, J., and Wedin, L. (1980). Perceptual and acoustic correlates of abnormal voice qualities.. *Acta Otolaryngol.*, 90:441-451.

Hasegawa, K., Sakamoto, T., and Kasuya, H. (1987). Effects of glottal noice on the quality of synthetic speech. *Proc. of ASJ Spring Meeting* (March 1987), pp. 205-206 (in Japanese).

Imaizumi, S. (1986). Acoustic measures of pathological voice qualities - roughness. *J. Phonetics*, 14:457-462.

Imaizumi, S. and Kiritani, S. (1989). A model of formant trajectories taking into account of the variations due to speaking rate. *Research Report No. PASL 01-5-1, Grant-in-Aid for Scientific Research on Priority Areas* (in Japanese).

Klatt, D.H. (1987). Acoustic correlates of breathiness: First harmonic amplitude, turbolent noise, and tracheal coupling. *J. Acoust. Soc. Am.*. 82(Sl):S91.

Koizumi, T., Taniguchi, S., and Hiromitsu, S. (1987). Two-mass models of the vocal cords for natural sounding voice synthesis. *J. Acoust. Soc. Am.*, 82(4):1179-1192.

Kruskal, J.B. (1964). Nonmetric multidimentional scaling: A numerical method. *Psychometrika*, 29:115-219.

Rosenberg, A.E. (1971). Effect of glottal pulse shape on the quality of natural vowels. *J. Acoust. Soc. Am.*, 49(2):583-598.

Rothenberg, M. (1981). Acoustic interactions between the glottal source and vocal tract. In: *Vocal Fold Physiology*, edited by K.N. Stevens and M. Hirano, pp. 305-328. Univ. of Tokyo Press, Tokyo.

Takane, Y., Young, F.W., and de Leeuw, J. (1977). Nonmetric individual differences multidimensional scaling: An alternating least squares method with optimal scaling features. *Psychometrika*, 42:7-67.

30

Some Acoustical, Perceptual, and Physiological Aspects of Vocal Quality

Ching-Kuen Lee and *Donald G. Childers

*Dept. of Electrical Engineering, Tatung Institute of Technology, Taipei, Taiwan, Republic of China, *Dept. of Electrical Engineering, University of Florida, Gainesville, FL 32601, USA*

For this study we investigated variations in vocal quality caused by changes in vocal fold vibratory patterns. Our purpose was to design an improved voice source excitation model for natural sounding speech synthesis. To accomplish our goal we examined the nature and extent of glottal excitation variations of several voice types, e.g., three voice registers: modal, vocal fry and falsetto, and breathy voice. We developed analysis and synthesis techniques to study the acoustical and perceptual characteristics of these four voice types. Using the knowledge gained from this study, we designed a vocal source model that incorporated some physiological aspects of vocal fold motion. The model was tested using speech synthesis and evaluated via listening tests.

Three categories of analysis techniques were developed to extract source-related features from speech and electroglottographic (EGG) signals. These included:

1. A new inverse filtering method for estimating the glottal volume-velocity waveforms from speech signals,
2. Methods for measuring the source features (the spectral slope, the amount of turbulent noise, and the temporal energy distribution) directly from speech signals, and
3. EGG waveform analysis methods for predicting the glottal vibratory phases and the glottal closure phenomena.

The analysis results showed a great diversity in temporal and spectral characteristics for glottal excitations of different voice types.

Based on the analysis results, four major factors were found to be important in characterizing the glottal excitations for different voice types: the glottal pulse width, the glottal pulse skewness, the abruptness of glottal closure, and the turbulent noise component. The significance of these factors for voice synthesis was studied. Existing voice source models were evaluated based on their capability to control these factors. Then an improved voice source model that accounted for certain physiological features of vocal fold physiology was proposed and evaluated.

The perceptual effects of the physiological glottal factors were studied by using the proposed voice source model with a cascade formant synthesizer. Synthetic voice samples were produced by systematically varying the source parameters under investigation.

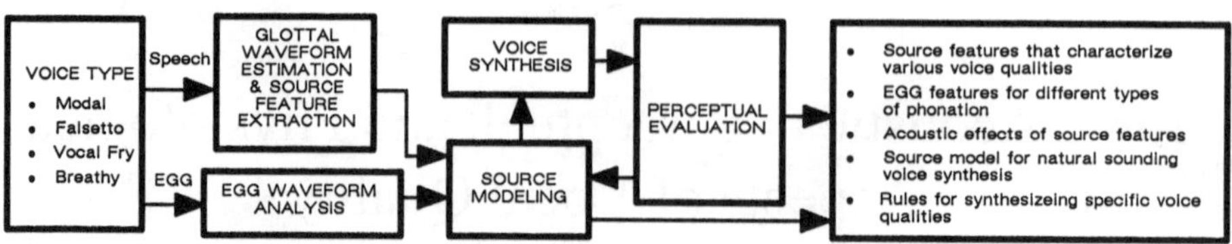

Fig. 1. Block diagram of the basic research scheme.

Listening tests were conducted to evaluate the auditory effects of the source parameters. The results showed that the sensation of vocal effort is closely related to the spectral slope of the source excitation. A source excitation with a steep-falling spectral slope results in hypofunctional or lax vocal quality, while a source excitation with excessive energy at high frequencies results in hyperfunctional or tense vocal quality. The perceptual evaluation also revealed that the existence of turbulent noise is essential for the vocal quality of breathiness. And a proper temporal characteristic of the turbulent noise source is important for producing a natural sounding breathy voice.

Considerable research has been conducted previously concerning the physiological, perceptual and acoustic characteristics of the four voice types we examined. Space limitations prohibit a proper literature survey of this material but a review will be provided upon request.

EXPERIMENTAL PROCEDURES

A summary of our research scheme appears in Figure 1. Both normal subjects (N1, N2, N3, N4, N5) with no history of vocal disorders or laryngeal pathology and patients (P1, P2, P3) with vocal disorders were used in this research. Two of the normal subjects (N1, N2) were accomplished mimics capable of imitating various voice types. The experimental tasks for each subject included:

1. Sustained vowels /i/ and /a/ using an Electro-Voice RE-10 microphone and a Brüel & Kjær model 4133 condenser microphone,
2. Counting from one to ten with comfortable pitch and loudness,
3. Counting from one to five with progressive increase in loudness,
4. Musical scale using *la*, and
5. Three sentences (*We were away a year ago. Early one morning a man and a woman ambled along a one mile lane. Should we chase those cowboys*?).

The EGG (Synchrovoice electroglottograph) and the acoustic speech waveforms were simultaneously digitized and stored on a computer disk for future analyses. All experiments were conducted inside an Industrial Acoustics Company (IAC) single wall sound room. The microphone was held at a fixed distance (6 inches) from the speaker's lips.

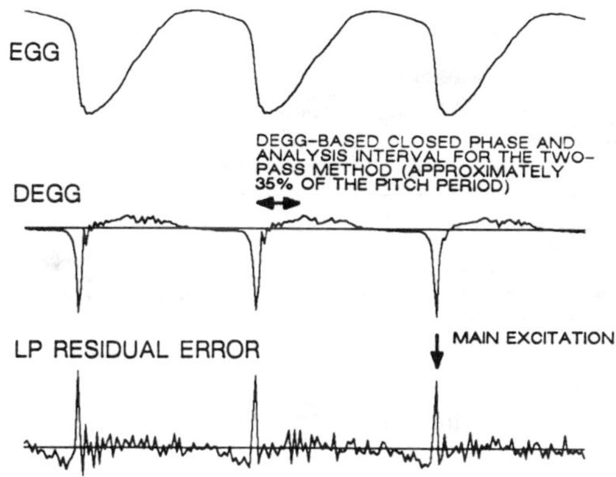

Fig. 2. Synchronized EGG, DEGG, and LP residual error.

The signal digitization was accomplished by a Digital Sound Corporation (DSC) model 200 stereo A/D and D/A system. The DSC-200 system has 16-bit accuracy. The signals were digitized with a sampling frequency of 10 kHz, with a 5 kHz anti-aliasing filter being used prior to digitization.

EXTRACTING SOURCE FEATURES

Inverse Filtering

Figure 2 illustrates that the peaks in the linear prediction (LP) error function occur nearly simultaneously with the negative peaks of the differentiated EGG (DEGG) signal, which correspond to the instants of glottal closure (Childers and Krishnamurthy, 1985; Childers et al., 1983; 1990). From these observations, we developed the "two-pass method" for accurate, automatic glottal inverse filtering, which works as well as the two-channel (speech and EGG) method (Krishnamurthy and Childers, 1986).

The basic idea of the two-pass method is first to identify the locations of the main pulses of the LP error signal derived in the first pass of the inverse filtering procedure. Then, using these main pulses as indicators of glottal closure, a "pseudo closed phase" is selected as the analysis interval for a pitch-synchronous covariance LP analysis to estimate the vocal tract filter, which in turn is used to obtain the desired glottal volume-velocity waveform. As with the EGG signal, the estimated LP pulses may not provide an exact indication for the instant of glottal closure. But, the key feature of the two-pass method is that it ensures the exclusion of the main pulse of the LP error signal from the analysis interval. This tayloring of the analysis interval increases the accuracy of the LP analysis.

A block diagram of the two-pass method is shown in Figure 3. In the first-pass procedure, a pitch-asynchronous (fixed frame) LP analysis is performed on the input speech signal $s(n)$. The estimated LP filter, $V_1(z)$, is used to derive the LP error signal, $q_1(n)$, by inverse filtering. For a voiced speech signal, the LP error function is characterized by a pulse train with the appropriate pitch period. The locations of these pulses are detected by a peak-picking method and are used as indicators of glottal closure. In the second-pass of the procedure, a pitch-synchronous covariance LP analysis is used to estimate an improved LP filter, $V_2(z)$. For each pitch period, the criterion for determining the analysis interval is to pick the samples starting one point after the instant of the main pulse. The

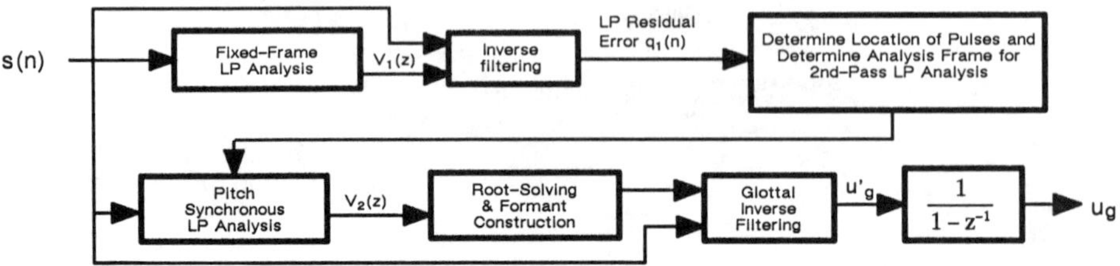

Fig. 3. Block diagram of the two-pass method for glottal inverse filtering analysis.

formant resonances of the vocal tract are estimated by solving the roots of the LP polynomial, and then shaping the formant structure by empirical rules, which include:

1. Discarding the roots with center frequencies below 250 Hz,
2. Discarding the roots with bandwidths greater than 500 Hz, and
3. Merging two adjacent roots.

The refined formant resonances are then used to construct the vocal tract transfer function, which is used in the final (second-pass) glottal inverse filtering procedure. The direct output of the glottal inverse filtering operation is a differential glottal volume-velocity $u'_g(n)$ (i.e., the equivalent driving function to the vocal tract filter), which represents the combined effect of the lip radiation and the glottal volume-velocity. A glottal volume-velocity waveform, $u_g(n)$, is derived by integration. The validity of the two-pass method was verified by testing it with synthetic speech signals. The synthetic speech signals were produced by a cascade formant synthesizer (Klatt, 1980) excited by stylized glottal pulses generated by the LF model (Fant et al., 1985). A typical result appears in Figure 4.

Source Features

Using the inverse filtered waveforms (glottal pulses) for the excitation voice types, modal, vocal fry, falsetto, and breathy, we measured the following features: 1) instant of maximum closing slope of the glottal pulse, 2) glottal pulse width, and 3) glottal pulse skewness (ratio of duration of glottal opening phase to duration of glottal closing phase).

For modal and vocal fry phonations, the instant of the maximum closing slope occurs near the instant of glottal closure, resulting in an abrupt termination of the glottal airflow. For falsetto and breathy phonations, the instant of the maximum closing slope occurs near the middle of the glottal closing phase, followed by a residual phase of progressive closure.

The glottal pulse widths were moderate (65% of the pitch period) for modal phonations and small (25% of the pitch period) for vocal fry. Falsetto and breathy voices had large pulse widths, often making it appear there was no closed phase. Glottal pulse skewness also varied with voice type. The ranking of voice type according to decreasing skewness was vocal fry, modal, falsetto, and breathy.

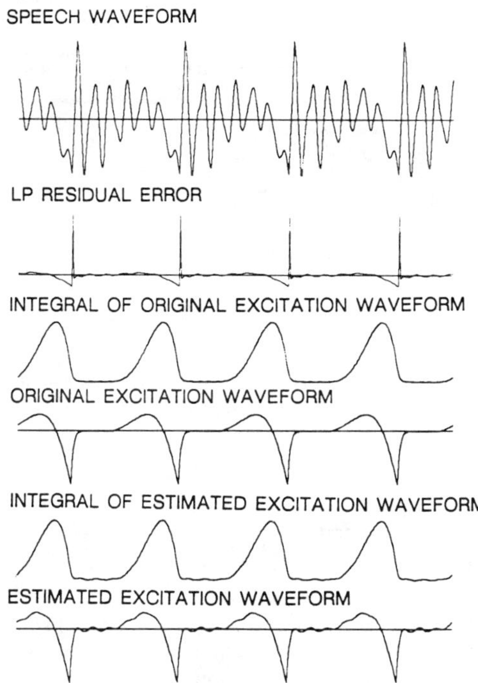

Fig. 4. An example of two-pass glottal inverse filtering.

We found that the glottal spectral characteristics for modal and vocal fry voices could be modelled well by a two-pole model (-12 dB/octave). On the other hand, an extra pole was required for falsetto and breathy phonations, yielding a steeper spectral slope of -18 dB/octave for the three-pole model. The glottal spectral model generally approximates the high-frequency portion of the spectrum of the glottal pulse better than the low-frequency characteristics. Since the glottal pulse is of finite duration, an exact model would be a finite impulse response filter possessing only zeros. We found that an all-pole model generally does not match the true data in the low-frequency region, thus giving an explanation for why larger errors occurred in the first formant estimates than in the higher formant estimates obtained by inverse filtering.

The harmonics in the speech signal below the first formant are often considered important for the perception of vocal quality (Holmes, 1973). This is presumably due to the high energy in these harmonics. We found that the glottal spectra of different voice types showed distinctive intensity relations between the fundamental and higher harmonics. We defined a parameter called the "harmonic richness factor" (*HRF*) to measure this relationship:

$$HRF = \frac{\sum_{i \geq 2} H_i}{H_1} \tag{1}$$

where H_i is the intensity of the ith harmonic and H_1 is the intensity of the fundamental frequency. We found that vocal fry was characterized by a high *HRF* (0 dB) followed by modal (-10 dB), breathy (-16 dB), and falsetto (-19 dB). Falsetto and breathy voices had a

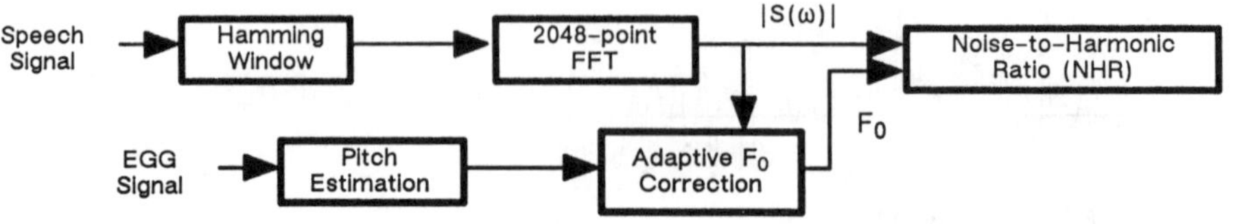

Fig. 5. Block diagram for computing the noise-to-harmonic ratio (NHR).

high intensity fundamental as well. These variations in harmonic relations appear to have little significance for speech intelligibility (phonetic identifiability) but affect the perceived vocal quality.

Measuring Source Features

The spectral tilt or slope of the glottal pulse can be measured without estimating the waveshape of the glottal pulse. The general spectral slope for a voiced phonation is determined by the combined contribution of the spectra of the glottal pulse and the lip radiation. This spectral slope may often be approximated as a two-pole spectrum, i.e., two real poles inside the unit circle. These poles are estimated using LP analysis of pre-emphasized speech. The results obtained are consistent with those obtained using inverse filtered speech. For falsetto and breathy voices, one pole is on the unit circle (or nearly so) and the other varies roughly from 0.2 to 0.9. The pole values are affected by the formants of the phonation, e.g., the same speaker with the same voice type usually had smaller pole values for an /i/ than for an /a/.

Turbulence at the level of the glottis has been noted to contribute to the perceptual quality of breathy voice (Hiraoka et al., 1984; Hillman et al., 1983; Isshiki et al., 1978; Yumoto et al., 1982). We modified the frequency-domain method of Hiraoka et al. (1984) as shown in Figure 5 to measure the noise-to-harmonic ratio (*NHR*). Our method uses an adaptive procedure to estimate F_0, which is crucial for identifying the higher harmonics. We measured the *NHR* for each ith harmonic and observed the behaviour of this ratio by plotting it along the frequency axis. We noted that breathy voices have more interharmonic noise above 2 kHz. So we defined the NHR for a high frequency region as

$$NHR_h = \frac{\sum N_i}{\sum H_i} \tag{2}$$

where N_i and H_i are the noise and harmonic components above 2 kHz respectively. We compared NHR_h to the *NHR* for 0-5 kHz and found that NHR_h is a better predictor of breathiness.

The temporal energy distribution of a speech waveform is related to the glottal excitation and has long been thought to affect vocal quality. Wendahl (1963) and Coleman (1963) established that the perception of vocal fry is related to the damping of the speech signal between glottal excitations. To measure the decay characteristics of a speech

Table 1: *Summary of the source-related features*

FEATURE		VOICE TYPE			
		MODAL VOICE	VOCAL FRY	FALSETTO	BREATHY VOICE
GLOTTAL WAVEFORM	Pulse Width	medium	very short	long	long
	Pulse Skewing	medium	high	low	low
	Abruptness of Closure	abrupt closure	very abrupt closure	progressive closure	progressive closure
GLOTTAL SPECTRUM	Spectral Slope	medium	flatter	steep-falling	steep-falling
	Harmonic Richness Factor	medium	high	low	low
SPEECH FEATURES	Spectral Tilt	medium	flatter	steep-falling	steep-falling
	Turbulent Noise	low	low	low	high
	Waveform Peak Factor	medium	high	low	low
EGG WAVEFORM FEATURES	Open Quotient	medium	low	high	high
	Closure Sharpness Factor	low	low	high	high

waveform during a single pitch period, a parameter called the waveform peak factor (*WPF*) was defined as

$$WPF = \frac{peak\ amplitude}{rms\ value} = \frac{MAX\,(|x_i|)}{\left(\frac{1}{N}\sum_{i=1}^{N} x_i^2\right)^{\frac{1}{2}}} \qquad (3)$$

where x_i is the amplitude in the ith sample point and N is the total number of sample points in one pitch period. Theoretically, the waveform peak factor, *WPF*, has a minimum value of 1 when the waveform is flat, and a maximum value $N^{1/2}$ when the waveform is an impulse. The *WPF* value of a speech waveform is related to the underlying glottal waveshape. For glottal waves with narrow pulses separated by long glottal closure, the *WPF* value is large and for pulses of long duration the *WPF* is near unity.

Although the average *WPF* values for sustained vowels vary somewhat with the type of vowel for the same subject and voice type, a general rule is that vocal fry, modal and

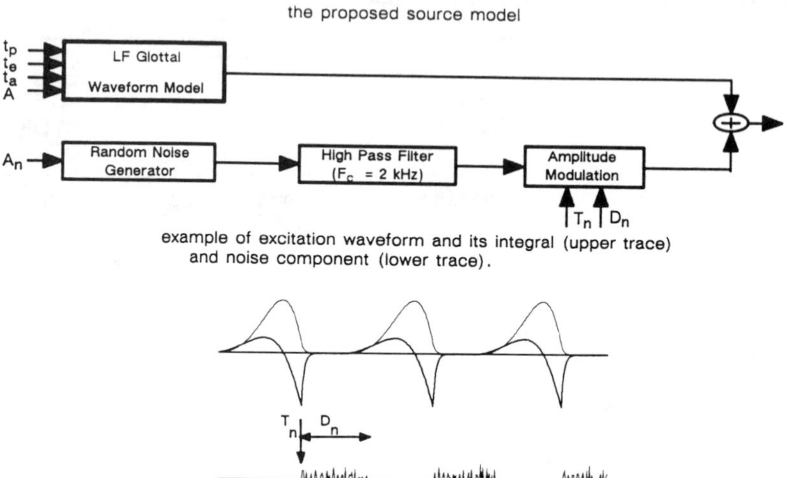

Fig. 6. Block diagram of the proposed source model and an example of the generated excitation waveform.

falsetto registers are characterized by high (4), medium (3), and low (2) values, respectively. Thus, our results imply that vocal fry register is characterized by a pulse-like excitation waveform with a long glottal closure, while falsetto register is characterized by a short glottal closure.

Finally, we also used the EGG and differentiated EGG (DEGG) to estimate the pitch period and open quotient (Childers et al., 1983). These results and all the others previously discussed are summarized in Table I. We used these source features to develop a new voice excitation model for producing natural sounding synthetic speech with desired vocal characteristics.

A NEW EXCITATION MODEL

Basically, researchers have used three types of excitation for speech synthesis, especially for formant synthesizers. These are:

1. Impulse excitation with a glottal shaping filter (Flanagan, 1957; Klatt, 1980; 1987; Rabiner, 1968),
2. Glottal waveforms obtained by inverse filtering (Holmes, 1973; Rosenberg, 1971) or glottal area waveforms (Yea et al., 1983) and
3. Excitation waveform models (Ananthapadmanabha, 1984; Fant et al., 1985; Fujisaki and Ljungqvist, 1986; Hedelin, 1984; Klatt, 1987; Rosenberg, 1971). We believe for various reasons that excitation waveform models are flexible, easy to use and produce natural sounding speech.

The four glottal factors we found important for characterizing several voice types were glottal pulse width and skewness, abruptness of glottal closure, and turbulent excitation. None of the above models has used all four of these characteristics. The first three glottal factors can be modeled with an existing waveform excitation model, e.g., the LF model (Fant et al., 1985). We obtain the required LF model parameters by using a least squares error criterion that minimizes the error between the inverse filtered excitation (not the volume-velocity waveform but its derivative) and the LF model waveform. The LF model parameters are adjusted iteratively until the least squares error is minimized. In this way we have tabulated values for the parameters t_c, t_p, t_e, t_a, OQ, and SQ for the LF model. Typically, these parameters may have wide ranges of values for various voice types. Turbulent excitation has been shown to be important for synthesizing certain sounds. We have added this form of excitation to the LF model as shown in Figure 6. The turbulent noise generator consists of a random number generator, a spectrum-shaping filter, and an amplitude-modulator. The amplitude-modulator simulates the amplitude fluctuations of the turbulent noise due to variations in airflow during vocal fold vibrations. We use a pitch-modulated square-wave with an adjustable duty cycle. Two parameters are used to control the starting position (T_n) and the duration (D_n) of the duty cycle. This model can synthesize breathy voices and voiced fricatives.

TESTING THE MODEL

A number of excitation waveforms were used to synthesize speech and formal listening tests were conducted using four judges who were either professional voice diagnosticians or voice scientists. The results were that the perception of vocal effort (hypo- and hyperfunction also known as lax voice and tense voice, respectively) is closely related to the SQ and the spectral slope of the glottal excitation waveform. A large SQ produces excessive energy at higher frequencies and results in the perception of tense or hyperfunctional vocal quality. A small SQ corresponds to a steep-falling spectral slope resulting in the perception of a lax or hypofunctional vocal quality.

Our conclusions regarding the turbulent noise source include:

1. The amplitude modulation of the turbulent noise is important for achieving naturalness for synthetic breathy voices. Our data suggests that a duty cycle in the range of 50% to 75% is preferred.
2. The location (within a pitch period) of noise production is not very critical; however, the perceptual naturalness is improved when the noise source simulates the natural manner of the human phonation, i.e., the noise source should be located near the point of maximum glottal closure.
3. High-pass filtering of the turbulent noise is not critical for perceptual breathiness because the effect of the noise in the low-frequency region is masked by strong harmonic components.
4. The degree of perceptual breathiness is primarily dependent on the noise-to-harmonic ratio at higher frequencies (above 2 kHz).

We believe this work has led to an improved understanding of the relationship between certain acoustical, perceptual, and physiological aspects of vocal quality.

ACKNOWLEDGEMENT

This work was supported by NIH grant NIDCD DC 00577.

REFERENCES

Anathapadmanabha, T.V. (1984). Acoustic analysis of voice source dynamics. *STL-QPSR* 2-3/1984:1-24. (Dept. of Speech Communication & Music Acoustics, Royal Institute of Technology, Stockholm).

Childers, D.G. and Krishnamurthy, A.K. (1985). A critical review of electroglottography. *CRC Critical Review, Bioeng.*, 12:131-164.

Childers, D.G., Hicks, D.M., Moore, G.P., Eskenazi, L., and Lalwani, A.L. (1990). Electroglottography and vocal fold physiology. *J. Speech and Hear. Res.*, 33:245-254.

Childers, D.G., Naik, J.M., Larar, J.N., Krishnamurthy, A.K., and Moore, G.P. (1983). Electroglottography , speech and ultra-high speed cinematography. In: *Vocal Fold Physiology: Biomechanics, Acoustics and Phonatory Control*, edited by I.R. Titze and R.C. Scherer, pp. 202-220. The Denver Center for the Performing Arts, Denver..

Coleman, R.F. (1963). Decay characteristics of vocal fry. *Folia Phoniatr.*, 15:256-263.

Fant, G., Liljencrants, J., and Lin, Q. (1985). A four parameter model of glottal flow. *STL-QPSR* 4/1985:1-13. (Dept. of Speech Communication & Music Acoustics, Royal Institute of Technology, Stockholm).

Flanagan, J.L. (1957). Note on the design of terminal-analog speech synthesizers. *J. Acoust. Soc. Am.*, 29:306-310.

Fujisaki, H. and Ljungqvist, M. (1986). Proposal and evaluation of models for the glottal source waveform. *Proc. ICASSP 86*, Tokyo, 3: 1605-1608.

Hedelin, P. (1984). A glottal LPC-vocoder. *Proc.ICASSP 84*, San Diego, California, 1.6.1-1.6.4.

Hillman, R.E., Oesterle, E., and Feth, L.L. (1983). Characteristics of the glottal turbulent noise source. *J. Acoust. Soc. Am.*, 74:691-694.

Hiraoka, N., Kitazoe, Y., Ueta, H., Tanaka, S., and Tanabe, M. (1984). Harmonic-intensity analysis of normal and hoarse voices. *J. Acoust. Soc. Am.*, 76:1648-1651.

Holmes, J.N. (1973). The influence of glottal waveform on the naturalness of speech from a parallel formant synthesizer. *IEEE Trans. Audio and Electroacoustics*, AU-21:298-305.

Isshiki, N., Kitajima, K., Kojima, H., and Harita, Y. (1978). Turbulent noise in dysphonia. *Folia Phoniatr.*, 30:214-224.

Klatt, D.H. (1980). Software for a cascade/parallel formant synthesizer. *J. Acoust. Soc. Am.*, 67:971-995.

Klatt, D.H. (1987). Review of text-to-speech conversion for English. *J. Acoust. Soc. Am.*, 82:737-793.

Krishnamurthy, A.K. and Childers, D.G. (1986). Two-channel speech analysis. *IEEE Trans. Acoust., Speech, and Signal Proc.*, ASSP-34:730-743.

Rabiner, L.R. (1968). Digital-formant synthesizer for speech synthesis studies, *J. Acoust. Soc. Am.*, 43:822-828.

Rosenberg, A.E. (1971). Effect of glottal pulse shape on the quality of natural vowels. *J. Acoust. Soc. Am.*, 49:583-590.

Wendahl, R.W. (1963). Laryngeal analog synthesis of harsh voice quality. *Folia Phoniatr.*, 15:241-250.

Yea, J.J., Krishnamurthy, A.K, Naik, J.M., and Childers, D.G. (1983). Glottal sensing for speech analysis and synthesis. *Proc. IEE Int. Conf. of Acoust. Speech and Signal Proc. 83*, Boston, Mass. 1332-1335.

Yumoto, E., Gould, W., and Baer, T. (1982). Harmonic-to-noise ratio as an index of the degree of hoarseness. *J. Acoust. Soc. Am.*, 71:1544-1550.

31

Insufficient Vocal Fold Closure as Studied by Inverse Filtering

Stellan Hertegård and *Jan Gauffin

*Dept. of Logopedics and Phoniatrics, Huddinge Hospital, Karolinska Institute, S-141 86 Huddinge. Sweden, *Dept. of Speech Communication and Music Acoustics, Royal Institute of Technology, S-100 44 Stockholm, Sweden*

There is great need in clinical practice to develop methods for quantification of glottal voice source behaviour. A potentially useful method is inverse filtering of the oral flow waveform recorded via the mask designed by Rothenberg (1973). The recording procedure is simple for the subject or patient and is non-invasive. After removal of the acoustic influence of the vocal tract with inverse filtering, the transglottal airflow during phonation is obtained. If the vocal folds close completely during phonation the airflow is presumed to be zero during the closed phase of the glottogram. Thus, the method can be used as an indirect way of describing insufficient vocal fold closure, as in the clinical studies by Fritzell et al. (1986). The shape of the waveform (the glottal volume velocity waveform) influences the acoustic output of the voice (Fant and Lin, 1991; Gobl and Karlsson, 1991). Gauffin and Sundberg (1989) have shown that the peak to peak amplitude of the glottogram is related to the voice source fundamental for male speakers and that the maximal negative amplitude of the differentiated glottogram can predict the sound pressure level (SPL) of a vowel. Holmberg et al. (1988) examined transglottal flow characteristics during soft, normal and loud phonation in 45 normals. They also described differences between males and females regarding the glottal volume velocity waveform.

The aim of the present study was to produce air flow glottograms and transglottal pressures on normal female and male subjects with the purpose of finding parameters related to the perceived degree of breathiness versus hupofunction and hyperfunction.

METHOD

Twenty-four female (age ranging from 21 to 49 years) and twenty male (age ranging from 24 to 57 years) normal speakers with normal larynxes served as subjects. None of the subjects had voice problems and none had extensive voice training.

The airflow at the mouth and the intraoral pressure were recorded on a TEAC MR30 FM tape recorder. The airflow was measured by means of a Rothenberg mask and a small catheter connected to a pressure transducer was held in the subjects mouth during the recording. The subjects produced the syllables /papapa:/ in a carrier phrase with their natural loud, normal and soft levels of vocal effort. The intraoral pressure during the /p/

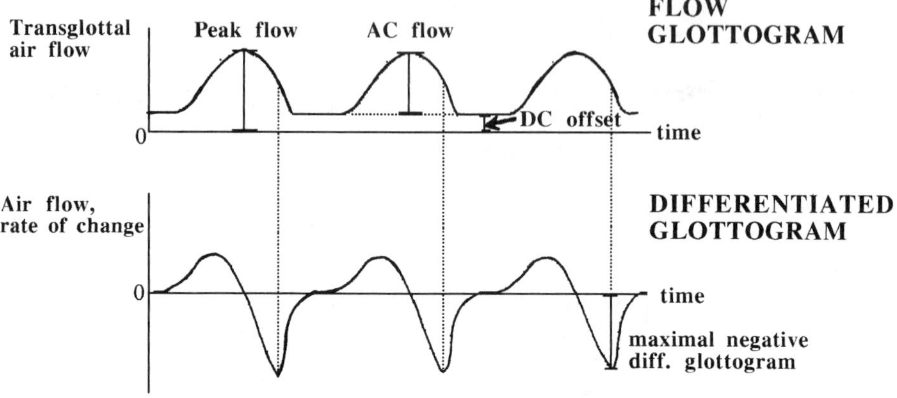

Fig. 1. Glottal volume velocity waveform, i.e., a flow glottogram, and the differentiated waveform.

occlusion was used as an estimate of the subglottic pressure for the following vowel (Löfquist et al., 1982; Rothenberg, 1973). An audio recording of identical speech material without the mask, was made at the same occasion on a Revox A77 tape recorder.

The inverse filtering was performed interactively on a computer. A midvowel section of the last syllable in /papapa:/ was analyzed. INA, a program written by J Liljencrants, was used for this purpose. The antifilter was adjusted so as to cancel the first and second formants to a maximally smooth flow glottogram, whereby a maximally even spectrum slope was obtained for the filtered signal. The signal was low pass filtered at 1.5 kHz. The differentiated flow glottogram and fundamental frequency (F0) were also computed. The transglottal airflow, the differentiated airflow glottogram (the maximal airflow declination rate) and the subglottal i.e transglottal pressure (Ps) were determined by means of recorded calibration signals. SPL was estimated from the differentiated air flow signal and corrected to a distance of 0.5 m from the mouth.

From the flow glottogram and the differentiated flow glottogram the following glottal parameters were extracted: Peak flow was the amount of flow from zero flow baseline to maximum flow; DC offset (or minimum flow) was the amount of flow from zero flow to the minimum flow during the most closed phase; AC flow (peak-to-peak flow) was the peak flow minus the DC offset. The maximum rate of decline of the airflow (the differentiated glottogram) was extracted as the maximum negative amplitude from the differentiated waveform (Figure 1). In addition to the above parameters, the DC/Peak Flow quotients (i.e., the DC Offset/Peak Flow] quotients) and the log10DC Offset/SPL quotients were computed.

The audio recordings without the mask were analysed perceptually by six experienced voice clinicians who rated the degree of breathiness, hyperfunction and hypofunction in the /papapa:/ syllables along a 7-point scale. The mean intra-reliability within .5 scale points was 95% and inter-reliability within 1 scale point was 81%.

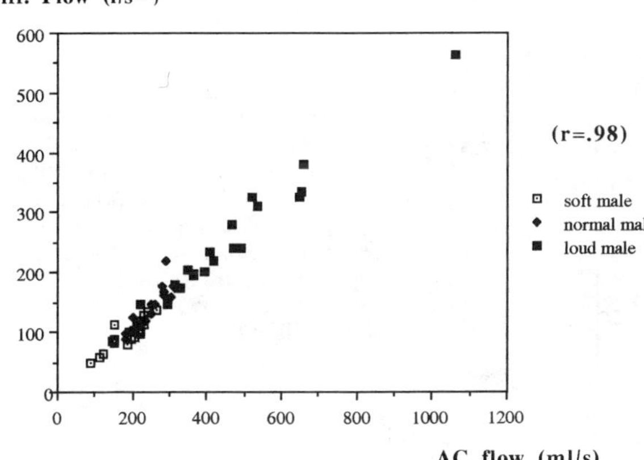

Fig. 2. Scatterogram showing the relationship between AC flow and the differentiated flow for male subjects. The soft, normal, and loud levels of vocal effort are marked in the figure.

RESULTS AND DISCUSSION

The DC/Peak Flow and the log10 DC/SPL quotients were calculated in order to test their degree of correlation to the perceptual degree of breathiness and hyperfunction. The DC/Peak Flow quotient was used by Fritzell et al. (1986) as a measure of "wasted air flow". The latter quotient was used to test the hypothesis that a high level of DC Offset results in a breathy voice quality, whereas a high level of SPL (which is related to the level of the higher harmonics in the voice) would conceal the perceptual impression of breathiness in the voice. In this study we assume that a DC Offset is an indication of incomplete vocal fold closure. However, it can not be ruled out that a small amount of DC Offset can be caused by vertical vocal fold movements during the closed phase of the glottis.

The mean values of each parameter for the male and female subjects are presented in Table 1. For each subject the mean value of three phonations was used. Included in the tables are the results of t-tests for each parameter, testing if there were any significant differences when the subjects changed from soft to normal and from normal to loud voice effort. To minimize the risk of bias due to multiple paired t-tests, a conservative level of significance was used ($p<0.005$).

The mean values for some of the parameters differ somewhat from those found by Holmberg et al. (1988). Thus, we found lower SPL values. Among the flow parameters the values of the differentiated flow and the minimum flow (DC offset) were lower in the present study. These differences might be related to different experimental situations and tasks for the subjects. Holmberg et al. (1988) measured SPL via a microphone fixed to the handle of the Rothenberg mask 15 cm from the mouth and in the present study the SPL was estimated from the differentiated flow, corrected for a distance of 50 cm to the mouth. We used the syllables /papapa:/ in a carrier phrase spoken as a sentence and Holmberg et al. (1988) used strings of sustained syllables [pae:], which probably is closer to sustained vowel phonation. However, differences in phonation between Swedish and American speakers cannot be ruled out. The relations between the parameters for soft and normal voice efforts and those for normal and loud voice efforts are very much similar in the two studies.

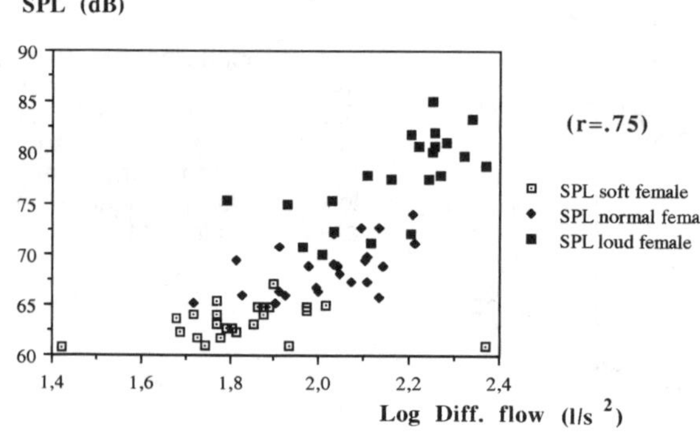

Fig. 3. Scatterogram showing the relationship between log10 Differentiated Airflow and sound pressure level (SPL) for female subjects. The soft, normal, and loud levels of vocal effort are marked in the figure.

In the present study as well as in the study by Holmberg et al. (1988), most subjects showed a DC offset even for loud voice effort, indicating incomplete vocal fold closure. We found diminishing DC offset levels with increasing levels of vocal effort, which would indicate a more effective vocal fold closure during phonation. Relatively few subjects in this study showed consistent complete vocal fold closure, expressed as zero DC offset during the most closed phase. No DC Offset was seen in only three out of 71 female phonations (i.e., 4%, 2 samples during loud voice and 1 during normal voice effort). One female subject showed no DC Offset both during normal and loud levels of vocal effort. Thirteen out of the sixty male phonations had zero DC offset (i.e., 22%, 9 samples with loud voice, 3 with normal voice and 1 with soft voice effort). The male subjects with zero DC offset during soft voice phonation also had zero offset during normal and loud voice phonation.

Södersten and Lindestad (1987; 1988) studied nine female and nine male normal speaking subjects using nasofiberoptic laryngostroboscopy during sustained [i:] vowel phonation. Some of their subjects also participated in the present study. They found complete closure of the vocal folds in 4% of the female phonations, which is in agreement with the results of this study. However, a higher population of males (67%) showed a complete closure. The relationship between glottal flow parameters indicating vocal fold closure and vocal fold vibration patterns obviously needs to be further examined.

The perceptual results showed that the degree of breathiness decreased and hyperfunction increased with increasing levels of vocal effort (Table 1). The mean values for both breathiness and hyperfunction were very low across all levels of vocal effort, with few subjects rated over 2 on a 7 point scale. This finding might be expected for normal speakers. The highest ratings for breathiness were found for the female subjects . Generally it was a rather lax or hypofunctional type of breathy voice quality that was produced in these cases.

The male-female differences were tested with analysis of variance. As expected, the females phonated on higher fundamental frequencies ($p<0.001$). The males generally produced 1 to 2 dB higher SPL values ($p<0.005$). The maximum rate of decline of the airflow (differentiated flow) was also higher for the males ($p<0.001$). The males also produced higher Peak flow and AC flow, which was expected because of the larger male larynx ($p<0.001$). The females had higher DC offset ($p<0.001$), which corroborates the

Table 1. *Mean values for male and female speakers for soft, normal, and loud levels of vocal effort. Each parameter is tested for differences when the subjects changed from soft to normal and from normal to loud effort.*

	MALE			FEMALE		
	Soft	Normal	Loud	Soft	Normal	Loud
SPL (dB)	64.9*	70.6*	78.8	63.3*	68.6*	77.6
Ps (cm H^2O)	4.2	5.85*	9.7	4.5*	6.2*	10.0
F0 (Hz)	111	117*	142	188	196*	227
Peak flow (ml/s)	270*	305*	505	215*	245*	310
AC flow (ml/s)	190*	255*	470	110*	155*	240
DC offset (ml/s)	80*	50*	35	105	90	70
Diff. airflow (l/s^2)	97.4*	142.8*	254.9	74.0	108.4*	153.3
DC offset/Peak flow	0.3*	0.15*	0.06	0.5	0.35*	0.2
log_{10}DC offset/SPL (ml/s/dB)	0.03*	0.025*	0.02	0.031	0.028	0.025
Perceptuall ratings:						
Breathiness	0.5	0.2	0.1	0.9	0.8*	0.2
Hyperfunction	0.1	0.2	0.4	0	0	0.3
Hypofunction	0.3*	0.15*	0	0.6	0.4*	0

* $p \leq 0.005$ on paired t-test.

findings by Holmberg et al. (1988). The DC Offset/Peak Flow and log10DC Offset/SPL quotient followed the ratings for breathiness, i.e., the females had higher values ($p<0.001$). There were no sex differences regarding the subglottal pressure (Ps), which also corroborate findings by Holmberg et al. (1988).

Correlations between different parameters from Table 1 were tested using the Pearson product moment correlation. The correlation between the AC Flow and the Differentiated Flow was generally very high ($r=0.98$ for male (Figure 2), and $r=0.87$ for the female subjects), which agrees with Holmberg et al. (1988). These findings differ somewhat from those in the studies by Gauffin and Sundberg (1989), who found that the amplitude (peak-to-peak) of the flow glottogram only for the trained singer increased parallel to the flow derivative with increasing vocal effort. This vocal behaviour was named flow phonation. The amplitude of the glottogram was not raised as much during loud voice phonation in the untrained subject, whose phonation was more pressed. The subjects in the present study did not seem to use this pressed phonation (they increased the AC flow and the differentiated flow in parallel). The low perceptual ratings for strain and hyperfunction support this assumption.

As shown in Figure 3, the correlation between log10 Differentiated Flow and SPL was lower ($r=0.75$ for the females). For the males the correlation was $r=0.86$. The log10 transformation was used because the SPL is the log10 transformation of intensity, the

Table 2. *(**a**) Mean values of perceived breathiness (Br) with corresponding DC Offset values in ml/s (DC) and corresponding DC Offset/Peak Flow quotient (DC/Peak).*
*(**b**). Samples with DC offset value of 50 ml/s or below (DC) and the corresponding mean values for breathiness (Br). Levels of vocal effort are shown in the table.*

	Table 2a						Table 2b			
	MALE			FEMALE			MALE		FEMALE	
Vocal effort	Br	DC	DC to Peak	Br	DC	DC to Peak	DC	Br	DC	Br
Soft	0	70	0.25							
	0	**133**	0.4							
Normal	0.05	60	0.15				25	0.15	45	0.15
	0.05	20	0.1				20	0.05		
	0.05	60	0.2							
	0.1	60	0.2							
Loud	0.1	40	0.1	0.1	50	0.35	40	0.1	50	0.1
	0	0	0	0	60	0.2	40	0.1	50	0.1
	0	0	0	0.1	60	0.15	0	0	0	0.1
	0	10	0	0.1	0	0	0	0	50	0
	0	**120**	0.2	0	**115**	0.3	0	0	45	0.05
	0.1	60	0.15	0	50	0.15	10	0		
	0	0	0	0	45	0.3	0	0		
	0	0	0				0	0		
	0	10	0.05				10	0		
	0	0	0				0	0		
	0	40	0.05				0	0.2		
	0	0	0							

underlying physical measure to which other parameters might be related (Isshiki, 1964). The reason for this lower correlation might be that many of the subjects used a slightly hypofunctional type of phonation and also had some DC offset (especially the female subjects). Most subjects produced slightly aspirated [pa] syllables during the speech task, which might have contributed to this. In many cases the result was a sinusoidal waveform which made a correct setting of the zeros during the inverse filtering difficult. This might have added some error to the differentiated airflow values. Furthermore, insufficient vocal fold closure and DC offset during phonation might result in energy losses through coupling effects to the subglottic space. This would also affect the differentiated airflow values.

In the present study an increase of the subglottal pressure by a factor of 2 was accompanied by an increase of the SPL with 12 to 13 dB for both male and female subjects. This finding corroborates the results of Holmberg et al. (1988). The correlation between the log10 subglottal pressure and the SPL was r=0.84 for both the males and the females. The log10 AC and SPL were also highly correlated (r=0.87 for the males and r=0.83 for the females).

Some relationships between the perceptual ratings and glottal parameters were also tested. The glottal parameters were DC Offset, DC/Peak Flow quotient and log10DC Offset/SPL quotient. The correlation between log10DC Offset/SPL quotient and breathiness for the female subjects was the highest (r=0.73). The DC/Peak Flow quotient also correlated well with breathiness for the females (r=0.69). Fritzell et al. (1986) found a correlation coefficient of r=0.83 between breathiness and DC/Peak Flow quotient. In their study they tested pathological voices with a large spread for perceptual ratings of breathiness.

The DC offset showed a lower correlation with breathiness for the female subjects (r=0.58). No high correlations were found for glottal parameters to strained voice quality. The low correlation between glottal parameters and hyperfunctional voice quality in general and between breathiness and the male glottal parameters might be explained by the fact that perceptual ratings in these cases were very low.

It was difficult for the voice clinicians to rate parameters precisely in normal subjects, who mostly rated below 1.5 on the 7 point scale. In Table 2a are shown only those phonation samples where all six judges' ratings were clustered within 0.5 scale points and the mean result for breathiness scored at 0.1 or below on the 7 point scale. The mean for breathiness for these samples was compared to some corresponding glottogram parameters of the same level of vocal effort, DC Offset and DC/Peak Flow quotient. In Table 2b is shown the result of the opposite operation comparing those samples of glottograms with DC offset of 50 ml/s or below to the perceptual ratings where the judges agreed within 0.5 scale points for breathiness.

These tables show a good correspondence between very low DC offset levels and low degree of perceived breathiness. Most cases with breathiness below 0.1 scale units also have DC offset values below 60 ml/s (Table 2b). This value might be a lower limit for what we can perceive as breathy voice quality. However, the correspondence even in these cases is not perfect. One female subject and two male subjects in Table 2a were not perceived as breathy, even though they had DC offsets over 100 ml/s. In the female case a possible explanation might be that the subject phonated at a high intensity level (85 dB for loud voice effort compared to the mean value of 77.6 dB for all the female subjects in loud voice effort). The high levels of higher harmonics might have masked the impression of breathiness in the voice. This is confirmed by the log10DC/SPL quotient, which as shown in the study corresponds fairly well to breathiness. In this case the value of this quotient (0.024) was lower than the mean value for all the female soft voice phonations (0.025).

The male samples are more difficult to explain. In one case the fundamental frequency was rather high (161 Hz). The SPL was 2 dB higher than the average, although the subglottal pressure and the AC flow were not. A spectrogram (bandwidth 300 Hz) revealed that the centre frequency of the first formant was low (around 550 Hz). Near this frequency there was a peak in the spectrum, possibly due to both the levels of the third and fourth harmonics. The other male sample had a very low fundamental frequency (around 85 Hz). The SPL-, subglottal pressure-, and AC flow values were somewhat higher than average. The spectrogram showed that the level of the fundamental seemed to determine his overall SPL. His voice quality was somewhat creaky, which might have affected the perceptual judgements.

In conclusion, the findings indicate that the relationship between breathiness and the glottal airflow parameters is rather complex. Probably other physiological and acoustical factors such as the harmonics to noise ratio (Kasuya and Ando, 1991) add important information. In addition, we do not yet know to what extent vertical movements of the vocal folds during the closed phase of the glottis can add to the DC offset in the flow glottogram. Considering the area of the vocal folds and possible vertical movements, the flow glottogram may be offset by up to 50 ml/s due to such vibratory movements

ACKNOWLEDGEMENTS

To Björn Fritzell for support and fruitful discussions and to Laurie Chapman for discussions regarding the statistical analysis.

REFERENCES

Fant, G. and Lin, Q. (1991). Comments on glottal flow modelling and analysis. In: *Vocal Fold Physiology: Acoustic, Perceptual and Physiological Aspects of Voice Mechanism,* edited by J. Gauffin and B. Hammarberg (this volume).

Fritzell, B., Hammarberg, B., Gauffin, J., Karlsson, I., and Sundberg, J. (1986). Breathiness and insufficient vocal fold closure. *J. Phonetics*, 14:549-553.

Gauffin, J. and Sundberg, J. (1989). Spectral correlates of glottal voice source waveform characteristics. *J Speech Hear. Res.*, 32:556-565.

Gobl, C. and Karlsson, I. (1991). Male and female voice source dynamics. In: *Vocal Fold Physiology: Acoustic, Perceptual and Physiological Aspects of Voice Mechanism,* edited by J. Gauffin and B. Hammarberg (this volume).

Holmberg, E., Hillman R., and Perkell, J. (1988). Glottal airflow and transglottal air pressure measurements for male and female speakers in soft, normal and loud voice. *J. Acoust. Soc. Am.*, 84:511-529.

Isshiki, N. (1964). Regulatory mechanisms of voice intensity variation. *J. Speech Hear. Res.*, 7(1):17-29.

Kasuya, H. and Ando, Y. (1991). Acoustic analysis, synthesis and perception of breathy voice. In: *Vocal Fold Physiology: Perceptual and Physiological Aspects of the Voice Mechanism,* Vol. 3. Edited by J. Gauffin and B. Hammarberg (this volume). Raven Press, New York.

Löfquist, A., Kitzing, P. and Carlborg, B. (1982). Initial validation of an indirect measure of subglottal pressure during vowels. *J. Acoust. Soc. Am.*, 72(2):633-635.

Rothenberg, M. (1973). A new inverse-filtering for deriving the glottal airflow waveform during voicing. *J. Acoust. Soc. Am.*, 53:1632-1645.

Södersten, M. and Lindestad, P.Å. (1987). Vocal fold closure in young adult normal-speaking females. *Phoniatric and Logopedic Progress Report*, 5:12-29. (Dept. of Logopedics and Phoniatrics, Huddinge Hospital, Karolinska Institute, Stockholm).

Södersten, M. and Lindestad, P.Å. (1988). Vocal fold closure and perceived breathiness in young adult normal-speaking males. *Phoniatric and Logopedic Progress Report*, 6:48-63. (Dept. of Logopedics and Phoniatrics, Huddinge Hospital, Karolinska Institute, Stockholm).

32

Acoustic Analysis, Synthesis, and Perception of Breathy Voice

Hideki Kasuya and Yuji Ando

Dept. of Electrical and Electronic Engineering, Faculty of Engineering, Utsunomiya University, Utsunomiya, 321 Japan

Breathy voice has proved to be associated with insufficient closure of the glottis (Fritzell et al., 1986), a psycho-acoustic impression of the extent of air leakage through the glottis (Hirano, 1981), an enhanced first harmonic level (Bickley, 1982; Hammarberg, 1986), and high frequency noise (Imaizumi, 1986; Hasegawa et al., 1987; Klatt, 1987). Problems still remain, however, with the significance of individual acoustic parameters for the perception of breathiness quality, specifically the contribution of glottal turbulence noise.

In this paper, we first investigate temporal and frequency characteristics of both glottal harmonics and noise components of breathy vowels and then the perceptual significance of selected acoustic parameters for breathiness quality, using speech synthesis. It will be shown from perceptual experiments that the frequency characteristics as well as the amount of turbulence noise are salient acoustic cues for perceived quality of breathiness.

ACOUSTIC MEASUREMENTS

Our acoustic measurements of a breathy vowel included an estimation of glottal harmonics and noise waveforms using a glottal inverse filter. This was followed by computation of the frequency spectra of the two components to observe their difference, if any, in breathiness quality. By averaging pitch-synchronously squared values of a noise signal over a number of pitch periods, the average instantaneous noise power level was also measured within a pitch period.

Materials and Methods

Two young females with no laryngeal disease produced the Japanese vowel /a/ for about two seconds in two different phonation styles: easy phonation and soft phonation. They habitually had hypofunctional voices with different degrees of breathiness. The voice signals were low-pass filtered at 4.5 kHz and digitized at a sampling rate of 40 kHz with an accuracy of 12 bits for the acoustic analyses described below.

An adaptive comb filter was first used to separate the noise from the harmonics, assuming additive glottal noise (Kasuya et al., 1986). The sampling rate of both signals was reduced to 10 kHz for further analyses. From an estimated noise signal, 11 PARCOR

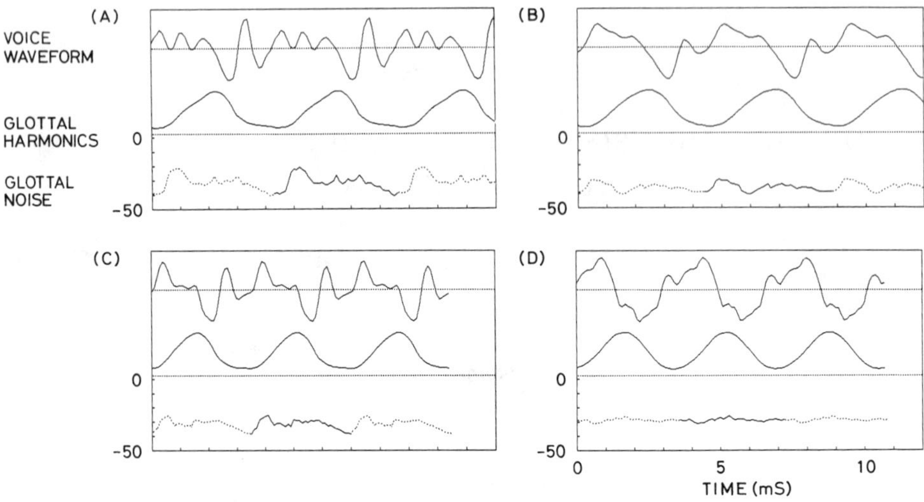

Fig. 1. Vowel waveforms, estimated glottal harmonics waveforms and average instantaneous power level of the differentiated glottal turbulence noise signal, for two types of phonations by two females. (A) and (C) are for easy phonations and (B) and (D) are for soft phonations. The zero level of the glottal harmonics waveform is arbitrary. The noise power level is normalized by the average power level of the differentiated glottal harmonics.

parameters were computed every 10 ms with a Hamming window of 20 ms over 20 frames, resulting in 20 sets of 11 PARCOR coefficients for each utterance. The first four formant frequencies and bandwidths were computed by solving an 11th-order polynomial with the filter coefficients converted from average values of 20 sets of the PARCOR parameters and used to constitute a vocal tract inverse filter. The reason for using the noise rather than the harmonics was that a mathematical model of the linear prediction analysis assumes either noise or single impulse excitation of the vocal tract (Markel and Gray, 1976). Each of the glottal harmonics and the noise signals was obtained as the output of the inverse filter.

To see the temporal characteristics of the average instantaneous power level of the glottal noise within a pitch period, the amplitude values of the glottal noise were squared and averaged pitch-synchronously over 100 pitch periods.

Results

Figure 1 illustrates four different sets of the waveforms: the original waveform of a breathy vowel and the estimated waveforms of the glottal harmonics and the glottal noise, obtained from the inverse filter. In the figure, the zero level of the glottal harmonics waveform is arbitrary since a phase distortion of a recording equipment was not calibrated at very low frequencies. The inverse filtered noise still included the radiation characteristic. The noise "waveform" in the figure is not a real waveform but shows the repetition of the average instantaneous power level (dB) of a single pitch period (indicated by a solid line) which was computed by averaging over 100 pitch periods squared values of the noise level at a same lag point from each of the pitch

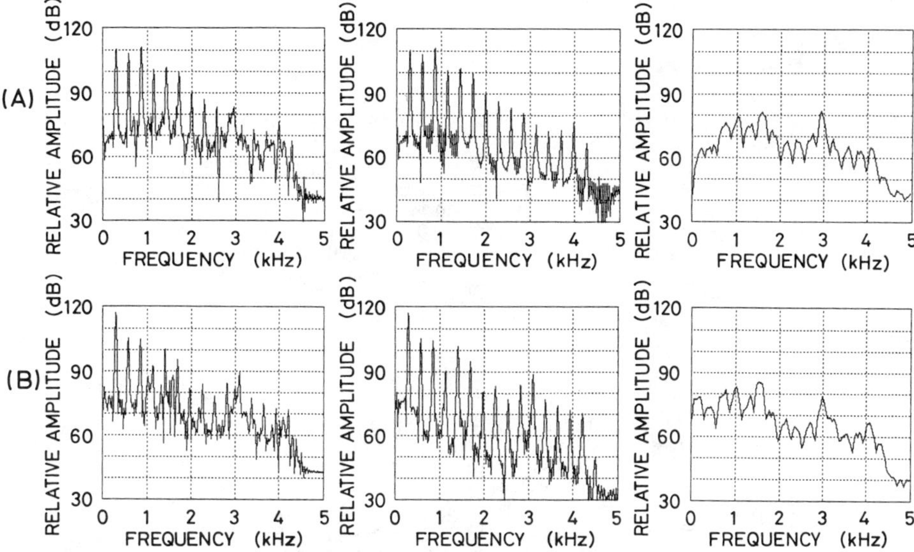

Fig. 2. Frequency spectra of the vowel /a/ phonated (A) easily and (B) softly by the same speaker. From the left are shown the spectra of the original vowel, the estimated harmonics and the estimated noise components. The noise spectra were obtained by averaging DFT spectra.

boundaries. The noise power level was normalized by an average value of a differentiated glottal harmonic signal within a period. In the figure, (A) and (C) are for the easy phonation of the two female speakers, and (B) and (D) for their soft phonations. The shape of the glottal harmonics waveform of a soft (hypofunctional) voice becomes similar to sinusoidal (Bickley, 1982; Fritzell et al., 1986; Hammarberg, 1986; Klatt, 1987). It is interesting to note that the noise energy revealed the maximum in the vicinity of the beginning of the opening phase and reached the smallest in the closing phase in most of the cases. In more hypofunctional (soft) phonation, however, one female speaker ((D) in Figure 1) had a rather flat energy distribution over a pitch period.

Figure 2 shows examples of the frequency spectra of a breathy vowel /a/ produced by a female speaker in the two phonatory conditions, (A) easy and (B) soft, where from the left are shown the spectra of the original vowel, the harmonics component and the vocal noise component. (A) and (B) in Figure 2 correspond to (C) and (D) in Figure 1, respectively. The noise spectrum is the average of 20 DFT spectra computed with a 25.6 ms Hamming window. The noise observed in each of the original breathy vowel spectra especially in a high frequency region (leftmost) was separated well from harmonic components (middle) by the comb filter. The average noise spectrum (rightmost) revealed the formant structure with relatively periodic energy dips resulting from application of the comb filter.

Figure 3 represents the frequency spectra of the glottal harmonics and the glottal noise components estimated from easy and soft phonations of the same speaker as the one in Figure 2. The spectra included the radiation characteristic. The glottal harmonics spectra

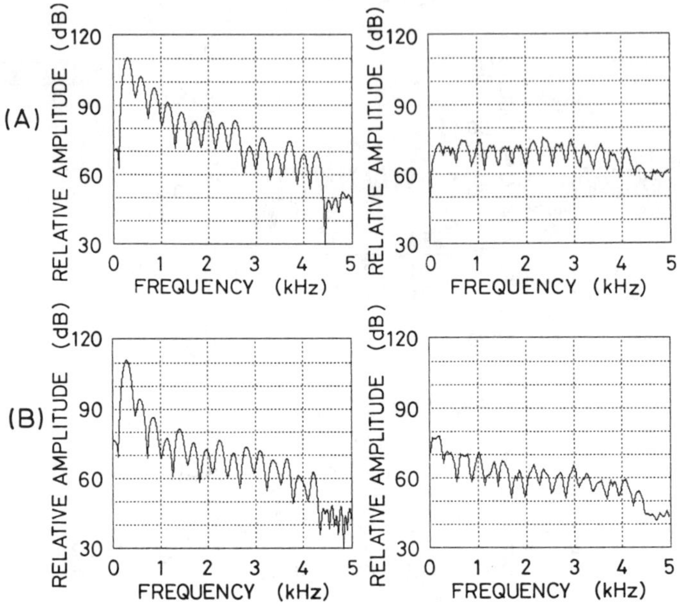

Fig. 3. Frequency spectra of the glottal harmonics (left) and the glottal noise (right) estimated with a glottal inverse filter. (A) for the easy phonation and (B) for the soft phonation. The speaker is the same as in Figure 2.

were obtained from differentiated glottal harmonics waveforms of three pitch periods, while the noise spectra were computed by averaging 20 DFT spectra obtained from each of the differentiated glottal noise signals of 25.6 ms duration with a frame shift of 25.6 ms. A Hamming window was used in both processings. The noise spectra again showed energy dips due to comb filtering. Differences in the two noise spectra were quite obvious.

SYNTHESIS MODEL

Figure 4 illustrates a synthesis model of sustained breathy vowels. An average (constant) pitch period sequence was perturbed using outputs of a random number generator whose magnitude and frequency characteristics were controllable. A sampling rate of 40 kHz was used in the entire synthesis system to enable accurate representation of jitter. Receiving a perturbed pitch period sequence, Klatt's model (Klatt, 1987) generated a differentiated glottal volume velocity waveform (differentiated glottal harmonics waveform). When synthesizing a hypofunctional voice the first harmonic (fundamental frequency component) level of the waveform was adjusted in the frequency domain on the basis of the Fourier series expansion, since Klatt's model lacked flexibility in simulating hypofunctional voice spectrum.

Meanwhile, a differentiated glottal turbulence noise signal was produced from a Gaussian random number generator through a spectral shaping circuit to adjust the

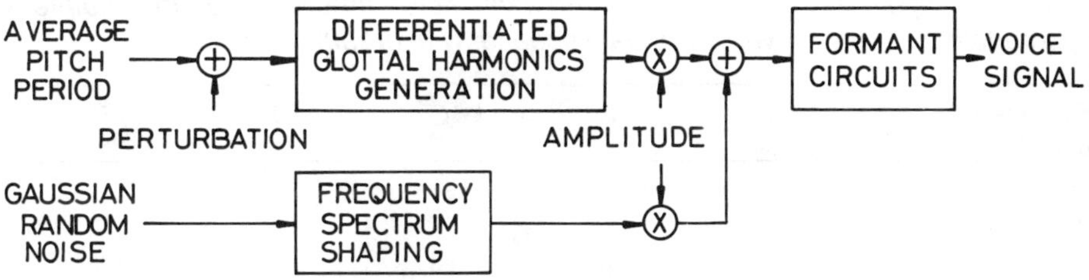

Fig. 4. A synthesis model used to simulate breathy vowels.

frequency characteristic of the noise. Both the glottal harmonics and noise components were modified in their amplitude to control the signal-to-noise ratio and then fed into a formant circuit.

PERCEPTION OF BREATHY VOICE

Method

To determine salience in breathy vowel perception, three acoustic parameters were investigated: the first harmonic (fundamental component) level, noise spectral shape and signal-to-noise ratio. The hypofunctional vowel with breathiness quality of the female speaker shown in Figures 1(D), 2(B), and 3(B) was simulated in terms of the three parameters. In this study, the pitch period sequence obtained from the original vowel was directly used in the synthesis to provide the same average and perturbation characteristics as the original. The first harmonic level was either 0 dB, the direct output of Klatt's model being in a good agreement with the original vowel spectrum in the high frequency region, or increased by 8 dB. The noise spectrum shape was adjusted by changing the bandwidth of a resonant frequency circuit at 0 Hz. The shape was either flat (corresponding to infinite bandwidth) or -10 dB at 3000 Hz. The signal-to-noise ratio was either 20 dB (identical to that of the original vowel), 23 dB or infinite (no noise).

Five vowel samples were synthesized with different combinations of the acoustic parameter values. These synthetic vowels were referred to as A, B,..., E, as shown in Table 1. Since vowel E has no noise, the noise spectrum is not specified in the table.

Two pairs of the original (O) and synthetic (S) vowels (O-S_i, O-S_j) were presented to eight subjects with normal hearing who were asked to judge which pair had more similarity. There were 20 possible combinations of two pairs. Each subject judged each of two original and synthetic vowel pairs four times.

Results

Figure 5 illustrates the similarity score of the five synthetic vowels to the original hypofunctional voice. The score was normalized so that a synthetic vowel attained a 100% score when it was always judged by all the subjects to be more similar to the original than any of the other vowels. Vowel A showed the highest similarity, whereas E had the lowest. E included no glottal noise at all. The similarity score of B with a flat

Table 1. *Synthesis conditions of three acoustic parameters used to simulate a hypofunctional (soft) vowel of a female speaker with breathiness quality.*

Synthesis conditions	A	B	C	D	E
1st harmonic level (dB)	+8	+8	+8	0	+8
Noise spectrum	-10	0	0	-10	
Noise level (SNR in dB)	20	23	20	20	∞

noise spectrum and with a slightly larger SNR value than the original was very close to that of vowel A. Vowel D, which had the same SNR value but a less enhanced first harmonic level than the original, was judged less similar to the original than A and B, both of which had the same first harmonic level as the original.

DISCUSSION

An accurate measurement of formant frequencies and bandwidths is often important in describing acoustic properties of a breathy voice. Since breathy vowels usually include some degree of glottal turbulence noise, an all-pole model can be applied to the noise better than to the harmonics. This approach worked well in our study. The formant structure was hardly seen in the harmonics spectra shown in Figure 2, especially for hypofunctional phonations, whereas the averaged noise spectra revealed clear formant structures.

The shape of turbulence noise spectrum depends largely upon the manner of phonation. It is apparent from Figure 3 that a largely hypofunctional voice includes a

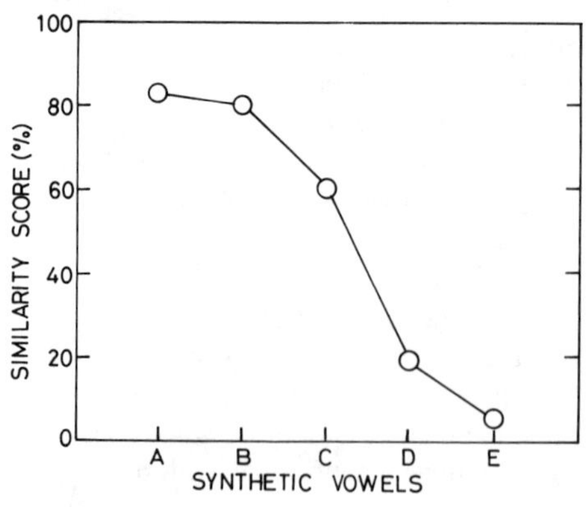

Fig. 5. Similarity scores of the five synthetic vowels with the original hypofunctional vowel in percent. Synthesis conditions of the vowels are given in Table 1.

comparatively large amount of turbulence noise in the low frequency region. Since the spectra shown in Figure 3 included the radiation characteristic, both of the glottal turbulence noise spectra in the hypofunctional voices tended to have less energy in the high frequency range.

We have evaluated the average power distribution of glottal turbulence noise over a cycle of vocal fold vibration in Figure 1 and observed that the turbulence noise was strong in the beginning of an opening phase and weak in a closing phase in most cases. These findings must be verified further by other measurements and theory.

Our perceptual experiments demonstrated that the spectral shape of glottal turbulence noise, the signal-to-noise ratio and the enhanced first harmonic level were important acoustic cues for perceived breathiness. It is interesting to note that a vowel with flat noise spectrum could have a similar degree of perceived breathiness as the original by increasing the SNR value. This implies that auditory masking affects the perception of the glottal noise.

SUMMARY

In addition to the enhanced first harmonic level, the spectral shape and the amount of glottal turbulence noise were important acoustic correlates of breathiness quality. Auditory masking effects may play an important role in the perception of breathy vowels.

The characteristic of the glottal turbulence noise distribution over the vocal fold vibratory period as measured in this research, needs further investigation for adequate interpretation.

ACKNOWLEDGEMENTS

This work was supported in part by a Grant-in-Aid (63860034) from the Ministry of Education, Science and Culture, Japan, and by Sound Technology Promotion Foundation.

REFERENCES

Bickley, C. (1982). Acoustic analysis and perception of breathy vowels. *MIT Working papers*, 1:71-81.

Fritzell, B., Hammarberg, B., Gauffin, J., Karlson, I., and Sundberg, J. (1986). Breathiness and insufficient vocal fold closure. *J. Phonetics*, 14:549-553.

Hammarberg, B. (1986). *Perceptual and Acoustic Analysis of Dysphonia.* Doctoral dissertation, Karolinska Institute, Dept. of Logopedics and Phoniatrics, Huddinge, Sweden.

Hasegawa, K., Sakamoto, T., and Kasuya, H. (1987). Effects of glottal noise on the quality of synthetic speech. In: *Proc. Spring Meeting of the Acoust. Soc. Japan.* 3-6-10: 205-206 (in Japanese).

Hirano, M. (1981). *Clinical Examination of Voice.* Springer-Verlag, Vienna.

Imaizumi, S. (1986). Acoustic measurement of pathological voice qualities for medical purposes. *Proc. ICASSP 86, Tokyo*, 3:677-680.

Kasuya, H., Ogawa, S., and Kikuchi, Y. (1986). An adaptive comb filtering method as applied to acoustic analyses of pathological voice. *Proc. ICASSP 86*, Tokyo. 1:669-672.

Klatt, D.H. (1987). Acoustic correlates of breathiness: First harmonic amplitude, turbulence noise, and tracheal coupling. *J. Acoust. Soc. Am.*, 82:S91.

Markel, J.D. and Gray A.H. (1976). *Linear Prediction of Speech.* Springer-Verlag, Berlin Heidelberg.

33

The Effect of Vocal Fold Surgery on the Speech Cepstrum

Yasuo Koike and Junji Kohda

Dept. of Otolaryngology, The University of Tokushima, School of Medicine, 3 Kuramoto, Tokushima, 770 Japan

The fundamental periodicity of the acoustic speech waveform is dependent upon the periodic vibration of the vocal folds. Since this vibration can be affected by various pathologic changes in the larynx, the regularity of the acoustic speech waveform can be sensitive to the existence of laryngeal pathology. Various acoustic indices showing the periodicity of the acoustic speech waveform have been applied to detect some laryngeal lesions such as glottic cancer. The cepstrum technique may be one of these acoustic indices suggesting the existence of laryngeal pathology.

Since cepstral peaks are affected by certain laryngeal diseases (Koike, 1986a), it was of interest to determine, then, if the effect of laryngeal pathology on the speech cepstrum can be eliminated by surgical treatment of the pathology. The purpose of the present study was to examine if such a change attributable to surgery takes place in the speech cepstrum, and to determine the characteristic changes in the cepstral display. Since the purpose of most surgeries for benign lesions in the larynx is to restore a normal voice, an assessment of the change in the cepstrum caused by a surgical operation may be a method for evaluating the success of the surgery.

Cepstrum analysis may be particularly useful for this type of evaluation, since it can be carried out objectively without the intervention of human judgement. The need for objective means for evaluating the effect of surgery does not require lengthy explanation. The effect on the speech cepstrum of surgery for laryngeal malignancy was not considered in the present article, since the objective of such operations is not restoration of a normal voice. For malignancy, assessment of vocal function may not be relevant to the success of the operation.

METHODS

The sexes, ages, and the pathologies of the subjects of the present study are listed in Table 1. The subjects were instructed to sustain the vowel /a/ at a comfortable pitch and loudness. A magnetic tape recording of the acoustic signal was made for each subject with an electret condenser microphone (Sony ECM-969) and a cassette-tape recorder (Sony TC-D5M). Recordings were made before and after the treatment for each patient.

Table 1. *The subjects' sex, type of vocal pathology, and age.*

Pathology type	Sex	Case No.	Age
Vocal nodule	f	1	19
	m	2	59
Vocal polyp	f	5,9	44,41
	m	3,4,6,7	50,38,42,73
		8,10,11,12	57,61,57,38
Polypoid	f	15,16	56,48
degeneration	m	13,14	63,62
Prolapsus			
ventriculi	f	17	53
Ventr. polyp	m	18	42
Papilloma	m	19	51
Granuloma	f	23	60
	m	20,21,22	39,60,58
Glottic cancer	m	24	78
Glottic Tbc	m	25	48
Unilateral	f	26	56
paralysis	m	27	56

Although surgery was performed on neither case #24 (glottic cancer) nor case #25 (glottic tuberculosis), the data from these patients were also included as a reference. A stable portion of the vowel /a/ of about 1 second in duration was adopted for analysis.

These materials were digitized with an analog to digital converter at a sampling rate of 10 KHz using a computer (PDP-11/73). An anti-aliasing filter was applied prior to the A/D conversion. The digitized data were stored on a floppy disk for each subject. The data were then analyzed with cepstrum analysis software (Signal Technology ILS). A 40 ms Hamming window was employed. The cepstrum is the power spectrum of the log spectrum of the speech wave, and is widely adopted for pitch detection. A detailed description of this analysis procedure is available elsewhere (Noll, 1964; Oppenheim, 1968). Five cepstra from five non-overlapping intervals were made for each utterance, and the one showing the most explicit periodicity was selected and employed for subsequent study.

Twenty-five of the 27 patients underwent laryngeal surgery. The method of surgery employed varied from patient to patient, depending upon the type of laryngeal pathology. Polyps or nodules were removed with conventional procedures under general anaesthesia. A "squeezing technique" (Koike, 1986b) was adopted for patients with polypoid degeneration. A median shift of the paralysed fold (modified Meurman's

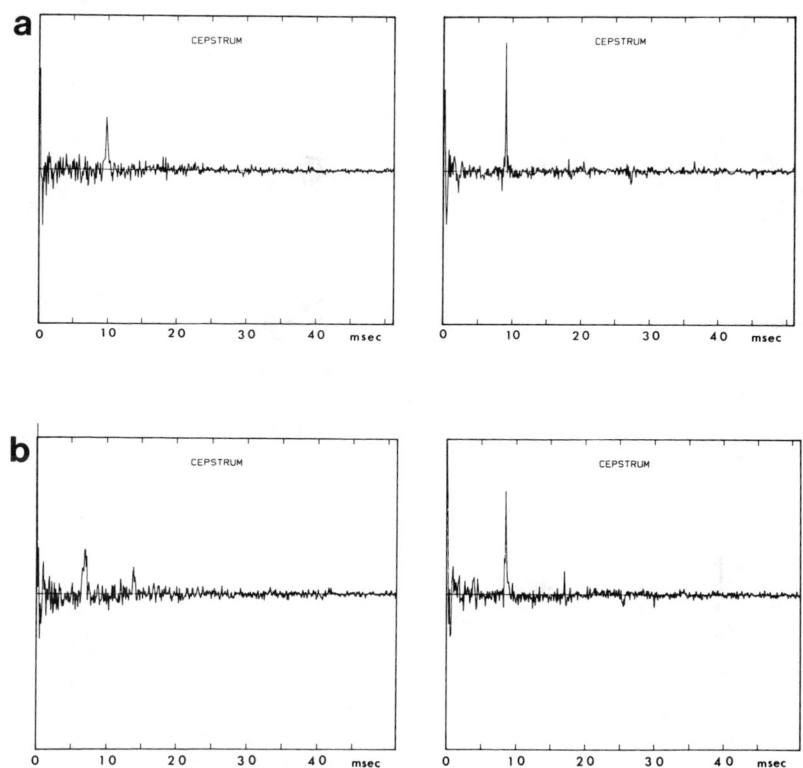

Fig. 1. (**a**) The cepstra of a patient with vocal polyp (case #10) before the surgery (*left*) and after surgery (*right*), with apparent lengthening of the cepstral peak after treatment. The abscissa is in "quefrency" in ms, and the ordinate is in arbitrary units. (**b**) The cepstra of a patient with unilateral recurrent nerve paralysis (case #27) before the surgery (*left*) and after surgery (*right*), with marked elongation of the dominant cepstral peak and an increase in the fundamental period after surgery.

Operation) was done for patients with unilateral recurrent nerve paralysis. Laser surgery was performed on the patient with papilloma. As was mentioned earlier, the patient with glottic cancer was given radio-therapy, and no surgery was performed. The patient with glottic tuberculosis was treated with antituberculous agents, and no surgery was attempted.

RESULTS

The most apparent effect of laryngeal surgery on the cepstra was a change in the size of the dominant cepstral peak. The position of the dominant peak, representing the fundamental period, was also often different after the surgery. The results were the same regardless of the type of surgery performed.

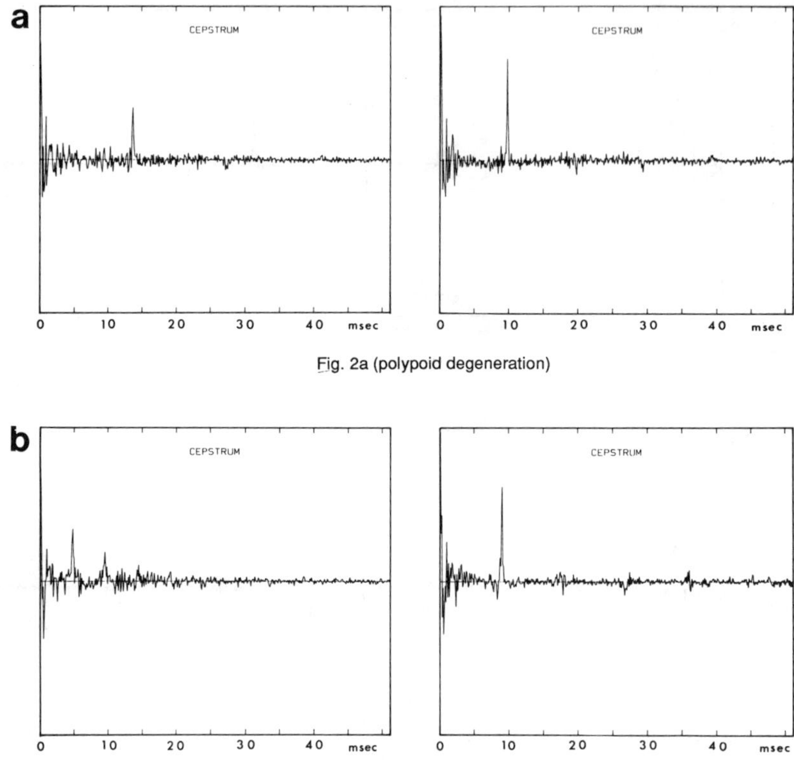

Fig. 2. (**a**) The cepstra of a patient with polypoid degeneration of both folds (case #13) before the surgery (*left*) and after surgery (*right*). The dominant cepstral peak is both lengthened and shifted to the left side on the quefrency scale after the operation. (**b**) The cepstra of a patient with glottic cancer (case #24) before radiation therapy (*left*) and after treatment (*right*). The dominant peak in the right tracing is shifted to the right side on the quefrency scale, indicating a downward shift of the fundamental frequency after the therapy.

Elongation of the Dominant Cepstral Peak

This effect is illustrated in Figure 1a, which is based on the data obtained from a patient with vocal polyp (case #10). The dominant peak observable in the cepstrum after the surgery (right tracing) was much taller than that for the speech wave recorded before the surgery (left tracing). The abscissa of this figure shows "quefrency" in ms, and the ordinate is cepstral energy plotted on an arbitrary scale.

This type of change in the cepstral peak corresponded well with the improvement in the perceived hoarseness of the patient's voice. In other words, there was invariably an explicit lengthening of the dominant cepstral peak, for the cases showing an apparent improvement in the perceived voice quality after the surgery. This type of cepstral change was not quite remarkable, however, for patients who had had a very low degree of hoarseness to begin with. The cepstral peaks for these patients had been generally quite tall even before the surgical intervention, and there was little room for improvement.

A similar elongation of the dominant cepstral peak was observed after surgery in the rest of the patients with vocal polyp or vocal nodule, though the degree of lengthening varied from patient to patient. The subjects with other benign lesions, such as papilloma or granuloma, also revealed an elevation of the dominant cepstral peak after the surgical treatments, including laser surgery. Here again, the extent of the cepstral change varied greatly from patient to patient, depending mainly upon how much the vibratory behaviour had been affected by these lesions before the surgical operation.

The median shift operation of the paralysed fold for patients with unilateral paralysis also yielded an elongation of the dominant cepstral peak, as seen in Figure 1b, even though the principle of this operation was entirely different from that of conventional endolaryngeal surgery. Case #25 with glottic tuberculosis revealed an elongation of the dominant cepstral peak as well, after the administration of antituberculous agents. With this case also, the change in the cepstral peak corresponded well with an improvement in the voice quality.

Decrease in the Fundamental Period

In addition to the lengthening of the dominant cepstral peak, an apparent shift of the fundamental frequency was generally observed in patients with polypoid degeneration of the vocal fold. Figure 2a shows this effect on the cepstral display. The dominant cepstral peak in the right tracing, which denotes the periodicity of the acoustic waveform after the surgery, is not only taller than that in the left tracing, but also considerably shifted to the left side, indicating a decrease in the fundamental period, i.e., an increase in the fundamental frequency. For this subject, the fundamental frequency was 74 Hz before surgery and 104 Hz after.

Increase in the Fundamental Period

Figure 2b shows the corresponding results for case #24 (glottic carcinoma) which involved radiation therapy instead of surgery. Here also we see a remarkable improvement in the regularity of laryngeal vibration. The dominant cepstral peak after the treatment (right tracing) is apparently taller than that before the therapy (left tracing). The tumour which had existed on the vocal fold completely disappeared after the irradiation, though some edema of the fold remained. The perceived voice quality of this patient was improved, and the cepstral change seemed to represent the restoration of regular vibratory motion of the fold fairly well.

In this particular case, in addition, an increase in the fundamental period, i.e., a lowering of the fundamental frequency from 216 Hz to 111 Hz, was also noted following the treatment. This type of downward shift of the fundamental frequency was also observed in patients with unilateral paralysis following the surgical repositioning (median shift) of the paralysed vocal fold, as seen in Figure 1b. Here also, this finding was in good agreement with the lowering of the perceived vocal pitch.

DISCUSSION

The data presented above show an appreciable difference in the dominant cepstral peak, attributable to laryngeal surgery. In most cases with benign lesions on or surrounding the vocal fold, an apparent lengthening of the dominant cepstral peak occurred following the surgery. This indicates that the periodicity of the acoustic speech waveform was improved after the surgical operation, implying that the regularity of the vocal fold vibration was restored. Since this type of change in the cepstral display was particularly clear when the pre-operative vibratory behaviour in the larynx had been remarkably distorted, the cepstrum analysis seems especially suited for the evaluation of the effect of surgery in moderate or severe cases with benign lesions.

The correspondence between the elongation of the dominant cepstral peak and an improvement in the perceived voice quality also seems noteworthy. Although the regularity of the speech signal can be revealed by the height of the dominant cepstral peak, the scale on the ordinate of the cepstral display is not linear. This makes quantitative analysis of the length of the peaks rather complicated. Quantitative measurement of the height of the cepstral peaks has not been attempted in the present study for this reason. The investigation of the relationship between the elevation of the dominant cepstral peak and the degree of perceived hoarseness, nevertheless, seems to be a worthwhile topic to pursue, since the cepstrum analysis can at least be performed objectively without human judgement.

The apparent upward shift of the fundamental frequency, found in the cases with polypoid degeneration, also seems to be an interesting finding. Although clinically it has been known that these patients in general have a lowered fundamental frequency, the post-operative recovery has not yet been sufficiently studied, mainly because of the difficulty in determining the fundamental frequency. Because the cepstrum analysis was originally designed to measure the fundamental frequency when it exists, it is an easy task to observe this shift on the cepstral display. This feature of the cepstrum seems to be convenient for measuring a downward shift of the fundamental frequency, as demonstrated in Figs 1b and 2b.

REFERENCES

Koike, Y. (1986a). Cepstrum analysis of pathological voices. *J. Phonetics*, 14:501-507.

Koike, Y. (1986b). Laryngomicrosurgery. In: *Illustrated Handbook of Otolaryngological and Head and Neck Surgery*, edited by Y. Honda et al., *Vol. 2*, pp. 88-93. Medical View, Tokyo.

Noll, A.M. (1964). Short-time spectrum and "cepstrum" techniques for vocal-pitch detection. *J. Acoust. Soc. Am.*, 36:296-302.

Oppenheim, A.V. (1968). Speech analysis-synthesis system based on homomorphic filtering. *J. Acoust. Soc. Am.*, 45:458-465.

34

Acoustic and Perceptual Characterization of Vocal Nodules

Paul H. Milenkovic, *Diane M. Bless, and *Linda A. Rammage

*Dept. of Electrical and Computer Engineering, University of Wisconsin-Madison, 1415 Johnson Drive, Madison, Wisconsin 53706, USA. *Dept. of Communicative Disorders, University of Wisconsin-Madison, Madison, Wisconsin 53706, USA.*

Perceptual evaluation is an important component of the clinical assessment of voice disorders. It is of scientific interest to determine quantifiable acoustic properties of the voice that underlie the perceptual judgements made by the clinician, and in turn to relate these acoustic properties to the underlying physiological mechanisms.

Vocal fold nodules are of particular interest in considering the problem of finding acoustic correlates of voice disorders. Their presence is a commonly occurring condition causing specific structural changes in the vocal folds. Nodules are a bilateral thickening of the vocal folds at the place of vibratory contact, occurring predominantly in adult females. Vocal nodules may interfere with the closure of the vocal folds during vibration (Peppard et al., 1988), increasing the degree of closed glottis leakage normally occurring in females (Bless et al., 1986). Nodules may introduce stiffness into the vocal folds, shortening the closed duration during the glottal vibratory cycle.

It has been noted anecdotally that the trained clinician can detect the occurrence of nodules with a high degree of accuracy by listening to speech. This implies that vocal fold nodules may have distinct acoustic characteristics. Our first objective was to conduct a listening trial to evaluate this claim under controlled conditions. Our second objective was to determine whether acoustic characteristics of vocal fold nodules may be determined by computer analysis of the acoustic speech waveform.

METHODS

Subject selection

We employed 38 female subjects with vocal fold nodules ranging in age from 18 to 40 years and 10 age matched female control subjects for our study. The subjects with nodules were recruited from a clinical patient population. The normal subjects were recruited by an advertisement in a local newspaper. In this manner we obtained naive subjects representative of the normal voice quality in the population at large.

Stroboscopic evaluation

A stroboscopic examination was conducted of each subject to confirm a diagnosis of nodules or to establish a subject as having normal vocal folds. The video tapes of the examination were evaluated subjectively, and a numerical score between 0 and 5 was assigned to the size of the posterior glottal chink during vocal fold closure for all subjects, and a score between 0 and 5 was assigned to the nodule size in the subjects with nodules.

Perceptual evaluation

An audio recording was made from each subject in a sound treated booth. The sound was transduced with a microphone placed six inches from the subject's lips and placed off axis to avoid air blast noise. The microphone output was recorded on a reel-to-reel tape recorder. The subject was asked to repeat the phrase *The blue spot is on the key* three times.

A perceptual test was conducted to determine if listening to this sentence could result in a reliable determination of the presence of vocal nodules. Four presentations of each subject making three repetitions of the test sentence *The blue spot is on the key* were dubbed onto a cassette to give the listener adequate opportunity to make a judgement. Two listeners with extensive clinical voice experience were presented the tape through headphones. The listeners gave their responses on a rating sheet where 0 denoted normal and 5 denoted the most severe acoustic effect of nodules.

Acoustic analysis

Digital recordings were made from the reel-to-reel analog tape of the middle repetition of the test sentence produced by each subject. The signal was anti-alias filtered by a 4-pole Butterworth filter with a 4 kHz corner frequency, and the signal was sampled with 12 bits resolution at a sampling rate of 8.33 kHz (sample interval of 120 μs) with an IBM PC computer and a Scientific Solutions Lab Master analog-to-digital converter card using the CSpeech software package.

We analysed the digital recordings with the following set of acoustic measures: LPC prediction gain, fundamental frequency (F0), jitter, shimmer, periodicity signal-to-noise ratio, signal-to-F0 ratio, and 2-4 kHz band pass periodicity signal-to-noise ratio. These measures were implemented in a computer program which operates automatically once furnished with indices of the starting and ending waveform position to analyse and with a starting value of the fundamental frequency.

Our acoustic measures were restricted to the word *spot* in the test sentence *The blue spot is on the key*. The analysis was applied to a 100 ms interval centred within the vowel portion of *spot*. This segment was selected because 1) it included the /a/ vowel and 2) we could obtain 100 ms of uninterrupted vowel from all of our subjects. We selected the /a/ vowel for our analysis because the elevated formant frequencies of this vowel reduce the interaction between the formants and the fundamental frequency.

The LPC prediction gain, the ratio of signal energy to energy in the LPC residual, is related to a formula for spectral flatness (Markel and Gray, 1976). A flat spectrum results in a low gain value. Davis (1976) employed the LPC derived spectral flatness measure for assessment of voice quality. Observations by Klatt (1987) suggest that glottal insufficiency broadens the formant peaks and thus flattens the speech spectrum.

We obtained the prediction gain by applying LPC analysis to the middle 20 ms of the vowel being analysed. The covariance method LPC analysis was applied to the speech waveform after applying a 6 dB/octave preemphasis (Markel and Gray, 1976).

Vocal jitter is the cycle-to-cycle fluctuation in pitch while shimmer is the cycle-to-cycle fluctuation in speech waveform amplitude. Elevated jitter and shimmer may result from unstable patterns of vocal fold oscillations induced by abnormalities in vocal fold structure. We derived values for fundamental frequency (F0), jitter, and shimmer using the algorithm described by Milenkovic (1987). The jitter measure was modified for use in sentence context speech where large swings in pitch may bias the jitter measure upward. Jitter was corrected by subtracting a bias term consisting of the difference between the maximum and minimum pitch periods divided by the number of pitch periods.

The voice periodicity signal-to-noise ratio (SNR) is the ratio of energy in the speech signal to the energy in the aperiodic component of the speech signal. Several different types of methods for measuring SNR and the related quantity HNR (harmonics-to-noise ratio) have been proposed (Yumoto, et al., 1982; Milenkovic, 1987; Muta, et al., 1988). The method developed for this study uses a pitch predictor (Atal, 1982) to extract the aperiodic component of the speech waveform. According to the periodicity model (Milenkovic, 1987), the speech waveform $s(t)$ can be expressed as

$$s(t) = p(t) + e(t) \tag{1}$$

where $e(t)$ is the aperiodic component and the periodic component $p(t)$ is

$$p(t) = Kp(t - t_p) \tag{2}$$

where t_p is the pitch period and K is the amplitude change between periods. If we compute

$$e_p(t) = s(t) - Ks(t - t_p) \tag{3}$$

and if we assume $p(t)$, $e(t)$, and $e(t\text{-}t_p)$ are uncorrelated we obtain

$$E(e_p^2(t)) = (1 + K^2)E(e^2(t)). \tag{4}$$

We derive accurate values of t_p that are updated every 4 waveform samples using the algorithm that computes jitter (Milenkovic, 1987). Computing sample values of $s(t\text{-}t_p)$ for pitch period values that are not an integer number of sample intervals T requires interpolating $s(t)$ between sample position $s(nT)$. We constructed our interpolator by computing sample values of a low-pass filter according to a method described by Crochiere and Rabiner (1983). We used a low-pass filter with the impulse response

$$h(t) = (0.54 + 0.46 \cos \frac{2\pi t}{t_f}) \; \frac{1}{\pi t} \sin \frac{\pi t}{t_b} \tag{5}$$

for $-t_f/2 < t < t_f/2$. This filter was determined by applying a Hamming window to an ideal low-pass filter (Oppenheim and Schafer, 1975). We used the interpolator to compute both the values of $s(t)$ as well as $s(t\text{-}t_p)$; in this manner the band-limiting artifact of the interpolator was applied equally to the two signals. For use with the 8.33 kHz sampling rate we chose $t_b = 0.16$ ms and $t_f = 0.96$ ms as a compromise between filter corner frequency, filter complexity, and frequency aliasing artifact.

The value of K was updated every four sample positions by minimizing the sum of $e_p(t)$ squared over overlapping eight sample intervals. Since K has values close to 1 for normal levels of voice shimmer, we divided our calculated value of $e_p(t)$ by the square root of 2 to obtain a signal with an RMS value close to the RMS value of $e(t)$ for use in our SNR calculation.

Table 1. *The scores of the two listeners*

	Listener 1		Listener 2	
	Normal subject	Nodule subject	Normal subject	Nodule subject
Judged normal	5	8	10	14
Judged nodule	5	30	0	24
Total	10	38	10	38

Table 2. *Mean values and standard deviations for the acoustic analysis*

	Normal subjects		Nodule subjects	
	M	S.D.	M	S.D.
LPC gain	7.94	5.37	8.25	5.51
F0 (Hz)	190	26	196	25
Jitter (ms)	0.019	0.014	0.026	0.023
Shimmer (SNR dB)	19.0	3.6	19.0	3.6
SF0 (dB)	9.8	4.4	7.5	3.7
2-4 kHz SNR (dB)	6.4	4.3	4.6	5.5

Klatt (1987) described glottal insufficiency as having the effect of reducing the periodic signal component at high frequencies while increasing the aperiodic noise at high frequencies resulting from aerodynamic turbulence. We made a second measure of SNR - bandpass SNR - restricted to the 2 to 4 kHz frequency band to measure this effect. The average bandpass energy for both $s(t)$ and the normalized $e_p(t)$ was determined by applying a Hamming window, computing the FFT, and by computing the sum of squares of the real and imaginary components of the FFT over a restricted frequency range. Energy values were averaged by moving the window in 10 ms increments over the 100 ms vowel interval prior to computing the bandpass SNR.

The female voice is described as having an elevated spectrum amplitude at the frequency value of F0 (Bickley, 1982; Klatt, 1987; Nittrouer et al., 1988) that is attributed to the increased closed glottis leakage and reduced closed glottis duration of females relative to males. It was of interest to describe the effect of nodules on this measure. We measured the ratio of total signal energy over the 100 ms interval to the energy in the fundamental, and we referred to this ratio as SF0. The measurement was made by computing cosine and sine waveforms that were modulated in frequency to track the changes in F0 that occur over the 100 ms analysis interval. The value of F0 is updated

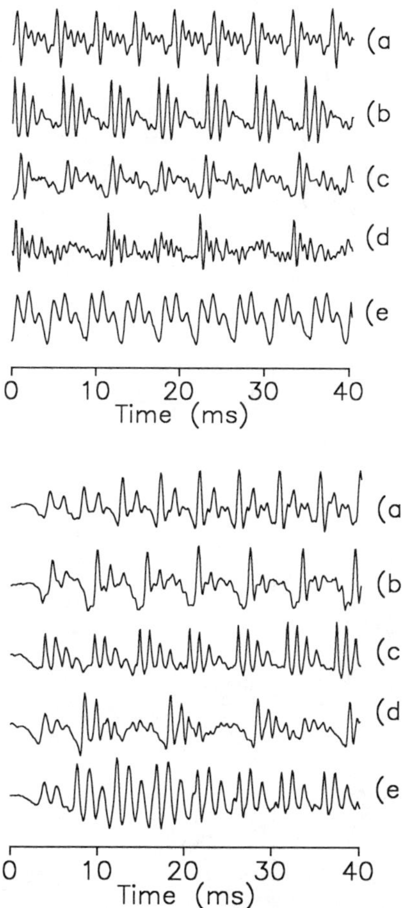

Fig. 1. Acoustic waveforms for sustained vowel portion of *spot*: (**a**) normal, (**b**) nodule, no outward acoustic symptoms, (**c**) nodule, double pulsing, (**d**) nodule, vocal fry, (**e**) nodule, elevated shimmer and slight degree of double pulsing.

Fig. 2. Acoustic waveforms for vowel onset portion of *spot*: (**a**) normal, soft attack, b) normal, hard attack, (**c**) nodule, no outward acoustic symptoms, (**d**) nodule, vocal fry, (**e**) nodule, irregular onset of voicing.

every four samples based on the pitch period value computed by the jitter algorithm. The speech signal was correlated with the cosine (in phase) and sine (quadrature phase) waveforms, and the energy at the fundamental was computed as the normalized sum of squares of the two correlations.

RESULTS

Table 1 shows the scores of the two listeners in correctly discriminating the subjects with nodules from the normal subjects. Listener 1 had an apparent lower threshold for making the judgement of nodules as evidenced by the fact that in only two instances had Listener 1 judged normal when Listener 2 had judged nodules.

The computer analysis of acoustic measures was applied to 30 of the subjects with nodules and all ten normal subjects; eight subjects with nodules were excluded from the analysis because they exhibited either vocal fry or marked double pulsing in the analysis

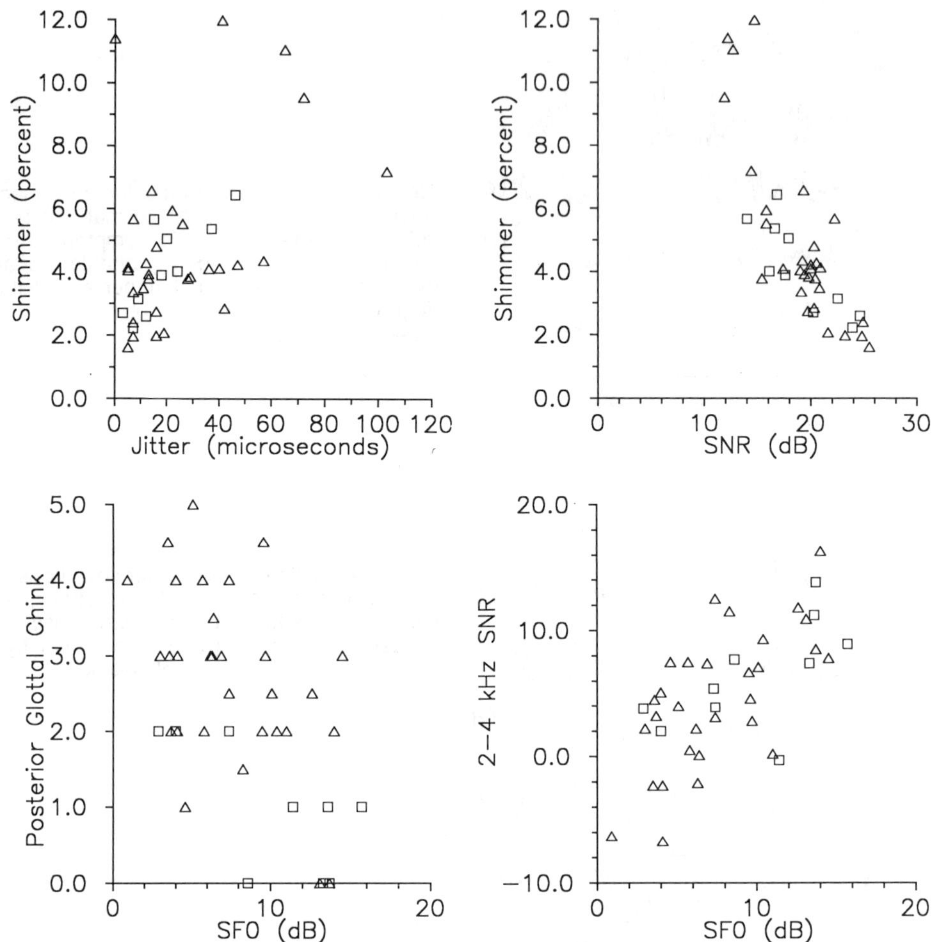

Fig. 3. Bivariate scatter diagrams for acoustic features of 10 normal subjects and 30 subjects with vocal nodules. Normal subjects are marked with the square while subjects with nodules are marked with the triangle. SF0 is the ratio of total signal energy to the energy in the fundamental. SNR is the ratio of energy in the speech signal to the energy in the aperiodic component of the speech signal.

interval as shown in Figure 1. These eight subjects exhibit shimmer values in excess of 20%, and they were removed as statistical outliers. The mean values and standard deviations of the results of the analysis are shown in Table 2. These data indicate that the means for normal and nodule voice lie within one standard deviation of each other for each measure. The acoustic measures for normals are consistent with those reported for other studies (Nittrouer et al., 1988; Peppard et al., 1988). One study (Milenkovic et al., 1986) described nodules as resulting in jitter levels 2 standard deviations above normal. This study did not screen for vocal fry or double pulsing.

Figure 3 presents a set of bivariate scatter plots. These plots give additional information regarding the distribution of values of the acoustic parameters for the two groups. The jitter-shimmer plot has 5 outliers which are exclusively nodule cases. The acoustic waveform for one of these outliers exhibiting elevated levels of shimmer is shown in Figure 1. Double pulsing is present in the waveform trace, but it is at a low level.

Five nodules cases were below a level of 0 dB for the 2-4 kHz SNR measure while one normal was right at 0 dB. Presumably, 0 dB is the minimum value for this measure because if the signal includes the aperiodicity noise, the noise power can be no greater than the signal power. Values below 0 dB are most likely an artifact of the analysis method. On the other hand, this artifact seemed to be selective for nodules cases.

Because double pulsing and vocal fry were selective for nodules, a visual inspection was conducted of the initial portions of the words *spot*, *on*, and *key* in the test sentence. This inspection uncovered ten nodule cases where the vowel onset was noted as being irregular. In Figure 2, examples are given of normal, irregular, and vocal fry onsets of the vowel in *spot*. A total of 24 nodule cases were selected according to the criteria of either 1) glottal fry or double pulsing, 2) excessive shimmer, 3) 2-4 kHz SNR below 0 dB, or 4) irregular oscillation pattern in the vowel onset. Some cases satisfied more than one of these criteria. The 24 cases include 4 instances which were missed by Listener 1 and 9 cases which were missed by Listener 2. No normals met these criteria.

The scatter plot for stroboscopic closed glottis gap size and SF0 (signal-to-F0) is part of Figure 3. Normals had gap sizes at or below a rating of 2. The correlation between gap size and SF0 was weak. The nodule cases with large gaps (in excess of 2) covered a wide range of SF0 values.

It appeared that subjects with nodules, even of large size, could produce vowel segments with normal acoustic measures. The primary acoustic trace, that we could identify, of nodules appears to be the intermittent occurrence of double pulsing ranging from levels detectable with the shimmer algorithm to vocal fry. Vowel onsets may have also been affected. The use of larger speech samples as well as the analysis of vowel onsets needs to be considered in order to more reliably detect nodules by acoustic methods.

ACKNOWLEDGMENTS

This work was funded in part by University of Wisconsin-Madison Graduate School Project No. 890377 and by NINCDS grant NS 24859.

REFERENCES

Atal, B. S. (1982). Predictive coding of speech at low bit rates. *IEEE Trans. Comm.*, 30:600-614.

Bickley, C. (1982). Acoustic analysis and perception of breathy vowels. *Speech Communication Group Working Papers* I:71-82. (Research Lab. of Electronics, MIT, Cambridge, MA.)

Bless, D.M., Biever D., and Shaikh, A. (1986). Comparisons of vibratory characteristics of young adult males and females. In: *Proc. of the Int. Conf. on Voice*, edited by M. Hirano and R.S. Hibi. Vol. II, pp. 46-54, Kurume, Japan.

Crochiere, R.E. and Rabiner, L.R. (1983). *Multirate Digital Signal Processing*. Prentice-Hall, Englewood Cliffs, NJ.

Davis, S.B. (1976). Computer evaluation of laryngeal pathology based on inverse filtering of speech. *SCRL Monograph* No. 13. (Speech Communications Research Laboratory, Inc., Los Angeles.)

Klatt, D.H. (1987). Acoustic correlates of breathiness: First harmonic amplitude, turbulence noise, and tracheal coupling. *J. Acoust. Soc. Am.*, 82(S1):91.

Markel, J.D. and Gray Jr., A.H. (1976). *Linear Prediction of Speech.* Springer-Verlag, Berlin.

Milenkovic, P., Bless, D M., and Ford, C.N. (1986). Profiles of voice disorders derived from a speech waveform periodicity model. In: *Proc. of the Int. Conf. on Voice*, edited by M. Hirano and R.S. Hibi. Vol.II, pp. 36-45, Kurume, Japan

Milenkovic, P. (1987). Least mean square measures of voice perturbation. *J. Speech Hear. Res.*, 30:529-538.

Muta, H., Baer, T., Wagatsuma, K., Murakoa, T., and Fukuda, H. (1988). A pitch-synchronous analysis of hoarseness in human speech. *J. Acoust. Soc. Am.*, 84:1292-1301.

Nittrouer, S., McGowan, R.S., and Beehler, D. (1988). Noise measurements of men's and women's voices. *J. Acoust. Soc. Am.*, 84(S1):83.

Oppenheim, A.V. and Schafer, R.W. (1975). *Digital Signal Processing.* Prentice-Hall, Englewood Cliffs, NJ.

Peppard, R.C., Bless, D.M., and Milenkovic, P. (1988). Comparison of young adult singers and nonsingers with vocal nodules. *J. Voice*, 2:250-260.

Yumoto, E., Gould, W.J., and Baer, T. (1982). Harmonics-to-noise ratio as an index of the degree of hoarseness. *J. Acoust. Soc. Am.*, 71:1544-1550.

35

Videostroboscopic Evaluation of Glottal Open Quotient, Related to Some Acoustic Parameters

Sören Fex, Anders Löfqvist, and Lucyna Schalén

Dept. of Logopedics and Phoniatrics, University Hospital, S-221 85 Lund, Sweden

The Open Quotient (OQ), the ratio open time to total time of the vibratory cycle of the vocal folds, has been extensively studied through the last decades. It has been reported that the OQ may vary with intensity and fundamental frequency of the voice (Sonesson, 1960). So far, analyses of the OQ included vibrations with as well as without complete glottal closure which should influence the interpretation of the results. The combination of microscope, stroboscope, and videotechnique offers a possibility for reliable recordings of the glottal behaviour during phonation, and also enables accurate measurements of maximal glottal width (Fex et al., forthcoming; Wendler and Köppen, 1988).

Our purpose was to evaluate the OQ in relation to acoustic voice characteristics and maximal glottal width.

METHODS

Initially 18 healthy volunteers were examined, eight males and ten females. Four females and one male had to be excluded as none of them closed the glottis completely during phonation. Recordings from seven males (mean age 34.2 years, range 21 to 61) and six females (mean age 29.5 years, range 22 to 39) were accepted for further analyses. Although none had professional vocal training, the majority were amateur singers. All were well motivated.

Indirect microlaryngoscopy was performed without anaesthetics during different types of phonation. First, subjects were instructed to phonate at a comfortable pitch and loudness. The phonations were made at different pitches, each at two loudness levels, "high" and "low". The experiments were terminated at the first sign of vocal fatigue.

The laryngeal mirror image was seen through an operation microscope (Zeiss OPMI 9) through which the stroboscopic light (Brüel & Kjær stroboscope 4914) was fed. To facilitate calculations, the stroboscope was changed so that one vocal fold vibration was seen per second instead of the original 1.4 vibrations per second. The magnified laryngeal mirror image was recorded on videotape (Sony U-matic video cassette recorder VO 5800 PS). A colour video camera (JVC GX-N7E) with a multi-system colour RGB monitor (JVC TM-150 PSN) was connected to the microscope.

The sound pressure of the voice was determined using an integrating sound level meter (Brüel & Kjær, type 2225) located 50 cm from the lips of the subjects. Background

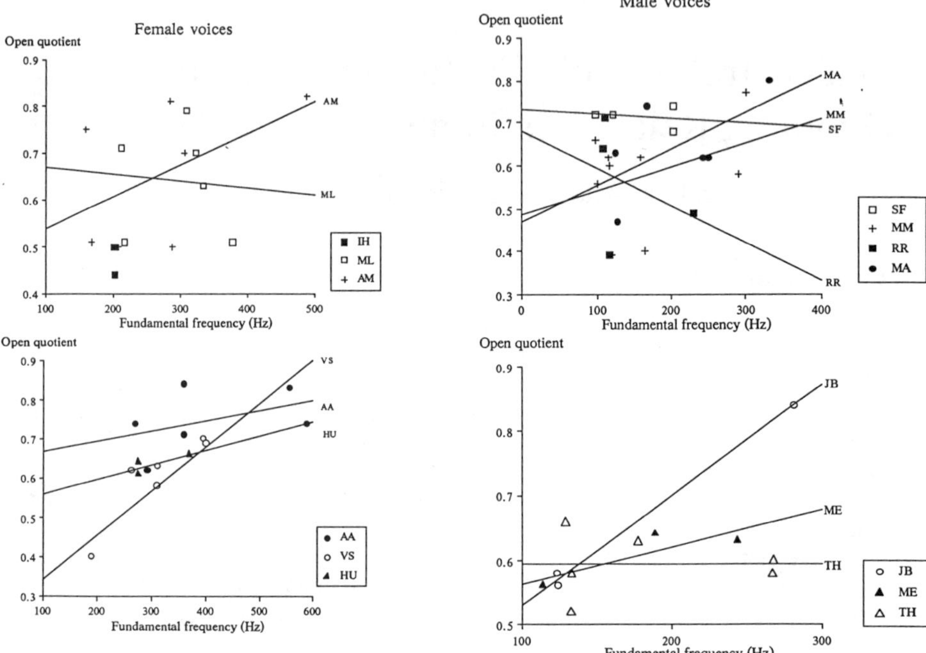

Fig. 1. Change of OQ in relation to F0. Individual regression lines indicated with initials. F0 values taken from acoustic analyses.

noise level was 35 dBA. The fundamental frequency of the voice was displayed on the stroboscope. The phonations were recorded on a reel-to-reel 2 track tape recorder (Revox A77). A dynamic Omni-directional microphone (Electrovoice) was attached to the microscope.

ANALYSES

All video-recordings were reviewed and only those phonations with total glottal closure observed during vocal fold vibration were accepted for further analysis. Thus, falsetto phonations were not included. A total of 153 phonations were measured, a mean of 11.8 per subject (4-28), with 65 on females, and 88 on males. The following measurements were made:

1. Open quotient (OQ). 25 double frames/s are shown in the PAL videosystem. The number of double frames per vibration during which the glottis was open were counted. Open quotient was thus the number of frames/50.
2. Maximal glottal width (G_m) (Titze, 1989) was measured directly from the monitor screen. The magnification factor was 11.8 and the maximal error about 2%.

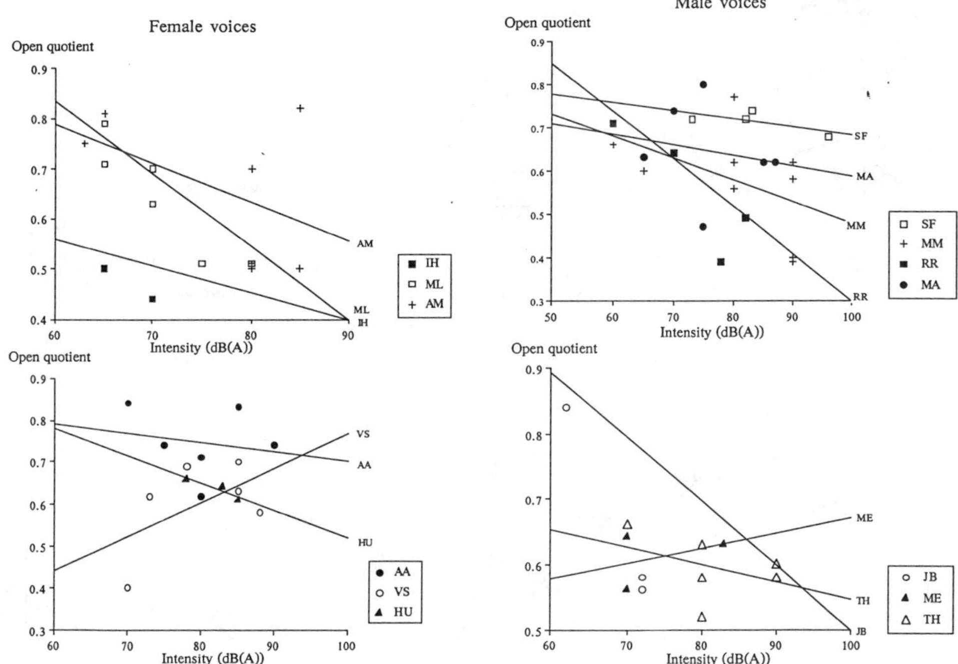

Fig. 2. Change of OQ in relation to intensity. Individual regression lines indicated with initials.

Acoustic analyses of selected phonations were performed from the sound tape using a computer program (Muta et al., 1988). From this program, the noise-to-signal ratio (in dB), N/S, was taken. The more negative this measure is, the less noise components there are in the voice. The fundamental frequencies of the phonations chosen for analyses were obtained. The time chosen for each acoustic analysis was 1 s. In total 30 measurements from females and 35 from males were obtained.

RESULTS

Relationships with the open quotient

Recordings from one female subject, (IH), were obtained only at frequencies 197 Hz and 204 Hz. Thus, it was not possible to analyse her OQ in relation to F0 variations. Among the remaining 12 subjects, in eight (four males and four females) there was a tendency for the OQ to increase with increasing F0 (Figure 1), irrespective of the intensity. The OQ varied between 0.32 and 0.90. In 11 subjects (five females, six males), there was a tendency for the OQ to decrease with increasing voice intensity. In one female and one male, the relationship between the OQ and the intensity was the opposite (Figure 2).

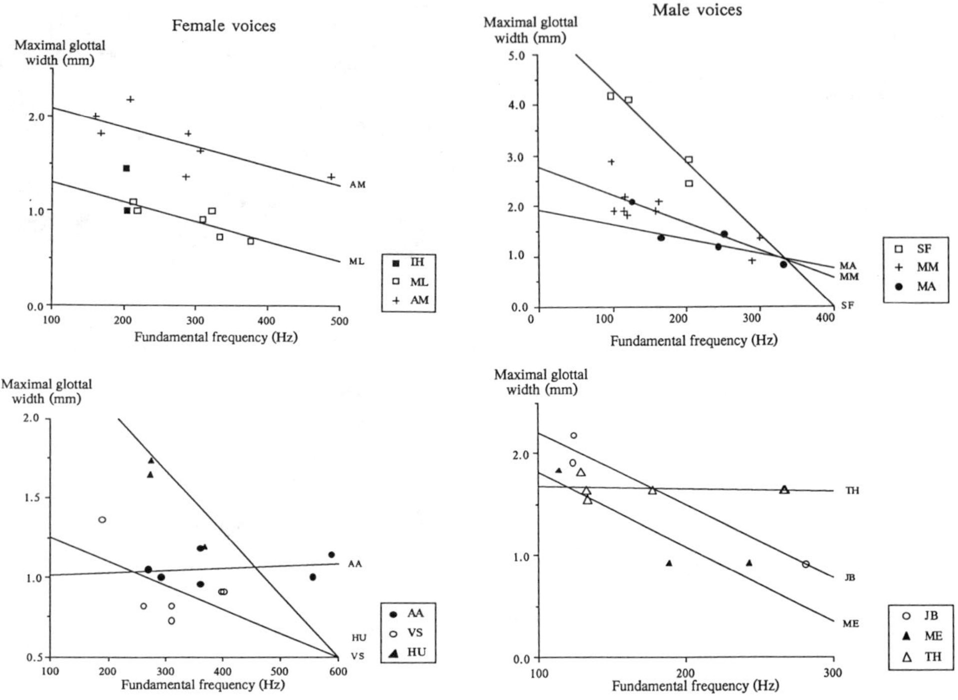

Fig. 3. Change of G_m in relation to F0. Individual regression lines indicated with initials.

No distinct relationship was found between OQ and G_m. In one male (RR), G_m measurements were not possible.

Relationships with maximal glottal width

No consistent relationship was found between G_m and intensity. In ten subjects (four females, six males), there was a tendency for G_m to decrease with increasing F0 (Figure 3). One male (RR) and one female (IH) were excluded for previously mentioned reasons.

Relationships with the N/S ratio

No consistent relationship was found between the OQ and the N/S ratio. In nine subjects (four females, five males), the N/S ratio tended to decrease with increasing intensity of the voice (Figure 4).

DISCUSSION

The results indicate that the OQ tended to increase with increasing F0 and to decrease with rising intensity of the voice. However, the OQ was not related in any obvious way to either N/S or G_m. Maximal glottal width tended to decrease with increasing F0 and the N/S ratio decreased with rising intensity.

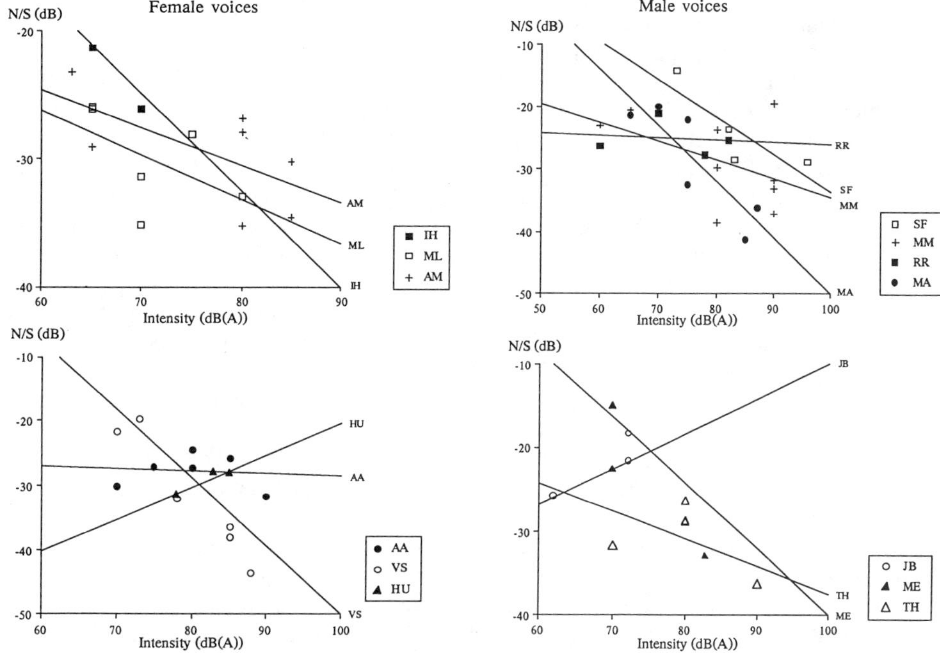

Fig. 4. Change of N/S in relation to intensity. Individual regression lines indicated with initials.

Considerable variation was found between and within the individuals suggesting that individuals used different strategies in vocal behaviour. Therefore, no statistical analyses were conducted.

To evaluate the OQ we used a video-stroboscopic technique. This optic method, like high-speed filming (Timcke et al., 1958), offers the possibility of determining the closure of the glottis during vibration and in that respect seems superior to transillumination (Sonesson, 1960) and inverse filtering (Holmberg et al., 1988). We also consider the accuracy of our measurements to be satisfactory due to the magnification from microscope and projection.

During stroboscopy not a real but a virtual image is seen. In other words, a vibration perceived in stroboscopic light is in reality an average based on many periods, where the number of cycles obviously differs depending on the fundamental frequency. It therefore seemed reasonable also to make the acoustic analyses over a long period. Thus, the measurements were averages of glottal vibrations during a time period of one second. It should be pointed out that the same procedure, averaging, is used when we hear; we do not perceive separate vibrations.

As many as five of 18 subjects, four of eight females and one of ten males, had to be excluded from our analyses since none of their recordings showed a complete closure of the vocal folds during phonation. These findings are in accordance with previous studies, reporting rather high incidence of incomplete glottal closure (Södersten and Lindestad, 1988). Our results also indicate some sex-related differences in glottal behaviour during phonation. However, the limited material does not allow for definite conclusions. The fact that it was possible to exclude phonations without complete closure should be considered advantageous when calculating the open quotient.

The increase of the OQ with frequency has been observed previously in humans (Sonesson, 1960) and in dogs (Moore and Berke, 1988) as well as a decrease in the OQ with the intensity in humans (Sonesson, 1960). Thus, our experiments confirm that an increase in frequency or intensity will alter the OQ in opposite ways. To clarify the interrelations between these three factors, a desirable test situation would be to have one factor fixed and the other two varying. Unfortunately, such a study design was not possible due to vocal fatigue in our test subjects. This illustrates the difficulty in collecting enough information for multifactoral analyses of interacting voice parameters.

The relationship between the OQ and the N/S was mixed. An increase in N/S would have been expected with increasing OQ, i.e., the voice would be more "noisy" with a large OQ. Usually, however, the N/S decreased with intensity.

The relationship between intensity and G_m was variable, most likely because people do different things when they increase the intensity. For example, a tighter glottal adduction at high intensities would be expected in many cases. This was also observed in some subjects which resulted in a negative relationship between intensity and glottal opening. The increased intensity with decreased glottal opening can be explained by other factors like increased subglottal pressure and fundamental frequency.

The decrease in G_m with rising frequency, which was observed here, seemed not to be related to a change in intensity, but might be explained by an increase in the vocal fold tension with rising frequency.

REFERENCES

Fex, S., Fex, B., and Hirano, M (forthcoming). A clinical procedure for linear measurement at the vocal fold level.

Holmberg, E.B., Hillman, R.E., and Perkell, J.S. (1988). Glottal airflow and transglottal air pressure measurements for male and female speakers in soft, normal, and loud voice. *J. Acoust. Soc. Am.*, 84:511-529.

Moore, D.M. and Berke, G.S. (1988). The effect of laryngeal nerve stimulation on phonation: A glottographic study using an in vivo canine model. *J. Acoust. Soc. Am.*, 83:705-715.

Muta, H., Baer, T., Wagatsuma, K., Muraoka, T., and Fukuda, H. (1988). A pitch-synchronous analysis of hoarseness in running speech. *J. Acoust. Soc. Am.*, 84:1292-1301.

Sonesson, B. (1960). On the anatomy and vibratory pattern of the human vocal folds. With special reference to a photo-electrical method for studying the vibratory movements. *Acta Otolaryngol.*, Suppl. 156.

Södersten, M. and Lindestad, P-Å. (1988). Vocal fold closure and perceived breathiness in young adult normal-speaking males. *Phoniatric & Logopedic Progress Rep. No 6*, pp. 48-65 (Karolinska Institutet, Huddinge Hospital, Stockholm).

Timcke, R., von Leden, H., and Moore, P. (1958). Laryngeal vibrations: Measurements of the glottic wave. *A.M.A. Arch. of Otolaryngol.*, 68:1-19.

Titze, I. (1989). On the relation between subglottal pressure and fundamental frequency in phonation. *J. Acoust. Soc. Am.*, 85:901-906.

Wendler, J. and Köppen, K. (1988). Schwingungsmessungen der Stimmlippen: Zur klinischen Relevanz der Stroboskopie. *Folia Phoniatr.*, 40:297-302.

36

Control of Laryngeal Vibration in Register Change

Bernard Roubeau, Claude Chevrie-Muller, and Catherine Arabia

Institut National de la santé et de la recherche Médicale, Groupe de Recherche sur le Langage, INSERM U3, Hôpital de la Salpêtrière, 75651 Paris Cedex 13, France

The use of different registers for voice production has been well described especially in singing. Such descriptions were first made using perceptual analyses and from the singer's proprioceptive experience (McGlone and Brown, 1968). Acoustic measurements and physiological investigations then permitted a better understanding of the laryngeal function in the different registers (Gay et al., 1972; Hirano, 1982; Childers et al., 1981).

In addition, the relationship of electroglottographic (EGG) patterns to the registers has been well described (Baer et al., 1983; Lecluse, 1977; Childers et al., 1981; Dejonckere, 1981). The typical aspect of the EGG signal in both registers is shown in Figure 1. As for the "shift" itself between vocal registers, it has been the object of a few studies (Askenfelt et al., 1980; Kitzing, 1982). A comprehensive study of the change from one type of register to another can provide data on the mechanical process and the neuromotor control of the larynx function. We present results of such a study here.

Regarding the different registers and the number of names used, "mechanism I" refers to a single mechanism similar to Hirano's analysis of 'chest', and 'mixed' registers and the term "mechanism II" is used for the 'falsetto' register.

METHODS

Ten male and nine female singers with different levels of vocal training participated in the study.

Recording

All the subjects were recorded on a two-track Revox tape recorder using an LEM microphone and a Frøkjær-Jensen EG 830 electroglottograph. An analog-to-digital conversion of the EGG signal was carried out using an IBM-AT3 microcomputer. This was followed by signal processing using the zero-crossing method. The sampling frequency was 10 kHz.

Next, a computer processing method (Guidet and Chevrie-Muller, 1983) provided synchronized displays of the EGG signal frequency (logarithmic scale) and of the amplitude (linear scale). To compare the amplitude variations from one subject to another, it was necessary to normalize the data by only considering relative amplitude values (Roubeau et al., 1987).

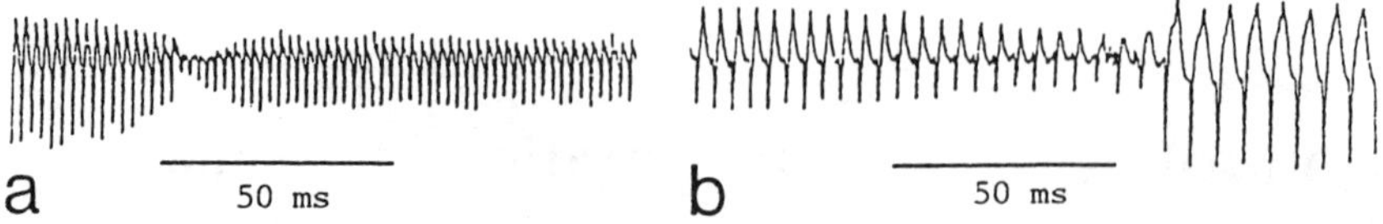

Fig. 1. EGG trace during glissandos. a) Ascending glissando; b) Descending glissando

Protocol

The subjects performed ascending and descending glissandos on the vowels /a, o/, and /i/. They were also asked to hold vowels at a constant pitch and to change the laryngeal mechanism without interrupting the production (held note or isoparametric tone). The pitches of the held notes could easily be produced using either of the two principal mechanisms.

Data Analysis

For each variable analyzed an average value was computed separately for the male and female subjects in each type of production (glissando, held note). The mean frequencies were calculated using logarithmic values.

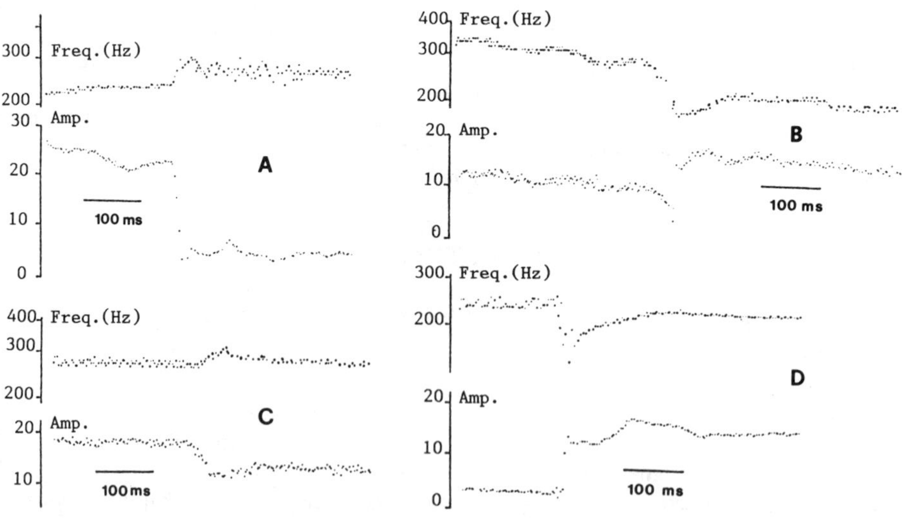

Fig. 2. Evolution of frequency and amplitude of the EGG signal during change of mechanism. (**a**) Ascending glissando (I-II); (**b**) Descending glissando (II-I); (**c**) Held note (I-II); (**d**) Held note (II-I).

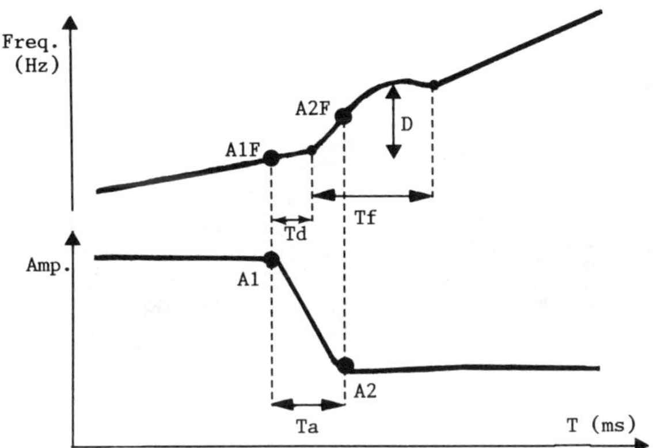

Fig. 3. Evolution of amplitude and frequency of the EGG signal during a mechanism change during an ascending glissando.

RESULTS

Analysis of the EGG trace

During ascending glissando (Figure 2a), the separate representation of both the amplitude and frequency of each EGG wave shows that when the vibratory mechanism changed, there was an abrupt decrease of the amplitude and a disturbance of the frequency curve. Here the shift was from "mechanism I" to "mechanism II". The modification of the shape of the waves, which is now well known, will not be analyzed here.

For descending glissando, the reverse pattern from that of the ascending glissando was seen (Figure 2b).

During held notes (Figures 2c and d), the phenomena were the same as those described for glissandos. The shift is characterized by a loss of frequency control in the upward direction during the change from "mechanisms I to II" (I-II) and in the downward direction going from "mechanisms II to I" (II-I).

Nine variables have been defined and measured in each shift (Figure 3). For the EGG amplitude, A1 is the EGG amplitude at the beginning of the shift, A2 is the EGG amplitude at the end of the shift, and A2/A1 is the ratio A2/A1.

For the EGG frequency, A1F is the frequency when the amplitude begins to change, A2F is the frequency when the amplitude becomes stable after the shift, and D (in semi tones) is the loss of frequency control during glissandos and held notes.

For the duration of the phenomena, Ta is the duration of amplitude readjustment during the mechanism change, Tf is the duration of frequency readjustment, and Td is the timing difference between the beginning of the amplitude readjustment and the frequency readjustment.

The amplitude of the EGG signal

The mean values of the normalized amplitude and of the ratio A2/A1 are given in Figure 4.

During the shift from I to II in glissandos (GL) or held notes (H.N.), the mean value A1 of the amplitude is always higher than A2 (thus the ratio is less than 1). One can ob-

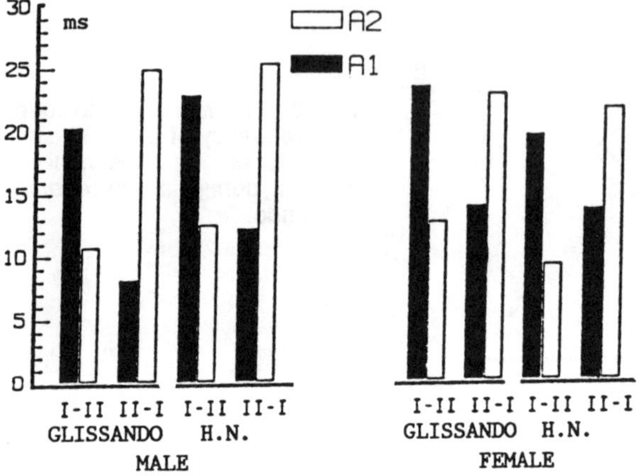

Fig. 4. Amplitude of the EGG signal before (A1) and after (A2) the change of mechanism for men and women during glissandos and held notes (H.N.), when changing from mechanism I to II or II to I.

serve the reverse phenomenon in a shift from II to I where the ratio A2/A1 is always greater than 1. It should be remembered that A2/A1 is the mean calculated from all A2/A1 values.

The t-tests confirmed that the ratio A2/A1 varied significantly as a function of direction of change (It was greater for I-II than for II-I) regardless of sex ($p<0.05$).

On the other hand, comparisons of glissandos with held notes in the same direction of change did not differ significantly for males and females. Comparisons of men's and women's productions for changes in the same direction did not differ significantly except for descending glissandos. The ratio A2/A1 for this glissando was much greater for men than for women.

Frequency location of the shift

The frequency at which the change in mechanism occurs was determined from A1F and A2F measured during the glissandos. The means, calculated from the logarithmic values, have been reconverted into Hz. The standard deviations are given in semitones in Table 1.

Table 1. *Mean values of starting frequency, A1F, and ending frequency, A2F, of the ascending and descending glissandos, GL I-II and GL II-I, respectively. Standard deviation, S.D., in semitones.*

Sex	Production	A1F (Hz)	S.D.	A2F (Hz)	S.D.
Male	GL I-II	238	3.8	318	6.3
	GL II-I	266	8.2	195	6.6
Female	GL I-II	312	4.5	345	4.5
	GL II-I	321	6.7	279	4.9

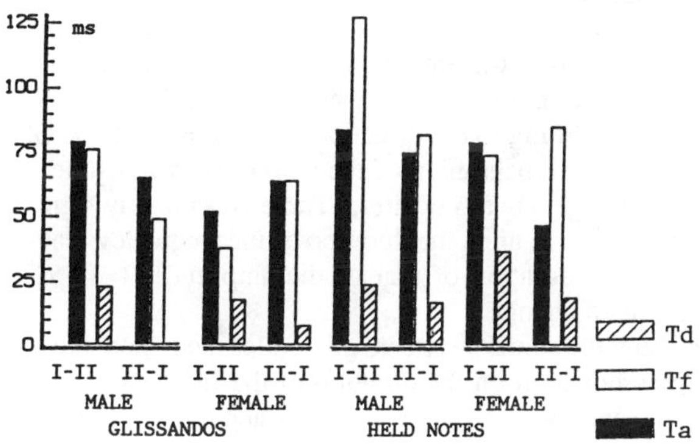

Fig. 5. Durations of the amplitude (Ta) and frequency (Tf) readjustments, and the timing difference (Td) between these readjustments, for glissandos and held notes (H.N.), when changing from mechanisms I to II or II to I.

The effect of sex and that of the type of glissando on the level at which there is a change of mechanism were tested. The frequency at which the shift began was significantly different for male and female subjects ($p<0.05$).

The frequency at which the shift began differed significantly for male and female subjects ($p<0.05$). For both the ascending and descending glissandos, the shift began at a lower frequency for men than for women. When comparing ascending and descending glissandos, however, the starting frequencies of the shift differed significantly for men and women ($p<0.05$).

Paired comparisons showed a significant difference ($t=2.973$, $df=43$, $p=0.005$) between the starting frequency (A1F) of the ascending glissando and the ending frequency (*A2F*) of the descending glissando for both men and women. Furthermore, the difference between the ending frequency (A2F) of the ascending glissando and the starting frequency (A1F) of the descending glissando were also significantly different ($t=2.623$, $df=34$, $p=0.025$). Thus, for a given subject the change I-II occurred in a higher frequency range than the change II-I did.

Loss of frequency control

The values of the variable D were measured in semitones during glissandos and held notes. No significant effect of the sex factor nor of type of production (glissandos or held note) could be observed in the D-values.

Duration of the readjustments

During glissandos, the delay (Td) (see Figure 5) between the beginning of the amplitude readjustment and that of the frequency was, on the average, always positive, i.e., the beginning of the amplitude readjustment preceded the beginning of that of the frequency. The t-test showed that the duration of readjustment of the amplitude (Ta) and of the frequency (Tf) did not significantly vary as a function of the direction of the glissando. For the ascending glissandos, the durations Ta and Tf were significantly longer for men than for women ($p<0.01$). As for the two variables describing the amplitude and frequency readjustments (Ta-Tf), no difference could be shown by the t-test. There is no significant difference between the durations of the amplitude and the frequency readjustments.

During held notes (Figure 5), no effect of the sex factor nor of the direction of the change could be demonstrated on the duration of the amplitude readjustment. As for the frequency readjustment, the longer duration in male subjects, when changing from I to II, might explain the significant difference according to the direction and the sex ($p<0.001$). Like the glissando, the delay (Td) between the beginning of the amplitude readjustment and that of the frequency were, on the average, always positive. There was not any significant effect of sex or direction of the change. In men, the duration of the frequency readjustment was significantly longer than the duration of that of the amplitude ($t=4.555$, $df=146$, $p=0.001$) regardless the direction of change.

A t-test comparison of readjustment durations between glissandos and held notes demonstrated an effect of the type of production on the duration of the frequency readjustment ($p<0.05$) but not on that of the amplitude regardless the sex and the direction of the change.

DISCUSSION

The method used in the present study permitted us to analyze the change of vibratory mechanisms in a sufficient number of productions (N=222) while also taking into account several factors: the type of production, the direction of the change, and the sex of the subject.

Neither any effect of the type of production nor of the sex of the subjects could be shown on the ratio (A2/A1) between the EGG amplitudes before and after the change of mechanism. This led to the idea that the change in the voice mechanisms might constitute an almost homogeneous physiological phenomenon. The only factor which influenced the ratio A2/A1 was the direction of the change (I-II versus II-I). In fact, increases and decreases of the amplitude seem to be related to the different motor processes.

In ascending glissandos, the ratio A2/A1 had an average of 0.6 while in the reverse case it reached at least 3.2. In a symmetrical process the figures would be 0.5 for I-II and 2.0 for II-I. This demonstrated asymmetry reflects differences in mechanical functioning. The progressive increase in vocal fold stretching and thinning during the rise in frequency, already existing in "mechanism I" (Hollien, 1974), is similar to the sudden phenomenon of the change from I to II.

Conversely, in the descending glissando the depth of thickness of the vocal folds is stable in "mechanism II" despite the decrease of frequency (Hollien, 1974). But when the change from II to I occurs, the muscular system is more relaxed than in the ascending modality and thus, there is a greater vocal fold thickness during the change. This phenomenon was more prominent in the descending glissando in men than in women for two additional reasons: (1) the greater size of the male larynx implies that men have a greater contact area during "mechanism I"; (2) the more frequent use of "mechanism II" by women leads to a more complete contact of the folds during that mechanism.

The change in EGG amplitude was an objective criterion for the onset of change, and the frequency level was measured in reference to changes in amplitude. It was possible from this criterion to determine the frequency area where the change occurred.

During ascending glissandos, the beginning of the change of the mechanisms (A1F) occurred significantly lower in men (238 Hz - A3, S.D. 3.8 semi-tones) than in women

(312 Hz - D 4, S.D. 4.5 semi-tones). These results were in agreement with those given, for men only, by Ocker et al., (1985). But, contrary to our two-tones difference between men and women, McGlone and Brown (1968) described a one-octave difference.

The end (A2F) of the mechanism change during ascending glissandos in men (318 Hz, E4, S.D.=6.3 semitones) did not significantly differ from that in women (345 Hz, F, S.D.=4.5, semitones). This again is in opposition with the results of McGlone and Brown (1968). The interval between the beginning and the end of the mechanism change was on the average greater in men (I-II: 238-318 Hz, II-I: 266-195 Hz) than in women (I-II: 312-345 Hz, II-I: 321-279 Hz); a parallel can be drawn with similar differences concerning the amplitude.

Moreover, the comparison of the upper limit of the "mechanism I" in ascending and descending glissandos (and the complementary comparison made in the reverse pattern of "mechanism II") demonstrated that the "mechanism I" is maintained up to a higher level in ascending and to a lower level in descending. This phenomenon which increases the instability of the system makes the change of mechanism much easier and confirms the overlapping of these mechanisms.

A brief upward loss of frequency control characterized the change from "mechanisms I to II" during glissandos and a similar but reverse pattern characterized the change from "mechanisms II to I". At the shift, the laryngeal tensions and the sub-glottic pressure are greater for a given frequency when in "mechanism I". The upward loss of frequency control is in fact due to the non immediate readjustment of these two parameters. With the change II-I, laryngeal tensions and subglottic pressure are weak and thus insufficient to maintain the frequency. Therefore, a loss of control of the frequency occurs in the downwards direction.

In the case of held notes, these losses of control are corrected at a later point in the production. The loss of frequency control is greater during the change II-I than the change I-II, regardless of the sex. Thus, a parallel could be drawn with changes in amplitude.

The duration of the amplitude readjustment was one of the parameters which was stable whatever the direction of change and the modality of production. This result was one more in favour of the homogeneity of the physiological phenomenon.

The timing of the frequency readjustment was not a stable parameter: for a held note the subject had to correct the jump or the drop of the frequency in order to return to the initial frequency which takes more time than in a glissando. For this last modality, the loss of control goes in the same direction as the process itself, thus the readjustment is easier. This was seen in the difference found between the amplitude and frequency readjustments only in held notes.

In conclusion, the concurrent analyses of the change of laryngeal mechanisms (the classical 'shift between registers') in different modalities of production (ascending and descending glissandos, held notes) and in subjects of both sexes permitted the demonstration of the homogeneity of the phenomenon. However, it was also possible to take into account this change of mechanism as a consequence of the mechanical constraints and the neuromotor control.

In future, the described basic phenomenon in laryngeal physiology must be used as a reference for the assessing training effects and pathological neuromotor and mechanical disturbances.

REFERENCES

Askenfelt, A., Gauffin, J., Sundberg, J., and Kitzing, P. (1980). A comparison of microphone and electroglottograph for the measurement of vocal fundamental frequency. *J. Speech Hear. Res.*, 23:250-273.

Baer, T., Titze, I.R., and Yoshioka, H. (1983). Multiple simultaneous measures of vocal fold activity. *Proc. of Int. Conf. on Physiology and Biophysics of Voice, May 4-7, 1983*. pp. 131-137.

Childers, D.G., Smith, A.M., and Moore, G.P. (1981). Relationship between electroglottograph, speech and vocal cord contact. *Folia Phoniat.*, 36:105-118.

Dejonckere, P.H. (1981). Comparison of two methods of photoglottography in relation to electroglottography. *Folia Phoniat.*, 33:338-347.

Gay, T., Strome, M., Hirose, H., and Sawashima, M. (1972). Electromyography of the intrinsic laryngeal muscles during phonation. *Ann. Otol. Rhinol. Laryngol.*, 81:401-409.

Guidet, C. and Chevrie-Muller, C. (1983). Methode de traitement du signal electroglottographique. Application au diagnostic des troubles de la phonation. *Innov. Tech. Med.*, 4:617-635.

Hirano, M. (1982). The role of the layer structure of the vocal folds in register control. *Vox humana*. University of Jyväskylä, Finland.

Hollien, M. (1974). On vocal registers. *J. Phonetics*, 2:125-143.

Kitzing, P. (1982). Photo- and electroglottographical recording of the laryngeal vibratory pattern during different registers. *Folia Phoniat.*, 34:234-241.

Lecluse, F.L.E. (1977). *Elektroglottografie*, Thesis Rotterdam, Drukkerig Elinkwijk, Utrecht.

McGlone, R.E. and Brown Jr., W.S. (1968). Identification of the 'shift' between vocal registers. *J. Acoust. Soc. Am.*, 46:1033-1036.

Ocker, C., Pascher, W. and Röhrs, M. (1985). Investigations of the vibration modes of the vocal cords during different registers. In: *Proc. Stockholm Music Acoustics Conf.*, edited by A. Askenfelt, S. Felicetti, E. Jansson, and J. Sundberg, pp. 239-246. Royal Swedish Acad. Music, No. 46, Vol. I, Stockholm.

Roubeau, B., Chevrie-Muller, C., and Arabia-Guidet, C. (1987). Electroglottographic study of the changes of voice registers. *Folia Phoniatr.*, 39:280-289.